② ₄

C.2

£9.99

Chronic Obstructive Pulmonary Disease

CRITICAL DEBATES

Chronic Obstructive Pulmonary Disease

CRITICAL DEBATES

EDITED BY

Mike Pearson

Director
Clinical Effectiveness and Evaluation Unit
Royal College of Physicians
London
and Consultant Physician
University Hospital Aintree
Liverpool

Wisia Wedzicha

Professor of Respiratory Medicine
Academic Unit of Respiratory Medicine
St Bartholomew's and Royal London Medical School
Dominion House
St Bartholomew's Hospital
London

Blackwell
Science

© 2003 by Blackwell Science Ltd
a Blackwell Publishing company
Blackwell Science, Inc., 350 Main Street, Malden, Massachusetts 02148-5018, USA
Blackwell Publishing Ltd, 9600 Garsington Road, Oxford OX4 2DQ, UK
Blackwell Science Asia Pty Ltd, 550 Swanston Street, Carlton South, Victoria 3053, Australia
Blackwell Wissenschafts Verlag, Kurfürstendamm 57, 10707 Berlin, Germany

First published 2003
Reprinted 2004

Library of Congress Cataloging-in-Publication Data
Chronic obstructive pulmonary disease: critical debates/edited by Mike Pearson, Jadwiga Wedzicha.
     p.   cm.
  Includes bibliographical references and index.
  ISBN 0-632-05972-9
  1 Lungs—Diseases, Obstructive.
  [DNLM: 1 Pulmonary Disease, Chronic Obstructive. WF 600 C5518 2003] I Pearson, Mike,
FRCP. II Wedzicha, Jadwiga Anna.
  RC776.O3 C47427
  616.2'4—dc21

                         2002151823

ISBN 0-632-05972-9

A catalogue record for this title is available from the British Library

Set in 10/13$\frac{1}{2}$ pt Sabon by SNP Best-set Typesetter Ltd., Hong Kong
Printed and bound in the UK by MPG Books Ltd, Bodmin, Cornwall

Commissioning Editor: Maria Khan
Managing Editor: Rupal Malde
Production Editor: Jonathan Rowley
Production Controller: Chris Downs

For further information on Blackwell Science, visit our website:
http://www.blackwellpublishing.com

Contents

List of Contributors

Peter Barnes *National Heart and Lung Institute, Imperial College, London, UK*

David Bellamy *James Fisher Medical Centre, Bournemouth, UK*

Demosthenes Bouros *Department of Thoracic Medicine, University General Hospital, Heraklion, Crete, Greece*

Martin Connolly *Platt Rehabilitation Unit 2, Manchester Royal Infirmary, Manchester, UK*

John Corless *St Helens and Knowsley NHS Trust, Merseyside, UK*

Mark Elliott *St James's University Hospital, Leeds, UK*

Michael Fitzpatrick *Respiratory Investigation Unit, Queen's University, Kingston, Ontario, Canada*

James Friend *Previously Aberdeen Royal Infirmary, Aberdeen, UK*

Roger Goldstein *University Health Network, Toronto, Canada*

Nick ten Hacken *Department of Pulmonary Diseases, University Hospital, Groningen, The Netherlands*

Gerard Koeter *Department of Pulmonary Diseases, University Hospital, Groningen, The Netherlands*

Walter McNicholas *University College Dublin, St Vincent's University Hospital, Elm Park, Dublin, Ireland*

Denis O'Donnell *Respiratory Investigation Unit, Queen's University, Kingston, Ontario, Canada*

Ronan O'Driscoll *Hope Hospital, Salford, UK*

Mike Pearson *University Hospital Aintree, Liverpool and Royal College of Physicians, London, UK*

Louise Restrick *Department of Respiratory Medicine, Whittington Hospital, London, UK*

Nikos Siafakas *Department of Thoracic Medicine, University General Hospital, Heraklion, Crete, Greece*

Mrinal Sircar *St James's University Hospital, Leeds, UK*

Eleni Tzortzaki *Department of Thoracic Medicine, University General Hospital, Heraklion, Crete, Greece*

Jørgen Vestbo *Department of Respiratory Medicine, Hvidovre University Hospital, Hvidovre, Denmark*

Thomas Waddell *University Health Network, Toronto, Canada*

Wisia Wedzicha *Academic Unit of Respiratory Medicine, St Bartholomew's and Royal London School of Medicine and Dentistry, St Bartholomew's Hospital, London, UK*

Johan Wempe *Department of Pulmonary Diseases, University Hospital, Groningen, The Netherlands*

Peter Wijkstra *Department of Pulmonary Diseases, University Hospital, Groningen, The Netherlands*

Preface

Increase in COPD; increase in smoking

COPD is a challenge to health systems across the world. As cigarette smoking increased during the 20th century so the prevalence of COPD increased in its wake. Acute exacerbations of COPD are the second most common cause of admission to UK hospitals. Over 5% of people aged over 60 in the UK are affected and seeking help to relieve their symptoms. Not all countries are as severely affected as the UK but in most countries across the world cigarette smoking is increasing and with it so is the prevalence of COPD. The World Health Organization predicts that by the year 2020, COPD will be the fourth most common cause of death worldwide.

Until quite recently there was little medical interest in COPD but a surge of interest has been stimulated by the development of simple measurements, and by inhaled drugs that relieve the symptoms at least in part. Although the damage caused by smoking cannot be reversed, the COPD patient's life quality can be significantly improved and in some cases their life expectancy improved too.

The research world has woken up to these possibilities and the burgeoning number of sessions at international meetings allocated to COPD is testament to the amount of new effort devoted to the disease. Now the pharmaceutical industry has developed a range of products of proven benefit; and more are on the way.

This book has an unusual format. It is not intended to be a textbook for the expert, and makes no attempt to be comprehensive in its coverage. Instead our contributors were asked to discuss COPD topics that the average clinician (doctors, nurses and allied health professionals) would be able to read easily and find interest in. The questioning format has allowed our contributors to select from the many issues that could be discussed and so inevitably some subjects have not been covered (so apologies if your pet concern is not described). Nevertheless we hope that there is plenty to interest all those who manage patients with COPD in primary and secondary care and they will be stimulated to want to know more about this all too common disorder. This is a rapidly developing field with many exciting and interesting developments that are being translated into direct patient care.

We hope that those who read this book are left with an enthusiasm that COPD is not a 'no-hope' disorder and will want to do more for their patients. Much can and should be done that will benefit not only the patients directly but also their families and thus society. But if we are to succeed we need not only to recognize what can be done, we also have to put into place systems that ensure it really is done.

Mike Pearson
Wisia Wedzicha

1: The aetiology and epidemiology of chronic obstructive pulmonary disease

John Corless

Introduction

Chronic obstructive pulmonary disease (COPD) is a leading cause of morbidity and mortality throughout the world. It is the fourth commonest cause of death in the United States after ischaemic heart disease (IHD), cancer and cerebrovascular disease. Unlike IHD and cancer, however, COPD suffers from an 'image problem'. Surely no other disease of similar impact can have as many different names—chronic obstructive airways disease, chronic obstructive lung disease, chronic bronchitis and emphysema, to name a few. Similarly, personal experience suggests that only a minority of patients know the name of the disease from which they suffer. The precise definitions used to diagnose the condition are open to contention and debate, based on assessment of symptoms and interpretation of spirometry. As the most important aetiological factor is smoking, the disease is often regarded as self-inflicted—and in turn, patients are at times viewed less sympathetically than those with malignancy, for example.

Despite the difficulties that arise from varying nomenclature and definitions, there is no doubt that COPD has a major impact on global health, particularly in the developed world. This chapter seeks to address the following issues:

- Does all COPD result from smoking?
- Other aetiological factors in the pathogenesis of COPD
- The global impact of COPD
- The natural history of COPD
- The future of COPD.

The aetiology of COPD

Does all COPD result from smoking?

The evidence that cigarette smoking is a major cause of lung cancer and COPD

Table 1.1 Annual mortality per 100 000 men. Adapted from [1].

	Never smokers	Current cigarette smokers	Ex-cigarette smokers	Current cigar/pipe smokers	Ex-cigar/ pipe smokers
COPD	10	127	57	51	40
Lung cancer	14	209	58	112	59
IHD	572	892	678	653	676

COPD, chronic obstructive pulmonary disease; IHD, ischaemic heart disease.

has been derived from a series of very different studies over many years. Although none of these have used the randomized controlled trial design that provides the 'gold standard' for evidence in most Cochrane reviews, it is widely accepted that cigarette smoking is the single most important risk factor for the development of COPD, even though a precise model of the mechanism has yet to be constructed. It is worth reviewing the strength of the evidence.

As late as 1948, there were experts prepared to argue that smoking was not harmful, but by 1950 the link to lung cancer seemed probable. Richard Doll and colleagues decided to commence a prospective longitudinal study to find out what other diseases might or might not be smoking-related. In 1951, all doctors in Britain were asked about their smoking habits, and 40 000 replied. These doctors were followed up for 40 years, with interim reports at 10 and 20 years that confirmed the link to cancer and showed that other conditions were also linked to smoking. The 40-year report [1] concentrated on the 34 439 males in the study, and at this time it was possible to establish the vital status of 99.7% of the 1951 cohort. A cause of death was obtained for 99% of the deaths, and of those who were alive, 94% completed a further questionnaire. Longitudinal studies are usually marred by a significant loss to follow-up, and the completeness of this study is remarkable. Although it was not a randomized, controlled trial, it is probably one of the most complete and devastatingly strong observational studies ever mounted.

Positive associations with smoking were confirmed for death from cancers of the mouth, oesophagus, pharynx, larynx, lung, pancreas and bladder. Details of mortality for COPD, lung cancer and ischaemic heart disease (IHD) are outlined in Table 1.1. Cigarette smoking increased the risk of death from COPD, lung cancer and from ischaemic heart disease. In each case, those who had ceased smoking had values that were intermediate between those of non-smokers and continuing smokers. Because ischaemic heart disease is so much more common, the total effects of cigarette smoking on the heart were similar to those on the lung. Thus, when expressed in terms of the population

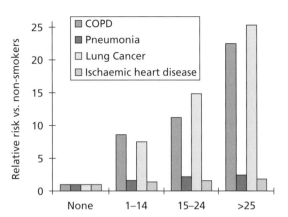

Fig. 1.1 Relative risks of current smoking—the risk in non-smokers for each condition has been set at 1, and values displayed for different intensities of smoking.

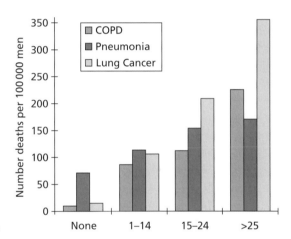

Fig. 1.2 Mortality of current smokers by amount smoked [1].

affected, there are an extra 320 deaths per 100 000 from ischaemic heart disease and 312 from COPD and lung cancer together.

The crude relative increase in ischaemic heart disease from these figures is 1.55 compared to 12.7 for COPD and 14.9 for lung cancer, and the much higher relative risk suggests a much closer and more complete causal link to pulmonary disease (Fig. 1.1). For heart disease, it is recognized that smoking is only one factor amongst several involved in the causation of disease. Genetic susceptibility (as shown by the strong influence of a history of heart disease amongst close relatives) and lipid control are two other strong predictors that may be as important as smoking.

The increased risks attributable to smoking are dose-dependent (Fig. 1.2). Not only is the number of deaths per 100 000 much increased for COPD and lung cancer, but there is also a significant increase in deaths from pneumonia, and many of the patients concerned could well have had COPD too. The

COPD effect may therefore be underestimated. This leaves approximately 5–10% of cases of COPD that are not directly attributable to smoking.

The authors were able to go further in their estimations of risk to show that for the average smoker, there was a loss of 7.5 years of life, increasing to 10 years for a smoker of more than 25 cigarettes per day. Another way of describing the data is to state that only 21% of smokers will attain the age of 85 years, compared to 41% of non-smokers. If a person ceases smoking, then the risks of death are reduced and there are discernible benefits even for those quitting when over 65 years of age.

As was noted above, this was an observational study and there were a number of potential confounding factors. Death certification could have been wrong—it is known that the reliability of death certificates is not good, and there were many changes in the lifestyle, wealth and personality of the population over the period studied. While it is possible that some of these factors could have affected survival, it is unlikely that they could have altered the huge relative risks observed.

These data were derived from a relatively privileged sector of the population; while this has an advantage in that there was no social class disease gradient to be taken into account, it also raises the possibility that the relative risks could be different in other parts of society. More recent data for the UK based on survival data from life-insurance work [2] show a very similar effect on loss of life expectancy—7 years between the ages of 30 and 70—suggesting that the Doll and Peto data can probably be extrapolated to the general population.

The size, completeness and length of this study make the links between smoking and both lung cancer and COPD irrefutable, and indeed many other studies since have confirmed and supported these conclusions.

How many non-smokers develop COPD? From the Doll and Peto figures, it would seem that of 285 deaths per 100 000 due to COPD, there were 10 individuals, or about 3%, who had never smoked and were labelled as having COPD. Similar figures are reported from cross-sectional studies of living patients, e.g. that 5–7% of their cohort were non-smokers [3]. Assuming that these cases of COPD do not result from incorrect recording of diagnosis or smoking status, other aetiological factors may exist. This is discussed later in the chapter.

Many other examples from other countries have confirmed the dose-related relationship between the risk of developing COPD and cigarette smoking [4]. They also confirm the lower incidence of COPD in those who smoke a pipe or cigars rather than cigarettes [5]. The incidence of COPD is consistently reported to be significantly lower in women, reflecting the lower prevalence of cigarette smoking amongst females, but the pattern is changing. In the UK, death rates from COPD in men have fallen, reflecting a change from a 65% rate of current smokers in 1970 to less than 30% in 2000, but the death rate in women is still rising [6] following the surge in female smoking after the second world war. In Denmark, where a high proportion of women have been smokers for many years, the percentage of deaths in women attributable to tobacco already approaches that of men [7]. This trend is likely to be seen in other European countries in the coming years.

Other aetiological factors in the pathogenesis of COPD

Asthma

A proportion of asthma patients develop an irreversible component that is usually attributed to airway remodelling. It is not known why some asthmatics progress to fixed airflow obstruction — but once they have, it is very difficult to differentiate them from patients with COPD on clinical or physiological grounds. Approximately 2% of asthmatics have a forced expiratory volume in 1 s (FEV_1) below 60% predicted. As asthma is so common, even this small percentage may explain many of those who are labelled as having COPD despite not having any history of exposure to cigarette smoke. In comparison, 10% of moderate smokers (21–40 pack-years) and over 22% of heavy smokers (>60 pack-years) will develop this severity of airway obstruction [8].

Bronchiolitis

An alternative mislabelling can occur with bronchiolitis. Bronchiolitis and bronchiolitis obliterans are general terms used to describe a non-specific inflammatory injury that primarily affects the small airways, often sparing the interstitium. This disorder is currently poorly understood. It is likely that a small proportion of patients with a diagnosis of COPD have a progressive, constrictive bronchiolitis that has not been recognized — hardly surprising, as there is no test other than histology with which to differentiate the cause of the airflow limitation.

Occupation

The precise role of occupation in the pathogenesis of COPD remains unclear. Epidemiological studies assessing the role of occupation in the development of COPD are difficult both to conduct and interpret [9]. Most of the evidence is derived from cross-sectional studies, in which it has been difficult to record dust exposure, or indeed cigarette exposure, reliably. There is no doubt that exposure to heavy dust loads leads to a productive cough, but this can be a normal physiological response to the particular burden that has to be cleared. There are cross-sectional studies of populations [10,11] that have described more COPD amongst those working in dusty jobs. But while cross-sectional studies can indicate associations, they cannot differentiate causality between the dust and other factors. Those in dustier jobs tend to be of lower social class and have a higher smoking prevalence, poorer nutrition and worse general health. Most data are available on coal miners, but even here the data are not conclusive. A UK legal ruling concluded that on the balance of probabilities, coal dust could cause emphysema and airway obstruction and thus miners are to receive compensation even with a smoking history [12]. There remains no mechanism to explain how coal dust (generally a remarkably inert substance) should compare with cigarette smoke (containing 10^{17} free radicals per puff), but legal cases are not science and conclude on a 'balance of probabilities'. Other studies have claimed similar effects from gold mining and for underground tunnel workers [13], although in the legal case which considered coal dust, the other rock dusts were excluded as likely causes.

Atmospheric pollution

If occupational dust can cause airway obstruction, then it is logical to examine the effects of pollution. A small additional contribution to COPD severity has been reported in patients who live in cities. However, these effects are small and remain contentious. High exposures to very small particles of less than $10\,\mu m$ (PM_{10}) have also been associated with an increase in both cardiac and respiratory deaths in cross-sectional population studies [14]. These exposures are many times less than the occupational exposures experienced by miners, and thus the question arises as to whether other components of pollution may be additive in causing these apparent effects. Ozone and diesel have also been associated with the development of COPD, but the latter claim must be balanced by the studies of miners in diesel pits (i.e. pits in which the underground trains that transported men and coal along the shafts were diesel-powered). Despite heavy exposures in quite enclosed environments, no adverse effects have been observed in these coal mines [15]. Indoor exposure to wood smoke and fumes from biomass fuels has also been implicated [16,17]. Paradoxically, while concerns in the popular press about the effect of outdoor pollutants on the lung have escalated in recent times, the levels of sulphur dioxide and black smoke have been dramatically reduced in most developed countries over the last 30 years. The situation regarding environmental pollution and COPD can best be described as confused—and of an order of magnitude less than any effect of smoking cigarettes.

Socio-economic status

Low socio-economic status correlates strongly with the development of

COPD. Men of social classes IV and V aged between 20 and 64 in the UK are 14 times more likely to die of COPD than men with professional occupations [18]. This seems to occur even when different smoking rates are taken into account. It is unclear whether this is due to nutrition, different patterns of respiratory infection exposure in early life, or environmental exposures.

Premature birth is more common amongst mothers of lower socio-economic group and in mothers who smoke. Smoking mothers produce smaller babies [19]. Prematurity is associated with early-life infections [20], and early-life infections are associated with COPD deaths 50 years later [21]. Precise mechanisms, or even a clear sequence of events that might cause this, are unknown, but it does seem increasingly likely that some of the later lung morbidity is due to failure to grow and develop properly both *in utero* and shortly thereafter.

In the Copenhagen City Heart Study, men in the lowest income/least education group had a forced vital capacity (FVC) that was 400 mL less than those in the highest group [22]. Even after control for smoking duration and quantity, the difference was still 363 mL. In females, the differences were smaller, at 259 mL (220 mL adjusted), but of similar pattern. The lowest socio-economic groups were more likely to have had an admission for COPD even after adjustment for smoking, so these differences would seem to be of clinical importance to patients.

Some of these changes may be due to effects of poor nutrition either precipitating or accelerating the development of COPD. Harik-Khan *et al.* [23] studied 458 men without COPD and followed them for a mean of 10.2 years. An inverse relationship between body mass index (BMI) and the risk of developing COPD was demonstrated. The relative risk of developing COPD was 2.76 times greater (95% confidence interval 1.15–6.59) in the lowest BMI tertile compared to the highest tertile. In rats, starvation has been shown to induce emphysematous changes within the lungs [24]. While this association has not been proven in humans, poor nutrition has been associated with pneumothorax [25] and pneumomediastinum [26].

Infections

Latent infection with viruses has been cited as a factor that may predispose to COPD. Double-stranded DNA viruses have the ability to persist in airway epithelial cells long after the acute infection has cleared. Expression of adenoviral genes produces a trans-activating protein that has been demonstrated to amplify the inflammatory response to cigarette smoke [27]. Thus far this remains speculation only.

The global impact of COPD

Any data on the prevalence of COPD must depend on the definition that is adopted. Early stages of COPD are not associated with symptoms, or only with 'smoker's cough' that is accepted as 'inevitable'. These individuals are unknown to the medical profession. Once symptoms develop, the COPD has typically become fairly advanced, with an FEV_1 that has already fallen to less than 60% of the predicted value or worse. Most studies will therefore underestimate the true prevalence and potential impact of the disease.

Historical variations in the terminology and International Classification of Diseases (ICD) codes used for COPD also create difficulties in compiling data on COPD. Until the late 1960s, the terms 'chronic bronchitis' and 'emphysema' were commonly used. Following the eighth revision of ICD codes, 'COPD' was used increasingly frequently in the United States, but often not in other countries, making comparison difficult. The current tenth revision of the ICD recognizes a broad band of 'COPD and allied conditions' (ICD-10 codes J42-46).

Morbidity

The World Bank and World Health Organization (WHO) predict that by 2020, COPD will be ranked fifth in terms of the worldwide burden of disease [27]. The WHO also estimates that 1.1 billion people currently smoke. Assuming that 14% of smokers develop COPD, one could estimate that 150 million either have or will develop COPD—a number equivalent to the entire population of Russia.

In the United Kingdom during 1999/2000, there were 28 million days of certified incapacity due to diseases of the respiratory system [30]. Over 10% of all acute medical admissions to hospital are due to exacerbations of COPD, and with an average length of stay of 10 days, these represent some 2.8 million hospital-bed days annually in the UK.

Morbidity from COPD is not confined to wealthy countries. Smoking prevalence is high and rising in many poorer regions, with China in particular likely to see huge death rates from smoking-related disease in the coming decades. Many of the statistics available in the UK or in the US are not collated in such countries, so that the effect of COPD can only be estimated. Some estimates of the global incidence of COPD in such countries are detailed in Table 1.2 [28,29].

But morbidity is not the only concern. Airflow limitation is associated with premature death, and the World Health Organization statistics attribute 2.74 million deaths worldwide to COPD in the year 2000. It is the fourth commonest cause of death in the USA, China and United Kingdom. In the United States,

Table 1.2 Prevalence of chronic obstructive pulmonary disease in poorer countries in 1990. Adapted from [28].

	Male/ 1000	Female/ 1000
China	26.20	23.70
Former socialist economies	7.35	3.45
Established market economies	6.98	3.79
Sub-Saharan Africa	4.41	2.49
India	4.38	3.44
Latin America and Caribbean	3.36	2.72
Other Asian countries and islands	2.89	1.79
Middle Eastern crescent	2.69	2.83
World	9.34	7.33

112 000 people died of COPD in 1998, and in the United Kingdom 32 000 people died of COPD in 1999 [30]. The latter figure represents 5% of all deaths in the country.

Health expenditure

The financial cost of COPD is very large. In 1993, it was calculated that it created annual costs of US$ 23.9 billion to the US economy. This included US$ 14.7 billion for direct medical costs, with the remainder representing costs resulting from morbidity and premature mortality [31]. The direct health costs of COPD in the UK have been estimated at £846 million (US$ 1.4 billion), accounting for 11% of all expenditure on prescription medications [32]. Typically, the expenditure on COPD is disproportionately distributed, with approximately 10% of patients accounting for 75% of expenditure.

In the UK (figures adapted from [33]), a typical primary-care group caring for a population of 100 000 will have:
- 1000 diagnosed cases of COPD
- 238 annual admissions due to COPD
- 55 deaths from COPD annually (25% below aged 65)
- General practitioner consultations costing £44 000 annually
- Drug therapy costing £718 per patient per year (asthma £198).

The natural history of COPD

The studies discussed above show that death from COPD is most commonly the result of smoking — but what of the processes that lead to these deaths? It is clear that a healthy individual has to pass through mild, then moderate and then severe stages of COPD to reach the stage at which COPD may cause death. But the processes by which this happens and the rate at which it develops require a different sort of study.

It is unclear what distinguishes individuals who develop clinically significant COPD from those who do not, despite a similar smoking history. In 1970, Thurlbeck showed that almost all smokers of more than 20 pack-years will have some emphysema detectable at post-mortem, although only about 15–20% had had any loss of lung function in life [34]. However, while an autopsy-based study can suggest likely causal factors and can add detail to information from longitudinal death certificate studies, it cannot detemine how the disease developed.

Cross-sectional studies of large populations can examine the manifestation of disease at stages of development in large numbers of people. The National Health and Nutrition Examination Survey (NHANES 3) [35] in the US questioned 34 000 people between 1988 and 1994. It reported that up to 24% of current smokers reported chronic cough. Airflow limitation (defined as $FEV_1/FVC <70\%$) among white males was present in 14.2% of current smokers, 6.9% of ex-smokers and 3.3% of those who had never smoked. Similar proportions were found in white females, while the incidence of airflow obstruction was lower in the black population. Other studies have also suggested ethnic variations in COPD incidence, with 15% of active white cigarette smokers and 5% of active Asian cigarette smokers developing clinically significant COPD [36]. Because the disease develops over many years, it is inevitable that the majority of the most severe disease cases are seen in the elderly, but the statistics from North America indicate that 50% are below age 65 and 22% are below 55, with a mean age at diagnosis of 53 years.

The heterogeneity of the disease is illustrated by the fact than even 'light' smokers can develop severe emphysema. Thus, deaths before the age of 50 in individuals claiming to only have smoked five cigarettes daily (equating to approximately nine pack-years) do occur, although such cases are unusual. Clearly, factors other than cigarette smoke alone must be involved (see below), whether acting through a separate mechanism or in synergy with cigarette smoke. More than 40 years ago, the 'Dutch hypothesis' [37] suggested that the risks of developing COPD were related to environmental exposures in combination with the genetic make-up of the individual. This concept may still be true today.

Rate of decline in lung function

Typically, FEV_1 reaches a peak at around age 20–25 and then gradually declines with age by approximately 20–30 mL/year. Little, however, is known about the lung function of existing individuals with COPD in the decades before the disease becomes apparent. It seems logical that patients with COPD may have reached their low FEV_1 by one of the following three routes.

1 An accelerated decline in lung function. In their classic paper that followed 800 London office staff with serial measures of FEV_1 over 8 years, Fletcher *et al.* [38] demonstrated that there is a range of FEV_1 decline per year from almost nil to over 100 mL per year. They suggested that those with a rapid decline were susceptible smokers. The average decline was 18 mL greater in a smoker than in a non-smoker, i.e. 54 mL vs. 36 mL/year. Some non-smokers showed a rapid decline in function, indicating that there are factors other than smoking to be considered, but there were many more rapid decliners amongst the smokers and it is only those with very rapid declines (i.e. of 70–100 mL per year) who can lose the 3 L or more of lung function that places them in the FEV_1 1-litre category that is seen with hospital admissions of patients in their sixties.

The rate of decline is not linear over a lifetime. In the young, FEV_1 may rise between 20 and 25, followed by a relative plateau, before falling at an initially slow but accelerating rate over the years. Thus, the average rate of fall in FEV_1 described in a cohort may be describing an average between small gains in the youngest and large falls in older subjects. This makes it difficult to compare different studies. There are few longitudinal studies to compare with that of Fletcher *et al.*

The US Lung Health Study [39] observed 4000 patients with mild COPD over 5 years with and without an anticholinergic bronchodilator. While the drug had no effect on rate of loss of FEV_1, the authors did note as a secondary end point that the rate of loss of FEV_1 was significantly less in those who quit smoking compared to those who continued. They also observed that those with bronchial hyperreactivity had an increased rate of loss compared to those without. Thus, both exogenous and endogenous factors may affect the rate of decline. As a generalization, the average fall in FEV_1 in susceptible smokers seems to be in the order of 60 mL per year (i.e. twice that of non-smokers) [40].

The cross-sectional studies of smokers and non-smokers have also found a greater loss of lung function amongst smokers. Many have applied linear regression analysis to the data in an attempt to determine the additional aetiological factors responsible. This must be viewed with caution—firstly because the rate of loss is not uniform, and secondly because the starting point for different cohorts is unknown. An analysis of decline in a Dutch community study [41] reported that there was a significant effect depending on when a person was born. Men born a generation later tended to be 2 cm taller and to have 360 mL more FEV_1—presumably a reflection of better socio-economic conditions and better conditions in childhood. Few studies include year of birth as a variable, and thus the cross-sectional analysis performed on the raw FEV_1 data would wrongly attribute this loss to another cause.

2 *Premature decline in lung function.* All parts of the human body deteriorate with increasing age, and the lung is no exception. Humans also age at different biological speeds, and perhaps one of the most promising areas for future research is the genetic basis of COPD. Accelerated loss of lung function in smokers with α1-antiprotease deficiency was first recognized by Laurell and Eriksson in 1963 [42]. This autosomal-recessive condition (ZZ phenotype) is found in 0.03% of the UK population. The lung is rendered susceptible to damage from neutrophil elastase, typically causing rapidly progressive emphysema in homozygotes who smoke. The heterozygotic state MZ is found in 3.9–14.2% of COPD patients, compared with 1.2–5.3% of controls (odds ratio 1.2–5.0). Other genetic predispositions are very likely to exist. Silverman *et al.* have reported a three-fold increased risk of developing COPD among first-degree relatives that is unrelated to α1-antiprotease status [43]. A family history of chronic bronchitis was shown by Carrozzi *et al.* to be associated with impaired FEV_1 in smokers [44]. Other postulated genetic mechanisms include polymorphisms in the tumour necrosis factor-α gene, the microsomal epoxide hydrolase gene and the glutathione S-transferase P1 gene.

3 *Impaired lung growth and therefore a decrease in the peak lung function attained.* Insults to the developing lung during childhood, including premature birth and infection, may have a role. In a study of 700 people with a mean age of 70, Shaheen *et al.* [45] reported that pneumonia before the age of two was associated with a mean reduction in FEV1 of 0.65 L in men, compared with controls. In women, the reduction was smaller and non-significant. In South Wales, children who had admissions for infections as children had an increased risk of dying 60 years later of COPD. Whether it is the infections themselves that are to blame or problems in utero is not known, but there is one study that suggests that poor nutrition in utero is a factor. Barker *et al.* noted that low birthweight was predictive of an increased risk of dying of COPD 60 years later [46].

It is of great concern therefore that women who smoke are known to have smaller babies with an increased incidence of prematurity—this may be placing their children at risk of COPD long before the children have a chance to make decisions for themselves.

The future of COPD

Despite the now well-documented health risks posed by smoking, the cigarette

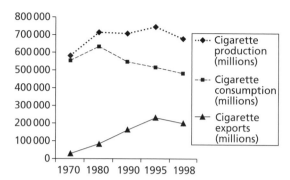

Fig. 1.3 Cigarette production and consumption in the USA, 1970–98. Source: World Health Organization.

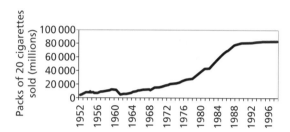

Fig. 1.4 Cigarette sales in China, 1952–98. Source: *China Statistical Year Book*, 1993, 1998; USDA, *China Tobacco Report*, 1999.

industry remains alive and well. Figure 1.3 outlines the current state of the industry in the United States. We are still surrounded by cigarette advertising. Governments have difficulty in reconciling the huge tax revenues they receive from cigarette sales and the outlay on health care that results from these sales. High-profile sports such as Formula One racing could not exist without cigarette advertising. The World Health Organization recently launched a counter-campaign with large posters in the style of 'Marlboro Man' proclaiming 'Bob—I've got emphysema'.

Even if the health message is beginning to have an impact in wealthy countries, cigarettes are heavily promoted in the Third World. The numbers of cigarette exports from the USA has doubled in the last 20 years. The WHO estimates that the number of smokers worldwide will increase from current numbers of 1.1 billion to 1.6 billion by 2025. Much of this growth will be in poorer countries. China in particular appears to have a grim future. Total cigarette consumption there has risen almost 10-fold in the last 50 years (Fig. 1.4), and the country will be reaping the whirlwind of subsequent respiratory disease for years to come.

The mortality figures discussed above describe a lower incidence of COPD in women than men. Recent large cross-sectional population-based studies in the US confirm this, but show a changing pattern emerging, with the prevalence of COPD almost equal in men and women [31,35]. This probably reflects the changing pattern of exposure to the most important risk factor, tobacco smoke.

References

1 Doll R, Peto R, Wheatley K, Gray R, Sutherland I. Mortality in relation to smoking: 40 years' observations on male British doctors. *BMJ* 1994; **309**: 901–10.

2 Health Education Authority. *The Smoking Epidemic: Years of Life Lost.* London: Health Education Authority, 1998.

3 Nisar M, Walshaw MJ, Earis JE, Pearson MG, Calverley PMA. Assessment of reversibility of airway obstruction in patients with chronic obstructive airways disease. *Thorax* 1990; **45**: 190–4.

4 Burrows B, Knudson RJ, Cline MG, Lebowitz MD. Quantitative relationships between cigarette smoking and ventilatory function. *Am Rev Respir Dis* 1979; **115**: 195–205.

5 US Surgeon General. *The Health Consequences of Smoking: Chronic Obstructive Pulmonary Disease.* Washington, DC: US Department of Health and Human Services, 1984 (Publication No. 84-50205).

6 Strachan DP. Epidemiology: a British perspective in COPD. In: Calverley PMA, Pride NB, eds. *Chronic Obstructive Pulmonary Disease.* London: Chapman-Hall, 1994.

7 Juel K. Increased mortality among Danish women: population based register study. *BMJ* 2000; **321**: 349–50.

8 Burrows B, Knudson RJ, Clein MG, Ribowitz MD. Quantitative relationships between cigarette smoking and ventilatory function. *Am Rev Respir Dis* 1979; **115**: 751–60.

9 Kromhout H, Vermeulen R. Application of job-exposure matrices in studies of the general population: some clues to their performance. *Eur Respir Rev* 2001; **11**: 80–90.

10 Bakke S, Baste V, Hanoa R, Gulsvik A. Prevalence of obstructive lung disease in a general population: relation to occupational title and exposure to some airborne agents. *Thorax* 1991; **46**: 863–70.

11 Kauffmann F, Drouet D, Lellouch J, Brille D. Twelve years' spirometric changes among Paris area workers. *Int J Epidemiol* 1979; **8**: 201–12.

12 Seaton A. The new prescription: industrial injury benefits for smokers? *Thorax* 1998; **53**: 535–6.

13 Ulvestad B, Bakke B, Melbostad E *et al.* Increased risk of obstructive pulmonary disease in tunnel workers. *Thorax* 2000; **55**: 277–82.

14 Dockery DW, Pope CA, Xu X *et al.* An association between air pollution and mortality in six U.S. cities. *N Engl J Med* 1993; **329(24)**: 1,753–9.

15 Ames R, Roger RB, Hall DS. Chronic respiratory effects of exposure to diesel emissions in coal mines. *Arch Environ Health* 1984; **39**: 389–94.

16 Dennis R, Maldonado D, Norman S, Baena E, Martinez G. Woodsmoke exposure and risk for obstructive airways disease among women. *Chest* 1996; **109**: 115–19.

17 Perez-Padilla R, Regalado U, Vedal S *et al.* Exposure to biomass smoke and chronic airway disease in Mexican women. *Am J Respir Crit Care Med* 1996; **154**: 701–6.

18 British Thoracic Society. *The Burden of Lung Disease.* London: British Thoracic Society, 2001.

19 Marsh MJ, Fox GF, Ingram D, Milner AD. The effect of maternal smoking during pregnancy on infant lung growth and development. *Proc Br Paediatr Assoc* 1994; **66**: 28.

20 Shaheen SO, Barker DJP. Early lung growth and chronic airflow obstruction. *Thorax* 1994; **49(6)**: 533–6.

21 Barker DJP, Godfrey KM, Fall C *et al.* Relation of birth weight and childhood respiratory infection to adult lung function and death from chronic obstructive lung disease. *BMJ* 1991; **303**: 671–5.

22 Prescot E, Lange P Vestbo J, Copenhagen City Heart Study Group. Socio-economic status, lung function and admission to hospital in the Copenhagen City Heart Study. *Eur Respir J* 1999; **13**: 1109–14.

23 Harik-Khan RI, Fleg JL, Wise RA. Body mass index and COPD. *Chest* 2002; **121**: 370–6.

24 Sahebjami H, Wirman JA. Emphysema-like changes in the lungs of starved rats. *Am Rev Respir Dis* 1981; **124**: 619–24

25 Corless JA, Delaney JC, Page RD. Simultaneous bilateral spontaneous pneumothoraces in a young woman with anorexia nervosa. *Int J Eat Disord* 2001; **30**: 110–12.

26 Aldridge SM, Glover SC, Johnson C. Spontaneous pneumomediastinum in two stowaways. *BMJ* 1986; **293**: 243.

27 Hogg JC. Role of latent viral infections in chronic obstructive pulmonary disease and asthma. *Am J Respir Crit Care Med* 2001; **164**: S71–5.

28 Murray CJL, Lopez AD. Evidence-based health policy: lessons from the Global Burden of Disease Study. *Science* 1996; **274**: 740–3.

29 Murray CJL, Lopez AD, eds. *The Global Burden of Disease: a Comprehensive Assessment of Mortality and Disability from Diseases, Injuries and Risk Factors in 1990 and Projected to 2020.* Cambridge, MA: Harvard University Press, 1996.

30 British Thoracic Society. *The Burden of Lung Disease: A Statistics Report from the British Thoracic Society* [2002]. URL: www.brit-thoracic.org.uk.

31 National Heart, Lung, and Blood Institute. *Morbidity & Mortality: Chartbook on Cardiovascular, Lung, and Blood Diseases.* Bethesda, MD: US Department of Health and Human Services, Public Health Service, National Institutes of Health, 1998. URL: www.nhlbi.nih.gov/nhlbi/seiin/other/cht-book/htm.

32 National Health Service Executive. *Burdens of disease: a discussion document.* London: Department of Health, 1996.

33 Bellamy D. Identification of individuals at risk [with COPD]. In: Wedzicha J, Ind P, Miles A, eds. *The Effective Management of Chronic Obstructive Pulmonary Disease.* London: Aesculapius Medical, 2001.

34 Thurlbeck WM. A pathologist looks at respiratory failure due to obstructive lung disease. *Chest* 1970; **58**: 408.

35 National Center for Health Statistics. *Current Estimates from the National Health Interview Survey, United States, 1995.* Washington, DC: Department of Health and Human Services, Public Health Service, Vital and Health Statistics, 1995 (Publication No. 96-1527).

36 Barnes PJ. Medical progress: chronic obstructive pulmonary disease. *N Engl J Med* 2000; **343**: 269–80.

37 Orie NGM, Sluiter HJ, De Vries K, Tammerling K, Wikop J. The host factor in bronchitis. In: Orie NGM, Sluiter HJ, eds. *Bronchitis: an international symposium.* Assen, The Netherlands: Royal Vangorcum, 1961: 43–59.

38 Fletcher CM, Peto R, Tinker C, Speizer FE. *The Natural History of Chronic Bronchitis and Emphysema: an Eight Year Study of Early Chronic Obstructive Lung Disease in Working Men in London.* Oxford: Oxford University Press, 1976.

39 Scanlon PD, Connett JE, Waller LA *et al.* Smoking cessation and lung function in mild to moderate chronic obstructive pulmonary disease. *Am J Respir Crit Care Med* 2000; **161**: 381–90.

40 Xu X, Dockery DW, Ware JH, Speizer FE, Ferris BG Jr. Effects of cigarette smoking on rate of loss of pulmonary function in adults: a longitudinal assessment. *Am Rev Respir Dis* 1992; **146**: 1345–8.

41 Xu X, Laird N, Dockery DW *et al.* Age, period, and cohort effects on pulmonary function in a 24-year longitudinal study. *Am J Epidemiol* 1995; **141**: 554–66.

42 Laurell CB, Eriksson S. The electrophoretic α_1-globulin pattern of serum in α_1-antitrypsin deficiency. *Scand J Clin Invest* 1963; **15**: 132.

43 Silverman EK, Chapman HA, Drazen JM *et al.* Genetic epidemiology of severe, early-onset chronic obstructive pulmonary disease: risk to relatives for airflow obstruction and chronic bronchitis. *Am J Respir Crit Care Med* 1998; **157**: 1770–8.

44 Carrozzi L, Rijcken B, Burney P *et al.* Family history for chronic lung diseases and epidemiological determinants of COPD in three European countries. *Eur Respir Rev* 2001; **11**: 49–54.

45 Shaheen SO, Barker DJ, Shiell AW *et al.* The relationship between pneumonia in early childhood and impaired lung

function in late adult life. *Am J Respir Crit Care Med* 1994; **149**: 616–19.

46 Barker DJP, Godfrey KM, Fall C *et al.* Relation of birth weight and childhood respiratory infection to adult lung function and death from chronic obstructive lung disease. *BMJ* 1991; **303**: 671–5.

2: Why do only some smokers develop COPD?

Nikos Siafakas, Eleni Tzortzaki and
Demosthenes Bouros

Are there cigarette smokers who are susceptible to COPD?

It is well known that less than 20% of smokers develop clinically significant chronic obstructive pulmonary disease (COPD) [1–3]. From a number of epidemiological studies, it has become apparent that there are susceptible smokers who will develop COPD [1,3]. However, the characteristics of such susceptible individuals are not known [4]. The questions 'Is there a distinct group of susceptible smokers?' and 'What is the distribution (bimodal or unimodal) of susceptible individuals?' are extremely difficult to answer on the basis of the current scientific knowledge.

According to a new working definition developed by the Global Initiative for Chronic Obstructive Lung Disease (GOLD) group, COPD is a '*disease state characterized by airflow limitation that is not fully reversible. The airflow limitation is usually progressive and results from an abnormal inflammatory response of the lungs to noxious particles and gases*' [5]. It is likely that the reason why fewer than 20% of smokers develop COPD is connected with an abnormal inflammatory response to noxious agents. COPD is the result of an environmental insult and a response by the host that is primarily genetically predetermined.

Another mystery concerning the pathogenesis of COPD is why some patients develop predominantly parenchymal disease (emphysema), while others mainly develop airways disease (chronic bronchitis). This suggests the possibility of subgroups of susceptible individuals, some primarily with defects at the level of the major airways and others with defects at the level of the parenchyma. Are these defects genetically determined? [4].

A brief summary of the pathogenesis of the disease will be presented here first, with a review of the current literature. The environmental insults (noxious agents) concerned will then be discussed, as well as possible genetic risk factors.

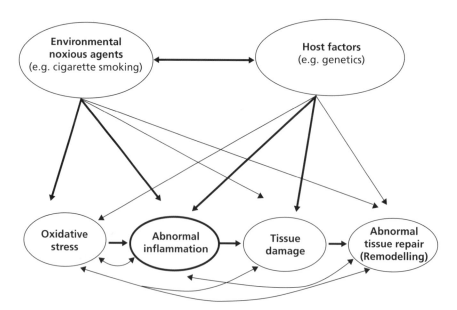

Fig. 2.1 Schematic presentation of the pathogenesis of chronic obstructive pulmonary disease (COPD) as a result of host exposure to environmental risk factors. Abnormal inflammation may play a significant role in the pathogenesis (for more details, see text).

What are the pathological processes that lead to the development of COPD?

Figure 2.1 is a schematic summary of the pathogenesis of COPD. Obviously, this schema has several limitations. A considerable proportion of the information is based on experimental animal studies; data from humans are limited by the number of subjects, the selection of patients and the tissues studied and methods used. There are therefore a number of missing links in our understanding of the pathogenesis of COPD, as shown in Fig. 2.1.

Oxidative stress

Cigarette smoke, the major environmental noxious agent, contains abundant amounts of oxygen-based free radicals, peroxides and peroxynitrite and results in severe oxidative stress in the lungs [6–9]. By oxidizing cellular proteins, lipids, DNA bases, enzymes and extracellular components such as matrix collagen and hyaluronic acid, these substances cause airway and parenchymal injury [10,11]. One of the consequences of the oxidative stress is chemotaxis, potent leucocyte adhesion and thus initiation of inflammation. The recruitment of inflammatory cells such as activated macrophages and neutrophils may also contribute to the oxidization by releasing specific enzymes [10–12].

Thus, cigarette smoke and the local release of oxidants initiate a vicious circle that may promote an 'abnormal' inflammatory response. For example, oxidants activate the transcription of nuclear factor-κB (NF-κB), which promotes genes of key inflammatory agents such as interleukin-8 (IL-8) and tumour necrosis factor-α (TNF-α) [13,14]. In addition, oxidants may oxidize antiproteases, resulting in a reduction of the antiprotease shield, and by activating matrix metalloproteinases may cause proteolysis [11,15]. Oxidative injury causes impairment to the barrier function of endothelial and epithelial cells [16,17]. Finally, if the oxidative stress is significant and prolonged, cells may undergo apoptosis or direct necrosis [18,19].

Inflammation

Many cells have been reported to be involved in the pathogenesis of COPD. However, their presence or activation in the affected tissues, or in fluids such as sputum or bronchoalveolar lavage (BAL), does not necessarily confirm their role in the process of disease development. The number of macrophages is increased in COPD [20]. Cigarette smoke also activates macrophages to release mediators, including IL-8, leukotriene B_4 (LTB_4) and TNF-α [21]. Thus, macrophages may orchestrate the inflammation process in COPD.

Neutrophils are the cells that have been studied most in COPD, but their role is not yet clear [22–24]. Neutrophils cause elastolysis by secreting neutrophil elastase, cathepsin G and proteinase 3 [25]. In addition, neutrophil proteases are mucus stimulants. Recruitment of neutrophils is the result of potent chemotaxis by IL-8, LTB_4 and increased adherence (Mac-1, E-selectin) [26]. Neutrophilic survival in the respiratory tract is increased in COPD by the increase of cytokines, such as granulocyte-macrophage colony-stimulating factor (GM-CSF). Although neutrophils are increased and/or activated in other diseases, such as cystic fibrosis, their elastolytic effect is not as prominent as in COPD. Other factors may therefore be involved in promoting the elastolytic activity of neutrophils in COPD [27].

T lymphocytes are increased in lung parenchyma, and in both peripheral and central airways in COPD [28,29]. In contrast to asthma, in which the CD4 cell is prominent in the airway, $CD8^+$ cells are increased in the airway mucosa in COPD patients and may cause cytolysis and apoptosis of alveolar epithelial cells [29,30]. Although there is an association between T lymphocytes and the amount of alveolar destruction and airflow limitation [28,31] the role of T cells in the pathogenesis of COPD is not yet certain.

Although eosinophils play an important part in the mechanisms of airway inflammation in asthma, their role in COPD is obscure. There are conflicting reports concerning their numbers in stable disease, but most reports have shown an increase during exacerbations [32–34]. Their interaction with neutrophils and their degranulation are also under investigation.

It has recently been shown that airway epithelial cells are of importance in secreting inflammatory mediators. Cigarette smoke activates epithelial cells to produce TNF-α and IL-8and may therefore initiate the abnormal inflammatory response [35]. Many inflammatory mediators may be involved in the pathogenesis of COPD; the most important ones that have been described are the lipid mediator LTB_4, the chemokine IL-8 and the cytokine TNF-α [21,33,35–37]. Other mediators that have been reported to have inflammatory effects in COPD include IL-5, GM-CSF, transforming growth factor-β (TGF-β), epidermal growth factor (EGF), endothelin-1 (ET-1) [33,38–40]. The inflammatory response in COPD may be up-regulated by a combination of the above mediators.

Tissue damage

The best-studied mechanism of tissue damage in COPD is that of protease–antiprotease imbalance. Proteases are enzymes that degrade matrix proteins. Elastin is an important target, but collagen, proteoglycans, laminin and fibronectin are also degraded [41–43].

The most potent proteases are the neutrophil elastase, cathepsin G and proteinase 3 and matrix metalloproteinases [44,45]. Neutrophils are the major providers of the above proteases, but other cells such as macrophages and airway epithelial cells may also contribute. The elastolytic activity of proteases is balanced by the antiproteases, such as α_1-antitrypsin. α_1-Antitrypsin is the major endogenous tissue antiprotease (plasma/lung parenchyma), and secretory leucoprotease inhibitor (SLPI) is the major antiprotease in the airways [41,46]. Clearly, in COPD there is an imbalance in the protease–antiprotease system in favour of proteases [47].

Tissue repair and 'abnormal' remodeling

Any incident of tissue damage is followed by a process of epithelial and parenchymal repair. This repair procedure is extremely complex and so far not fully understood. In the airways, the repair (remodeling) process includes repair of the tight junctions, cell migration, cell differentiation and metaplasia, mitosis and hyperplasia of basal cells and mitotic redifferentiation, among other processes [48]. It has been shown that smoke impairs lung repair mechanisms [49,50] and disrupts procedures that are able to restore the tissue structure. This may lead to peribronchial fibrosis and narrowing, particularly at the site of small airways. Fibronectin and TGF-β produced by the epithelial cells are involved in the normal repair processes, but there may be an excess of factors that cause fibrosis and abnormal remodeling [39,51].

In summary, the pathogenesis of COPD is extremely complex, and until the mechanisms that are involved become more clear, it is difficult to understand why only 20% of smokers develop COPD.

What is the evidence for cigarette smoke increasing susceptibility to COPD?

Among the risk factors that have been related to COPD, cigarette smoke is the best studied and is a consistent finding in numerous studies [1,52,53]. In all recent guidelines on COPD, cigarette smoking has been regarded as the best-established risk factor for the development of the disease [54,55]. In addition, passive cigarette smoking has been related to chronic cough and sputum and is also a candidate risk factor for the development of airflow limitation [53,56,57].

However, from the above epidemiological studies, it is apparent that not all smokers develop clinically significant COPD, and also that there is no direct dose–effect relationship. A passive smoker may develop the disease, whereas a heavy smoker may not. These observations have led to the hypothesis that there are smokers who are susceptible to COPD.

Longitudinal epidemiological studies have suggested that a more important factor than the dose (pack/years) is the timing of the exposure to cigarette smoke [58,59]. This is summarized in the epidemiological model of COPD risk shown in Fig. 2.2. Although COPD is a disease of middle/late adult life, events that occur during early life may play a significant role. For example, active or passive smoking during adulthood, when the lungs are fully developed, may make an individual susceptible to developing COPD (Fig. 2.2). An additional effect during maturation of the respiratory system could be maternal smoking during pregnancy (Fig. 2.2a). Finally, there is a well-known third phase in adult life, in which the susceptible smoker is characterized by a rapid decline in forced expiratory volume in 1 s (FEV_1) (Fig. 2.2d). The timing of exposure to cigarette smoke is thus crucial and may have different and/or additive effects. Cigarette smoke may cause changes before birth (lower initial lung volume), during growth (lower maximal attained volume), in the plateau phase (earlier start of decline) and during the late phase, with an accelerated decline [1,60,61]. However, the epidemiological model discussed above may partly explain the fact that not all smokers develop COPD.

Do risk factors act in combination in the development of COPD?

A combination of exogenous risk factors could be an alternative hypothesis to

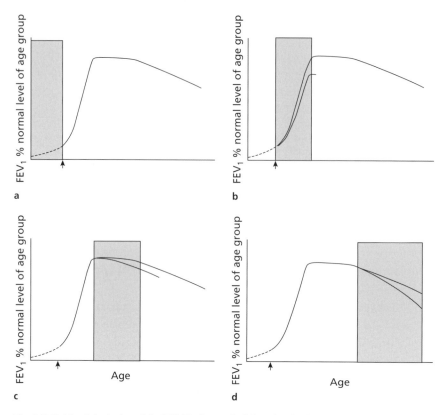

Fig. 2.2 Epidemiological model of COPD during the life cycle. Shaded area indicates changing function: (a) during pregnancy; (b) during lung growth (age 0–20); (c) during the plateau phase (age 20–40); and (d) during lung function decline (age > 40). Adapted with permission from [3].

explain why there are susceptible smokers. Exposure to a mixture of known noxious agents, such as active plus passive smoking, and environmental pollution and occupational pollution could cause COPD. However, current data do not support the hypothesis of combinations of these risk factors as the basis for the existence of susceptible smokers [3]. A number of other risk factors have been proposed that may play a role in the development of COPD.

Some studies have suggested a link between severe childhood respiratory infections and COPD in adult life [62]. However, this association is rather weak, because it is not easy retrospectively to exclude the possibility that these infections result from lung function impairment, rather than being the cause of it. Nevertheless, viral infections may directly contribute to the development of COPD by incorporating viral DNA into the airway cells. This could alter their genetic material and thus their response to subsequent exposure to cigarette smoke. In fact, increased levels of adenoviral DNA have been found in

COPD patients in comparison with control individuals [63]. Incorporation of adenoviral DNA in animal epithelial cells has also been shown to amplify the inflammatory response on exposure to cigarette smoke [64,65]. A possible scenario might therefore be that susceptible smokers are those in whom a viral infection early in life leads to an excess load of adenoviral DNA in the epithelial cells. These cells might then orchestrate an 'abnormal' inflammatory response to cigarette smoke. However, results of this type have not been reproduced by other investigators in humans.

What is the role of nutritional factors in the susceptibility to COPD?

Nutrition may play a role in the development of COPD, especially where oxidants and antioxidants are involved. Protective dietary factors concerned include the antioxidant vitamins C and E, magnesium and fish oils. In addition to the endogenous enzymatic antioxidant systems, the antioxidant vitamins C and E may enhance host defences against the oxidative stress of cigarette smoke. Fish oil contains highly polyunsaturated ω-3 fatty acids that act as competitive inhibitors of arachidonic acid metabolism. Fish oil may therefore down-regulate the inflammatory potency of lipid mediators such as LTB_4 and provide protection against COPD [66,67].

It is possible that smokers who develop COPD have dietary deficiencies in the nutritional elements mentioned above. However, this hypothesis is not supported by longitudinal studies [68] and would not explain the whole problem, since there are so many confounding factors between diet and cigarette smoking (alcohol intake, etc.).

What is the place of the Dutch hypothesis in COPD?

A relationship between increased airway reactivity, atopy and the development of COPD was first proposed by Orie *et al*. in 1961 [69]. In other words, smokers with hyperreactive airways could be the susceptible ones who will develop COPD. This hypothesis is still open to debate, as it is not clear whether hyperresponsiveness is the cause or the effect of the decrease in FEV_1 in smokers. Airways reactivity and atopy are complex disorders related to a number of genetic and environmental factors leading to allergic inflammation (asthma). This inflammation, however, has recently been shown to be different from that caused by cigarette smoke [70]. In addition, other investigators have suggested that the hyperresponsiveness seen in smokers is the result of abnormal geometry of the airways caused by prolonged smoking, leading to 'reactivity'. In addition, the majority of the studies investigating FEV_1 decline have tested airways reactivity at the end of the study (after the initiation of smoking)

[71,72] and only a few have tested it at the beginning [73,74]. Recently, two studies that reported an association of hyperresponsiveness in subgroups of smokers lacked statistical analysis of the smoking status [75,76]. When the smoking status was accounted for [77,78], the association between reactivity and smoking was not significant. In conclusion, the Dutch hypothesis has failed to clarify the issue of the susceptible smoker, which is still open to debate.

How do genetic factors modify COPD?

It is most likely that the answer to the mystery of why only a minority of smokers develop COPD is to be found in the field of genetics. Familial aggregation has been reported in COPD [79,80], but it is difficult to exclude confounding factors. In addition, COPD is a disease of middle age—by which time parents or grandparents are rarely still alive, so that it is difficult to conduct classical hereditary studies. It is also likely that many genetic factors interact to increase or decrease the risk of developing COPD. Thus, Mendel's laws of inheritance of 'susceptibility' to cigarette smoke could be ruled out [81].

α_1-Antitrypsin

The only established genetic risk factor for COPD is homozygosity of the α_1-antitrypsin (α_1-AT) gene. α_1-AT is a potent antiprotease produced by the liver. Numerous investigations have assessed the risk associated with heterozygous genotypes. The common gene variants are M, S and Z, and their frequencies are reported to be 0.93, 0.05, and 0.02, respectively.

The MM genotype is considered normal. The MS genotype shows a mild reduction in α_1-AT (approximately 80% of normal); MZ has reduced α_1-AT (about 60% of normal); levels in the SZ genotype are even lower (about 40% of normal); and in ZZ they are less than 15% of normal. Large studies have compared subjects with the MZ genotype with those with the MM genotype and found no significant difference in pulmonary function or symptoms in non-smokers [80]. There are conflicting results in smokers, as it has been shown that MZ smokers have a greater loss of elastic recoil than MM smokers [87] and a rapid decline in FEV_1 [88]. Homozygous ZZ patients have a very low α_1-antitrypsin level and show a rapid decline in FEV_1 even without smoking [82,83]. In smokers who are homozygous Z patients, COPD is developed at a younger age [84,85]. However, this homozygous state is rare in the general population (one in 5000 live births) [86] and as a genetic risk factor can therefore explain less than 1% of COPD cases.

In addition to the mutations that affect the level of serum α_1-AT, other mutations have been described that affect its function [89]. One of these is a mutation in the 3' region of the α_1-AT gene [90,91]. However, this mutation is not specific for COPD, as it has also been found in bronchiectasis [90,91]. Other investigators have proposed that the 3' mutation allele might be in disequilibrium with an α_1-antichymotrypsin deficiency allele [92], while others again have suggested that the 3' mutation may affect the acute-phase response, leading to inadequate up-regulation of α_1-AT during acute inflammation [93]. This could be also true during the acute oxidative stress of cigarette smoking. Thus, not only the level but also the structure and function of α_1-AT are genetically predetermined and may predispose to COPD in smokers.

α_1-Antichymotrypsin (α_1-ACT)

α_1-ACT is an acute-phase reactant with antiprotease properties produced by the liver. α_1-ACT deficiency is present only in 1% of the general population in Sweden, and is transmitted with autosomal-dominant inheritance [94]. Two mutations in the α_1-ACT gene have been associated with a reduced α_1-ACT serum level [95], but the relationship between low α_1-ACT or defective functioning of α_1-ACT and COPD is not as clear as it is for α_1-AT.

Blood group antigens

An association between the ABO locus and COPD has been reported, with the type A blood group being associated with impaired lung function [96]. Others have failed to confirm any relationship between ABO alleles and pulmonary function [97,98].

Although the ABO antigens in respiratory secretions may have a protective role [99,100] and might be responsible for the defect in susceptible smokers, these observations have not been confirmed in airflow obstruction [97,98,101]. Similarly, the Lewis blood system was investigated in airflow limitation, and it was shown that Lewis-negative subjects were at greater risk [102]. Blood group antigens have been associated with recurrent infections that may lead to COPD. However, the role of ABO, Lewis and secretor genes remains unclear in the pathogenesis of COPD.

Vitamin D-binding protein (VDBP)

VDBP is a protein secreted by the liver that is able to bind vitamin D and endotoxin and to act as macrophage-activating factor or chemoattractant enhancer of C5a [103,104]. Thus, it can regulate the inflammatory response or diminish antioxidative capacity of the host. A reduced frequency of the 2–2 genotype of VDBP was reported in COPD patients in one study [105], but this was not replicated [99].

α_2-Macroglobulin

α_2-Macroglobulin is a protease inhibitor and its serum deficiency is rare. The α_2-macroglobulin gene is located on chromosome 12, and its sequence has been identified. However, there have only been case reports of patients with COPD and α_2-macroglobulin polymorphism [106].

Cytochrome P450$_{1A1}$

A study has reported that the high-activity allele of CYP1A1 was associated with susceptibility to centrilobular emphysema and lung cancer, but this was not linked to cancer alone in the absence of emphysema [107].

Cystic fibrosis transmembrane regulator (CFTR)

The frequency of the CFTR gene has been examined in chronic bronchitis. The study found that none of the known mutations of CFTR were associated with COPD [108].

Human leucocyte antigen (HLA) locus

A significant decrease in the HLA-Bw16 allele was found in COPD patients with a low FEV_1 value and an increase in HLA-B7 antigen [99]. However, it is not clear whether these associations are due to variations in the HLA genes themselves, or whether there is any relation to susceptibility to COPD.

Immunoglobulin deficiency

Selective IgA deficiency has been found to segregate with COPD in three generation pedigrees [109]. Other investigators have studied the role of IgA or IgG deficiency in the aetiology of COPD in relation to recurrent infections [110,111].

Extracellular superoxide dismutase (EC-SOD)

EC-SOD is an important extracellular antioxidant enzyme in the lung that attenuates tissue damage produced by oxygen radicals from cigarette smoke. Polymorphism in the EC-SOD gene has been reported in 2% of the general population [112]. However, it is not known whether this variant of the gene plays a role in the pathogenesis of COPD.

Secretory leucocyte proteinase inhibitor (SLPI)

SLPI is produced by airway epithelial cells; it is able to inhibit neutrophil elastase [113] and is thought to be a potent antiproteinase in the airways. Polymorphisms of the *SLPI* gene have been detected, but no mutations have been reported [114]. This suggests that structural alterations in *SLPI* may not be involved in the pathogenesis of COPD.

Other candidate genes

A mutation in the cathepsin G gene, a serine protease, has been found, but it was not associated with COPD [115]. In addition, a relationship has been reported between polymorphism in the gene for microsomal epoxide hydrolase and susceptibility to emphysema [116].

DNA microsatellite instability (MSI) in COPD

Microsatellites of DNA are short tandem nucleotide repeats, commonly found throughout the genome. Microsatellite instability has been correlated with high mutational rates [117]. Studying MSI might therefore be a useful technique for identifying the locus of potentially altered genes.

This method had been applied to sputum cells of COPD patients, and it was shown that this defect can be detected [118]. Recently, sputum cells from groups of smokers without COPD and smokers with COPD were tested for MSI [119]. The two groups had similar smoking histories. MSI was detected in 24% of COPD patients, but in none of the non-COPD smokers. These results suggest that MSI may be part of the complex genetic basis of COPD and could serve as a marker of genetic alteration caused by smoking, leading to the development of COPD. MSI may therefore be an index of the susceptible smoker [119]. However, more studies are needed to verify these results.

In conclusion, there must be a number of genetically predetermined host factors that characterize the susceptible smoker.

Conclusions

COPD is a common disease, and the major risk factor for it—cigarette smoking—has been identified. However, only a minority of smokers develop clinically relevant disease. Although significant progress has been made in understanding the pathogenesis of COPD, it remains unclear why only a few smokers develop COPD. The cornerstone of the pathogenesis of COPD is the response of the host (the smoker) to an environmental risk factor (cigarette smoke). The main effect of this response has been described as 'abnormal inflammation', but the various pathways involved are not clear. Oxidative stress, inflammation, tissue damage and tissue repair (remodeling) are parts of the complex procedure leading to COPD.

An epidemiological model has been proposed in which the emphasis is on the timing of the exposure to cigarette smoke (before birth, during lung growth, etc.). There is evidence that respiratory adenoviral infection in early life could be an important factor that characterizes the susceptible smoker. Airway hyperresponsiveness has failed to clarify the whole picture and is still a topic of debate. Differences in nutritional elements, such as vitamins or fish oil, could play a role in providing protection against the effects of oxidative stress, but cannot fully explain the existence of susceptible individuals. Genetic differences are therefore the most likely parameters for identifying susceptible smokers. The only well-established genetic risk factor so far is the α_1-antitrypsin gene; other candidate genes are being investigated.

In conclusion, there are as yet no definitive answers to the basic question of why only a few smokers develop COPD. It is most likely that a number of genes are involved, affecting various pathways in the pathogenesis of the condition — but as this review shows, the genetic basis of the disease is only beginning to be elucidated. Understanding the genetic basis of COPD should lead to better methods of prevention and treatment in the future.

References

1 Fletcher C, Peto R, Tinker C, Speizer FE. *The Natural History of Chronic Bronchitis and Emphysema*. Oxford: Oxford University Press, 1976.

2 Burrows B, Bloom JW, Traver GA, Cline MG. The course and prognosis of different forms of chronic airways obstruction in a sample from the general population. *N Engl J Med* 1987; **317**: 1309–14.

3 Rijcken B, Britton J. Epidemiology of chronic obstructive pulmonary disease. *Eur Respir Monogr* 1998; **7**: 41–72.

4 Siafakas NM, Postma DS. Future research in chronic obstructive pulmonary disease. *Eur Respir Monogr* 1998; **7**: 299–302.

5 Global initiative for Chronic Obstructive Lung Disease. *Global Strategy for the Diagnosis, Management and Prevention of Chronic Obstructive Pulmonary Disease*. National Heart Lung and Blood Insitute and World Health Organisation Workshop publication no. 2701; 2001.

6 Rahman I, Morrison D, Donaldson K, MacNee W. Systemic oxidative stress in asthma, COPD, and smokers. *Am J Respir Crit Care Med* 1996; **154**: 1055–60.

7 Pryor WA. Biological effects of cigarette smoke, wood smoke and the smoke from plastics: the use of electron spin resonance. *Free Radic Biol Med* 1992; **13**: 659–76.

8 Ludwig PW, Hoidal JR. Alterations in leukocyte oxidative metabolism in cigarette smokers. *Am Rev Respir Dis* 1982; **126**: 977–80.

9 Repine JE, Bast A, Lankhorst I. Oxidative stress in chronic obstructive pulmonary disease. *Am J Respir Crit Care Dis* 1997; **156**: 341–57.

10 Kao RC, Whener NG, Skubitz KM, Gray BH, Hoidal JR. Proteinase 3: a distinct human polymorphonuclear leukocyte proteinase which produces emphysema in hamsters. *J Clin Invest* 1988; **82**: 1963–73.

11 Hautamaki RD, Kobayashi DK, Senior RM, Shapiro SD. Requirement for macrophage elastase for cigarette smoke-induced emphysema in mice. *Science* 1997; **277**: 2002–4.

12 Hoidal JR, Jeffery PK. Cellular and biochemical mechanisms in chronic obstructive pulmonary disease. *Eur Respir Monogr* 1998; **7**: 84–91.

13 DeForge LE, Preson AM, Takeuchi E *et al*. Regulation of interleukin 8 gene expression by oxidant stress. *J Biol Chem* 1993; **268**: 25568–76.

14 Sellak H, Franzini E, Hakim J, Pasquier C. Reactive oxygen species rapidly increase endothelial ICAM-1 ability to bind neutrophils without detectable upregulation. *Blood* 1994; **83**: 2669–77.

15 Pardo A, Selman M. Proteinase–antiproteinase imbalance in the pathogenesis of emphysema: the role of metalloproteinases in lung damage. *Histol Histopathol* 1999; **14**: 227–33.

16 Marui N, Offermann MK, Swerlick R *et al*. Vascular cell adhesion molecule-1 (VCAM-1) gene transcription and expression are regulated through an antioxidant-sensitive mechanism in human vascular endothelial cells. *J Clin Invest* 1993; **92**: 1866–74.

17 Andreoli SP, Mallett C, McAteer JA, Williams LV. Antioxidants defense mechanisms of endothelial cells and renal tubular epithelial cells in vitro: role of the glutathione redox cycle and catalase. *Pediatr Res* 1992; **32**: 360–5.

18 Trevani AS, Andoegui G, Giordano M *et al*. Neutrophil apoptosis induced by proteolytic enzymes. *Laboratory Invest* 1996; **74**: 711–21.

19 Smyth MJ, Trapani JA. Granzymes: exogenous proteinases that induce target cell apoptosis. *Immunol Today* 1995; **16**: 202–6.

20 Di Stefano A, Capelli A, Lusuardi M *et al*. Severity of airflow limitation is associated with severity of airway inflammation in smokers. *Am J Respir Crit Care Med* 1998; **158**: 1277–86.

21 Keatings VM, Collins PD, Scott DM, Barnes PJ. Differences in interleukin-8 and tumor necrosis factor-α in induced sputum from patients with chronic obstructive pulmonary disease or asthma. *Am J Respir Crit Care Med* 1996; **153**: 530–4.

22 Saetta M, Turato G, Facchini FM *et al*. Inflammatory cells in the bronchial glands of smokers with chronic bronchitis. *Am J Respir Crit Care Med* 1997; **156**: 1633–9.

23 O'Shaughnessy TC, Ansari TW, Barnes NC, Jeffery PK. Inflammatory cells in the airway surface epithelium of bronchitic smokers with and without airflow obstruction. *Eur Respir J* 1996; **9**: 14S.

24 Majori M, Gabrielli M, Cuomo A *et al*. Cellular inflammation in chronic obstructive bronchitis. *Eur Respir J* 1995; **8**: 227S.

25 Witko-Sarsat V, Halbwachs-Mecarelli L, Schuster A *et al*. Proteinase 3, a potent secretagogue in airways, is present in cystic fibrosis sputum. *Am J Respir Cell Mol Biol* 1999; **20**: 729–36.

26 Di Stefano A, Maestrelli P, Roggeri A *et al*. Upregulation of adhesion molecules in the bronchial mucosa of subjects with chronic obstructive bronchitis. *Am J Respir Crit Care Med* 1994; **149**: 803–10.

27 Stockley RA, Cellular mechanisms in the pathogenesis of COPD. *Eur Respir Rev* 1996; **6**: 264–9.

28 Flinkelstein R, Fraser RS, Ghezzo H, Cosio MG. Alveolar inflammation and its relation to emphysema in smokers. *Am J Respir Crit Care Med* 1995; **152**: 1666–72.

29 Liu AN, Mohammed AZ, Rice WR *et al*. Perforin-independent CD8(+) T-cell-mediated cytotoxicity of alveolar epithelial cells is preferentially mediated by tumor necrosis factor-alpha: relative insensitivity to Fas ligand. *Am J Respir Cell Mol Biol* 1999; **20**: 849–58.

30 Saetta M, Di Stefano A, Turato G *et al*. CD8+ T-lymphocytes in peripheral airways of smokers with chronic obstructive pulmonary disease. *Am J Respir Crit Care Med* 1998; **157**: 822–6.

31 O'Shaughnessy TC, Ansari TW, Barnes NC, Jeffery PK. Inflammation in bronchial biopsies of subjects with chronic bronchitis: inverse relationship

of CD8+ T-lymphocytes with FEV$_1$. *Am J Respir Crit Care Med* 1997; **155**: 852–7.

32 Lacoste JY, Bousquet J, Chanez P. Eosinophilic and neutrophilic inflammation in asthma, chronic bronchitis and chronic obstructive pulmonary disease. *J Allergy Clin Immunol* 1993; **92**: 537–48.

33 Mueller R, Chanez P, Campbell AM *et al.* Different cytokine patterns in bronchial biopsies in asthma and chronic bronchitis. *Respir Med* 1996; **90**: 79–85.

34 Saetta M, Di Stefano A, Maestrelli P *et al.* Airway eosinophilia in chronic bronchitis during exacerbations. *Am J Respir Crit Care Med* 1994; **150**: 1646–52.

35 Wyatt TA, Heires AJ, Sanderson SD, Floreani AA. Protein kinase C activation is required for cigarette smoke-enhanced C5a-mediated release of interleukin-8 in human bronchial epithelial cells. *Am J Respir Cell Mol Biol* 1999; **21**: 283–8.

36 Zakrzewski JT, Barnes NC, Costello JF, Piper PJ. Lipid mediators in cystic fibrosis and chronic obstructive pulmonary disease. *Am Rev Respir Dis* 1987; **136**: 779–82.

37 Yamamoto C, Yoneda T, Yoshikawa M *et al.* Airway inflammation in COPD assessed by sputum levels of interleukin-8. *Chest* 1997; **112**: 505–10.

38 Balbi B, Bason C, Balleari E *et al.* Increased bronchoalveolar granulocytes and granulocyte/macrophage colony-stimulating factor during exacerbations of chronic bronchitis. *Eur Respir J* 1997; **10**: 846–50.

39 Vignola AM, Chanez P, Chiappara G *et al.* Transforming growth factor-beta expression in mucosal biopsies in asthma and chronic bronchitis. *Am J Respir Crit Care Med* 1997; **156**: 591–9.

40 Chalmers GW, Mocleod KJ, Sriram S *et al.* Sputum endothelin-1 is increased in cystic fibrosis and chronic obstructive pulmonary disease. *Eur Respir J* 1999; **13**: 1288–92.

41 Drost EM, Selby C, Lannan S, Lowe GD, MacNee W. Changes in neutrophil deformability following in vitro smoke exposure. mechanism and protection. *Am J Respir Cell Moll Biol* 1992; **6**: 287–95.

42 Robbins RA, Gossman GL, Nelson KJ *et al.* Inactivation of chemotactic factor inactivator by cigarette smoke: a potential mechanism of modulating neutrophil recruitment to the lung. *Am Rev Respir Dis* 1990; **142**: 763–8.

43 Janoff A. Reduction of the elastase in inhibitory capacity of alpha-1-antitrypsin by peroxides in cigarette smoke; an analysis of the brands and the filters. *Am Rev Respir Dis* 1982; **126**: 25–30.

44 Morrison HM, Welgus HG, Stockley RA, Burnett D, Campbell EJ. Inhibition of human leukocyte elastase bound to elastin: relative ineffectiveness and two mechanisms of inhibitory activity. *Am J Respir Cell Mol Biol* 1994; **41**: 442–7.

45 Shapiro SD. Matrix metalloproteinase degradation of extracellular matrix: biological consequences. *Curr Opinion Cell Biol* 1998; **10**: 602–8.

46 MacNee W, Wiggs B, Belzberg AS, Hogg JC. The effect of cigarette smoking on neutrophil kinetics in human lungs. *N Engl J Med* 1989; **321**: 924–8.

47 MacElvaney NG, Crystal RG. *Proteases and Lung Injury*. Philadelphia: Lippincott-Raven, 1997.

48 Puchelle E, Zahm JM. Repair processes of the airway epithelium. In: Lenfant CL, ed. *Airways and Environments—from Injury to Repair: Lung Biology in Health and Disease*. New York: Dekker, 1996: 157–82.

49 Nakamura Y, Romberger DJ, Tate L *et al.* Cigarette smoke inhibits lung fibroblast proliferation and chemotaxis. *Am J Respir Crit Care Med* 1995; **151**: 1497–503.

50 Osman M. Cigarette smoke impairs elastin resynthesis in lungs of hamsters with elastase-induced emphysema. *Am Rev Respir Dis* 1985; **132**: 640–3.

51 Shoji S, Ertl RF, Linder J, Romberger DJ, Rennard SI. Bronchial epithelial cells produce chemotactic activity for bronchial epithelial cells: possible role for fibronectin in airway repair. *Am Rev Respir Dis* 1990; **141**: 218–25.

52 US Surgeon-General. *The Health Consequences of Smoking: Chronic Obstructive Lung Disease*. Washington, DC: US Department of Health and Human Resources, 1984 (Publication No. 84-50205).

53 Buist AS, Vollmer WM. Smoking and

other risk factors. In: Murray JF, Nadel JA, eds. *Textbook of Respiratory Medicine*. Philadelphia: Saunders, 1994: 1259–87.

54 Siafakas NM, Vermeire P, Pride NB *et al.* Optimal assessment and management of chronic obstructive pulmonary disease (COPD). *Eur Respir J* 1995; **8**: 1398–420.

55 American Thoracic Society. Standards for the diagnosis and care of patients with chronic obstructive pulmonary disease (COPD) and asthma. *Am Rev Respir Dis* 1987; **139**: 225–44.

56 Leuenberger P, Schwartz J, Ackermann-Liebrich U *et al.* Passive smoking exposure in adults and chronic respiratory symptoms (SAPALDIA Study). *Am J Respir Crit Care Med* 1994; **150**: 1222–8.

57 Dayal HH, Khuder S, Sharrar R, Trieff N. Passive smoking in obstructive respiratory disease in an industrialized urban population. *Environ Res* 1994; **65**: 161–71.

58 Burrows B, Cline MG, Knudson RJ, Taussig LM, Lebowitz MD. A descriptive analysis of the growth and decline of the FVC and FEV_1. *Chest* 1983; **83**: 717–24.

59 Weiss ST. Early life predictors of adult chronic obstructive lung disease. *Eur Respir Rev* 1995; **5**: 303–9.

60 Tager IB, Segal MR, Speizer FE, Weiss ST. The natural history of forced expiratory volumes: effect of cigarette smoking and respiratory symptoms. *Am Rev Respir Dis* 1988; **138**: 837–49.

61 Sherrill DL, Lebowitz MD, Knudson RJ, Burrows B. Smoking and symptom effects on the curves of lung function growth and decline. *Am Rev Respir Dis* 1991; **144**: 17–22.

62 Burrows B, Knudson RJ, Lebowitz MD. The relationship of childhood respiratory illness to adult obstructive airway disease. *Am Rev Respir Dis* 1977; **115**: 751–60.

63 Matsuse T, Hayashi S, Kuwano K *et al.* Latent adenoviral infection in the pathogenesis of chronic airways obstruction. *Am Rev Respir Dis* 1992; **146**: 177–84.

64 Keicho N, Elliott W, Hogg J, Hayashi S. Adenovirus E1A upregulates interleukin-8 expression induced by endotoxin in pulmonary epithelial cells. *Am J Physiol* 1997; **272**: L1046–52.

65 Vitalis TZ, Kern I, Croome A *et al.* The effect of latent adenovirus 5 infection on cigarette smoke-induced lung inflammation. *Eur Respir J* 1998; **11**: 664–9.

66 Shahar E, Folsom AR, Mlnick SL *et al.* Dietary ω-3 polyunsaturated fatty acids and smoking-related chronic obstructive pulmonary disease. *N Engl J Med* 1994; **331**: 228–33.

67 Sharp DS, Rodriguez BL, Shahar E, Hwang L, Burchfiel CM. Fish consumption may limit the damage of smoking on the lung. *Am J Respir Crit Care Med* 1994; **150**: 983–7.

68 Miedema I, Feskens EJM, Heederik D, Kromhout D. Dietary determinants of long-term incidence of chronic nonspecific lung disease. The Zutphen study. *Am J Epidemiol* 1993; **138**: 37–45.

69 Orie NG, Sluiter HJ, DeVries K, Tammeling GJ, Witkop J. The host factor in bronchitis. In: Orie NGM, Sluiter HJ, eds. *Bronchitis: an International Symposium*. Assen, Netherlands: Royal Vangorcum, 1961: 43–59.

70 Jeffery PK. Structural and inflammatory changes in COPD: a comparison with asthma. *Thorax* 1998; **53**: 129–36.

71 Barter CE, Campbell AH. Relationship of constitutional factors and cigarette smoking to decrease in 1-second forced expiratory Volume. *Am Rev Respir Dis* 1976; **113**: 305–14.

72 Sparrow D, O'Connor G, Colton TH, Barry ChL, Weis ST. The relationship of nonspecific bronchial responsiveness to the occurrence of respiratory symptoms and decreased levels of pulmonary function. *Am Rev Respir Dis* 1987; **135**: 1255–60.

73 Parker DR, O'Connor GT, Sparrow D, Segal MR, Weiss ST. The relationship of nonspecific airway responsiveness and atopy to decline of lung function. *Am Rev Respir Dis* 1990; **141**: 589–94.

74 Campbell AH, Barter CE, O'Connell JM, Huggins R. Factors affecting the decline of ventilatory function in chronic bronchitis. *Thorax* 1985; **40**: 741–8.

75 Frew AF, Kennedy SM, Chan-Yeung M. Methacholine responsiveness, smoking and atopy as risk factors for accelerated

FEV$_1$ decline in male working populations. *Am Rev Respir Dis* 1992; **146**: 878–83.

76 Villar MT, Dow L, Coggon D, Lampe FC, Holgate ST. The influence of increased bronchial responsiveness, atopy, and serum IgE on decline in FEV$_1$: a longitudinal study in the elderly. *Am J Respir Crit Care Med* 1995; **151**: 656–62.

77 Rijcken B, Schouten JP, Xu X, Rosner B, Weiss ST. Airway hyperresponsiveness to histamine is associated with accelerated decline of FEV$_1$. *Am J Respir Crit Care Med* 1995; **151**: 1377–82.

78 O'Connor GT, Sparrow D, Weiss ST. A prospective longitudinal study of methacholine airway responsiveness as a predictor of pulmonary-function decline. The Normative Aging Study. *Am J Respir Crit Care Med* 1995; **152**: 87–92.

79 Oswald NC, Harld JT, Martin WJ. Clinical pattern of chronic bronchitis. *Lancet* 1953; **ii**: 639–46.

80 Tager IB, Rosner B, Tishler PV, Speizer FE, Kass EH. Household aggregation of pulmonary function and chronic bronchitis. *Am Rev Respir Dis* 1976; **114**: 485–92.

81 Sandford AJ, Weir TD, Pare PD. Genetic risk factors for chronic obstructive pulmonary disease. *Eur Respir J* 1997; **10**: 1380–91.

82 Black LF, Kueppers F. Alpha$_1$-antitrypsin deficiency in nonsmokers. *Am Rev Respir Dis* 1978; **117**: 421–8.

83 Janus ED, Phillips NT, Carrell RW. Smoking, lung function and alpha$_1$-antitrypsin deficiency. *Lancet* 1985; **i**: 152–4.

84 Brantley ML, Paul LD, Miller BH *et al.* Clinical features and history of the destructive lung disease associated with alpha$_1$-antitrypsin deficiency of adults with pulmonary symptoms. *Am Rev Respir Dis* 1988; **138**: 327–36.

85 Tobin MJ, Cook PJL, Hutchinson DCS. Alpha$_1$-antitrypsin deficiency: the clinical and physiological features of pulmonary emphysema in subjects homozygous for Pi type Z. A survey by the British Thoracic Association. *Br J Dis Chest* 1983; **77**: 14–27.

86 O'Brien ML, Buist NRM, Murphey HW. Neonatal screening for alpha$_1$-

antitrypsin deficiency. *J Pediatr* 1978; **92**: 1006–10.

87 Tattersall SF, Pereira RP, Hunter D, Blundell G, Pride NB. Lung distensibility and airway function in intermediate alpha$_1$-antitrypsin deficiency. *Thorax* 1979; **34**: 637–46.

88 Tarjan E, Magyar P, Vaczi Z, Lantos A, Vaszar L. Longitudinal lung function study in heterozygous PiMZ phenotype subjects. *Eur Respir J* 1994; **7**: 2199–204.

89 Owen MC, Brennan SO, Lewis JH, CarrellRW. Mutation of antitrypsin to antithrombin: α_1-antitrypsin Pittsburgh (358 met→arg), a fatal bleeding disorder. *N Engl J Med* 1983; **309**: 694–8.

90 Kalsheker NA, Hodgson IJ, Watkins GL *et al.* Deoxyribonucleic acid (DNA) polymorphism of the α_1-antitrypsin gene in chronic lung disease. *BMJ* 1987; **294**: 1511–14.

91 Poller W, Meison C, Olek K. DNA polymorphisms of the α_1-antitrypsin gene region in patients with chronic obstructive pulmonary disease. *Eur J Clin Invest* 1990; **20**: 1–7.

92 Kalsheker NA, Watkins GL, Hill S *et al.* Independent mutations in the flanking sequence of the alpha$_1$-antitrypsin gene are associated with chronic obstructive airways disease. *Dis Markers* 1990; **8**: 151–7.

93 Cruickshank AM, Hansell DT, Burns HJG, Shenkin A. Effect of nutritional status on acute phase protein response to elective surgery. *Br J Surg* 1989; **76**: 165–8.

94 Eriksson S, Lindmark B, Liljia H. Familial α_1-antichymotrypsin deficiency. *Acta Med Scand* 1986; **220**: 447–53.

95 Poller W, Faber JB, Scholz S *et al.* Missense mutation of α_1-antichymotrypsin gene associated with chronic lung disease [letter]. *Lancet* 1992; **339**: 1538.

96 Cohen BH, Ball WC, Brashears S *et al.* Risk factors in chronic obstructive pulmonary disease (COPD). *Am J Epidemiol* 1977; **105**: 223–32.

97 Higgins MW, Keller JB, Becker M *et al.* An index of risk for obstructive airways disease. *Am Rev Respir Dis* 1982; **125**: 144–51.

98 Vestbo J, Hein HO, Suadicani P,

Sorensen H, Gyntelber F. Genetic markers for chronic bronchitis and peak expiratory flow in the Copenhagen Male Study. *Dan Med Bull* 1993; **40**: 378–80.

99 Kauffmann F, Kleisbauer JP, Cambon D *et al*. Genetic markers in chronic airflow limitation: a genetic epidemiologic study. *Am Rev Respir Dis* 1983; **127**: 263–169.

100 Cohen BH, Bias WB, Chase GA *et al*. Is ABH non-secretor status a risk factor for obstructive lung disease? *Am J Epidemiol* 1980; **111**: 285–91.

101 Abboud RT, Yu P, Chan-Yeung M, Tan F. Lack of relationship between ABH secretor status and lung function in pulp-mill workers. *Am Rev Respir Dis* 1982; **126**: 1089–91.

102 Horne SL, Cockcroft DW, Lovegrove A, Dosman JA. ABO, Lewis and secretor status and relative incidence of airflow obstruction. *Dis Markers* 1985; **3**: 55–62.

103 Yamamoto N, Homma S. Vitamin D-binding protein (group-specific component) is a precursor for the macrophage-activating signal factor from lysophosphatidyl-choline-treated lymphocytes. *Proc Natl Acad Sci USA* 1991; **88**: 8539–43.

104 Kew RR, Webster RO. Gc-globulin (vitamin D-binding protein) enhances the neutrophil chemotactic activity of C5a and C5a des Arg. *J Clin Invest* 1988; **82**: 364–9.

105 Kueppers F, Miller RD, Gordon H, Hepper NG, Offord K. Familial prevalence of chronic obstructive pulmonary disease in a matched pair study. *Am J Med* 1977; **63**: 336–42.

106 Poller W, Barth J, Voss B. Detection of an alteration of the α_2-macroglobulin gene in a patient with chronic lung disease and serum α_2-macroglobulin deficiency. *Hum Genet* 1989; **83**: 93–6.

107 Cantlay AM, Lamb D, Gillooly M *et al*. Association between the CYP1A1 gene polymorphism and susceptibility to emphysema and lung cancer. *J Clin Pathol Mol Pathol* 1995; **48**: M210–14.

108 Entzian P, Muller E, Boysen A *et al*. Frequency of common cystic fibrosis gene mutations in chronic bronchitis

patients. *Scand J Laboratory Invest* 1995; **55**: 263–6.

109 Webb DR, Condemi JJ. Selective immunoglobulin A deficiency and chronic obstructive lung disease. *Ann Intern Med* 1974; **80**: 618–21.

110 Bjorkander J, Bake B, Oxelius VA, Hanson LA. Impaired lung function in patient with IgA deficiency and low levels of IgG_2 or IgG_3. *N Engl J Med* 1985; **313**: 720–4.

111 O'Keefe S, Gzel A, Drury R *et al*. Immunoglobulin G subclasses and spirometry in patients with chronic obstructive pulmonary disease. *Eur Respir J* 1991; **4**: 932–8.

112 Sandstrom J, Nilsson P, Karlsson K, Marklund SL. Tenfold increase in human plasma extracellular superoxide dismutase content caused by a mutation in heparin-binding domain. *J Biol Chem* 1994; **268**: 19163–6.

113 Sallenave JM, Shulmann J, Crossley J, Jordana M, Gauldie J. Regulation of secretory leukocyte proteinase inhibitor (SLPI) and elastase-specific inhibitor (ESI/Elafin) in human airway epithelial airway cells by cytokines and neutrophilic enzymes. *Am J Respir Cell Mol Biol* 1994; **11**: 733–41.

114 Abe T, Kobayashi N, Yoshimura K *et al*. Expression of the secretory leukoprotease inhibitor gene in epithelial cells. *J Clin Invest* 1991; **87**: 2207–15.

115 Ludecke B, Poller W, Olek K, Bartholome K. Sequence variant of the human cathepsin G gene. *Hum Genet* 1993; **91**: 83–4.

116 Smith CA, Harrison DJ. Association between polymorphism in gene for microsomal epoxide hydrolase and susceptibility to emphysema. *Lancet* 1997; **350**: 630–3.

117 Charlesworth B, Sniegowski P, Stephan W. The evolutionary dynamics of repetitive DNA in eukaryotes. *Nature* 1994; **371**: 215–20.

118 Spandidos DA, Ergazaki M, Hatzistamou J *et al*. Microsatellite instability in patients with chronic obstructive pulmonary disease. *Oncol Rep* 1996; **3**: 489–91.

119 Siafakas NM, Tzortzaki EG, Sourvinos G *et al*. Microsatellite DNA instability in COPD. *Chest* 1999; **116**: 47–51.

3: How should COPD be diagnosed?

Mike Pearson

What is COPD? Is it to do with cough and sputum?

'Chronic bronchitis' was the term commonly used throughout the UK in the 1950s for the syndrome we would now describe as chronic obstructive pulmonary disease (COPD). The Americans were inclined to describe it as 'emphysema', and there were many other synonyms in use until, in the last decade, general agreement developed that we should use the umbrella term 'COPD' and accept that it includes a series of subsidiary components (Table 3.1). It is important to recognize that some of the early studies worked with definitions that are different from those we use today and that therefore one must be cautious before extrapolating some of the earlier studies to current practice.

The productive cough that occurred particularly in smokers and in those working in dusty jobs was shown in the 1950s to be primarily a large-airway problem. Several studies demonstrated an increase in mucosal goblet cells, and the Reid index defined the increased thickness of the mucosa pathologically [1]. The definition of chronic bronchitis used today is that produced by the Medical Research Council (MRC) for epidemiological surveys and not for clinical purposes [2]. The definition restricted chronic bronchitis to 'a productive cough for more than 3 months of the year in each of two successive years'. Thus, chronic bronchitis is related to the productive cough and not to any level of airflow limitation. This symptomatic definition has been used in many epidemiological studies, in which it has been of considerable value, but it is less helpful in managing individuals in clinical practice. For example, patients with bronchiectasis and/or with chronic asthma — very different pathological processes — would be included. However, this is of little consequence in large, population-based surveys, since bronchiectasis is sufficiently uncommon for it not to confound the results unduly.

Cough and sputum are common in smokers. The prime cause is the need to clear the increased inhaled particulate load from the airways and to respond to the toxic chemicals within the smoke. Cigarette smoke consists of a particulate fume containing particles of less than $0.5\,\mu m$ in size [3], as well as many highly irritant chemicals. The 'full-strength' cigarettes of the 1950s contained 40 mg per cigarette or more, while the lowest-tar filter cigarettes of the 1990s had as little as 1 mg. Smokers are much more likely to fulfil the MRC definition, with the incidence rising from 10% in young adults to over 50% in those aged over 50 years. Dusty occupations such as mining yield dust that contains mostly larger particulates, of which only the minority smaller than 10 μm are inhaled. The effects of smoking and dust inhalation on the prevalence of cough are additive at all ages [4]. In many cases, those who cease to be exposed to dust or who stop smoking stop having a productive cough [5]. But do the cough and sputum represent disease, or are they simply a normal lung defence against the increased particulate and toxic burden in the large airways? In other words, does the reported symptom help to define the disease or simply describe a potential cause of the disease?

The Global Initiative for Obstructive Lung Disease (GOLD) initiative suggests that chronic sputum production is an early part of the COPD process and should be used to define an at-risk population. Cough and sputum indicate a cohort who should be targeted for lung function measurements. They are also a marker of the prevalence of cigarette smoking and thus a useful public health measure.

It is still unclear whether cough and sputum are part of the process that leads to obstruction or an entirely separate phenomenon. Physiologically, the mucosal thickening in the large airways contributes little to the overall limitation of airflow [6] — and in most patients with moderate to severe reductions in their forced expiratory volume in 1 s (FEV_1), it is widespread small-airway disease [7] and loss of elastic recoil leading to expiratory collapsibility of the subsegmental airways in those with emphysema [8] that is responsible.

Fletcher and Peto suggested that chronic sputum production does not affect life expectancy and by implication should be considered a separate process from conditions leading to airflow limitation, which does reduce both the quality and quantity of life [9]. More recently, Vestbo *et al.*, in a large population study in Copenhagen [10], showed that those with cough and sputum do suffer some loss of life expectancy, suggesting that the separation is less than complete. There are small but quite subtle changes in lung mechanics and airflow in patients with chronic sputum production [11], but it is not known whether these are permanent or whether they reverse on ceasing exposure.

However, when applied to the individual patient, a label of 'chronic bronchitis' is less helpful. It is possible to have a cough and regular sputum production without any decrement in airflow, and it is also true that a third or more of patients with severe airflow obstruction have no sputum [12]. Detecting a non-specific symptom should make the clinician consider COPD, but only in the context of a differential diagnosis that may include many other conditions. On the other hand, the absence of cough and sputum is not helpful in excluding COPD. Symptoms are not a substitute for measuring airflow in all cases of suspected COPD.

Can COPD be diagnosed on symptoms and signs?

The first section described the limitations of making a diagnosis from cough and sputum alone. In more severe disease, there is a much wider range of symptoms and signs, which are well described. The classic textbook descriptions of the 'pink puffer' and the 'blue bloater' refer to two of the more severe manifestations of end-stage COPD. But even these extreme states are not exclusive to COPD, and the overlap with other causes of respiratory and sometimes cardiac insufficiency is significant. It is worth considering how the COPD patient progresses from rude health to these severe manifestations over a period of up to 40 years or more.

The young 25-year-old smoker has no symptoms or measurable signs, despite a decade of smoking. Large epidemiological studies can demonstrate small statistically significant decrements in lung function, but the magnitude (25 mL) is too small to be detectable in the individual [13]. Although the disease process is already active, the exercise ability of young people is usually limited by the cardiovascular system, and the in-built respiratory reserve (about 30% of respiratory function) is never called upon. Only a minority of these smokers will even report a smoker's cough.

It is only when the continuing damage from smoking erodes the respiratory reserve and lung function becomes abnormal that patients begin to notice the first signs of breathlessness—in their 40s or 50s. Even at this stage, only a minority will report cough and sputum, and breathlessness on heavy exertion may be the only symptom. Those who do not have a heavy task or who do perform active physical exercise will be unaware that their maximum performance is becoming limited. There are likely to be few detectable signs at rest, and even a wheeze on auscultation can only be elicited on forced expirations. Many smokers succeed in hiding (or denying) breathlessness either by blaming 'normal ageing', or by avoiding breathlessness by giving up heavy exertion (e.g. retiring from competitive sport), or by avoidance of activity (e.g. using the car).

When the changes in lung function become moderately severe (an FEV_1 of 50% predicted for age and gender), breathlessness on moderate exertion is difficult to conceal, since it interferes with everyday activity. More than half of continuing smokers will report troublesome cough and phlegm, and the mechanical changes consequent on hyperinflation change the configuration of the chest. As the disease progresses, the degree of exercise restriction increases and the clinical signs become more obvious. The limited airflow is audible as expiratory wheezing, and there is prolongation of the expiratory (compared to inspiratory) phase of the breathing cycle—often observable from across the room. The hyperinflation leads to an elevation of the ribcage and the apparent barrel-shaped chest—although in fact a barrel-shaped chest (defined as an anteroposterior diameter that exceeds the lateral diameter) is actually more common in kyphosis. It is not known whether the extreme pink puffer and blue bloater characteristics are actually distinct variants or part of a continuum of disease. In the former, the features of a pink, thin individual with rapid shallow breathing and a prominent ribcage demonstrate the dyspnoea and weight loss common in severe disease, while the cyanosis and fluid retention with swollen ankles and a raised jugular venous pressure show the problems of hypoxia and pulmonary hypertension that are also common late features.

Thus, the signs change over the years, and it is not possible to apply a common rule at all ages. Moreover, none of the features are specific to COPD. Any cause of pulmonary hypertension can lead to hypoxia and fluid retention. Wheeze can occur in asthma and in left heart failure. Cough may be part of asthma or bronchiectasis, or may be due to gastric reflux. Breathlessness is a feature of heart as well as chest disease. Thus, symptoms either singly or in combination can make the clinician suspect COPD, but are rarely sufficient for a firm diagnosis.

The only way of confirming that airflow limitation is present is to measure it. Just as no doctor would diagnose hypertension without measuring blood pressure, or diabetes without measuring blood sugar, so no patient should be diagnosed as having COPD without a positive confirmation that airflow limitation is present—i.e. spirometry must be done [14].

Can COPD be distinguished from asthma?

The sceptic might ask, 'Is there any benefit in making this distinction'? Both conditions are forms of airflow limitation that are treated by inhaled bronchodilators. Both have an element of inflammation, so that particularly in the more severe cases, the patients receive inhaled steroids. If the treatment is the same, why bother making a distinction?

However, the causes and pathological processes underlying the two conditions are quite different. The natural history and the outcomes of treatment are very different, and thus guidelines suggest that both the management plan and the monitoring of treatment should not be the same.

Differentiation can be made in terms of clinical presentation, physiology, and pathology.

COPD is rarely present under the age of 40. Thus, younger patients with wheezing and airflow obstruction are almost always going to have asthma or occasionally one of the less common causes of airway obstruction, such as bronchiolitis. In patients over the age of 40, the overlap between the two con-

Table 3.1 A comparison between asthma and COPD.

	COPD	Asthma

History and symptoms	Onset in mid-life
	Symptoms slowly progressive
	Long smoking history
	Less likely to have a family
	  or atopic history, but
	  remember that these are
	  common features
	Dyspnoea during exercise
		Onset early in life (often childhood)
		Symptoms vary day to day
		Non-smoker or variable smoking
		History allergy, rhinitis,
		  and/or eczema
		Family history of asthma
		Dyspnoea immediately after
		  exertion

Lung function	Reduced FEV_1 and FEV_1/FVC
	  ratio
	Largely irreversible airflow
	  limitation
		Largely reversible airflow limitation
		Function may be normal
		  between attacks

Pathology	Neutrophils CD8+T lymphocytes Parenchymal destruction Mucus metaplasia Little or no effect of steroids	Eosinophils and mast cells CD4+Th_2 lymphocytes Thickened basement membrane Fragile epithelium Steroids inhibit inflammation

COPD, chronic obstructive pulmonary disease; FEV_1, forced expiratory volume in 1 s; FVC, forced vital capacity.

ditions is considerable. Both are common—asthma affects up to 5% of the adult population across all age groups [15], and symptomatic COPD affects 5% of the population aged over 65 [16].

In younger patients, the classical asthma history of acute breathlessness and wheezing interspersed with periods of complete wellness, especially if coupled with a history of waking coughing and wheezing in the night, makes the diagnosis relatively straightforward. In asthma patients over the age of 40, there is often chronicity secondary to airway remodelling that has led to a non-reversible element, and the symptom pattern is less clear cut. Even the classical nocturnal worsening of symptoms is a poor discriminator. Breathlessness on exertion, wheezing, cough productive of sputum (especially in current smokers), are common in both COPD and asthma. Perhaps because of this lack of specificity, the descriptive definitions used in management guidelines make little reference to symptoms.

Table 3.1 (adapted from the GOLD document [17]) shows that while there are symptom and history features that may point to either asthma or to COPD, there is no cardinal feature that differentiates between the two. Because atopy and asthma are common, inevitably a significant number of COPD patients will also have a similar history. Similarly, a significant number (25% or so) of asthma patients smoke.

COPD was defined by the British Thoracic Society Guidelines [18] in terms of an abnormal airflow obstruction—a reduced FEV_1 and FEV_1/forced vital capacity (FVC) ratio—that remains largely unchanged over time. The more recent GOLD guideline from the WHO [17] includes additional reference to the inflammation present in COPD. While there is no dispute that the inflammations in asthma and COPD are entirely different, the distinction in clinical practice is academic, as it is not practical to collect and examine tissue routinely. The procedures are too invasive to be justifiable other than for research studies, since the relevance to better clinical care has yet to be demonstrated.

Because it is unusual to have a pathological sample, clinical medicine has to rely on physiology. But here too, there is no absolute definition of reversibility. If a patient's obstructed lung function is shown to return to the normal range simply by administering a bronchodilator, then the diagnosis of asthma is almost certain. COPD is effectively excluded by normal values. Unfortunately, in older patients, the reversibility of the airway obstruction is partial even in asthma, and the unanswered question is what the smallest level of reversibility that diagnoses asthma to be present.

The differentiation is further complicated as COPD varies so much in its clinical manifestations over the 40–50-year time course. Most patients with mild disease (an FEV_1 of above 60% of that predicted) are likely to report few or no symptoms, because they have simply lost their respiratory reserve of function. They rarely present to a doctor. In contrast, a fall of FEV_1 from 100% to 70% in an asthmatic over the course of a few hours will almost certainly be reported as tightness and wheezing. The difference probably reflects the accommodation to the chronic situation in COPD. Thus, if the FEV_1 in a symptomatic patient is near normal, the diagnosis is more likely to be asthma than COPD. If a reversibility test returns the lung function to the normal range, then asthma is confirmed—although an element of coincident COPD cannot be excluded.

As COPD progresses to moderate impairment, with an FEV_1 of around 50% of predicted, chronic symptoms of exertional dyspnoea are likely, although this will be modified by the demands placed on the person concerned—e.g. by their occupation—and the opportunity to use mechanical aids or avoid the activity involved. Over half of patients with moderate COPD will exhibit a significant response of 200 mL to bronchodilators. In a few, FEV_1 values will not return to normal, but changes of 300–400 mL are strongly suggestive of an asthmatic component. Up to 20% of patients will also show a 200-mL or more response to an oral steroid trial (30 mg/day for 2 weeks). Does this make them asthmatic—or is the term 'COPD with an asthma element' more appropriate? Chronic asthma patients can show an identical picture, and it is extremely difficult to separate patients on clinical or physiological grounds.

At the severe end of the COPD spectrum, with an FEV_1 in the range of 35% of predicted, chronic symptoms are always present. A patient with acute asthma and an FEV_1 that has fallen to this level over a few hours is likely to be in ex-

tremis and is easily differentiated. A few patients with chronic asthma have values in this range, but they are relatively few in number, and the probability is that a patient with an FEV_1 of 35% predicted is likely to have COPD rather than asthma. In severe disease, the level of response to bronchodilators is often small and the potential for confusion with the 'asthmatic element' is less.

Thus, in patients with chronic symptoms, the lower the FEV_1, the less the response to bronchodilators, the older the patient, and the heavier the smoking history, the more likely is the diagnosis to be COPD. But this is an inexact science, and there are as yet no figures to help make this an objective exercise. But until a simple pathology test is found, it is the best that can be done in the practical clinical situation.

Why is it necessary to record spirometry in COPD rather than rely on peak expiratory flow?

Adding peak flow measurement to the assessment of asthma control introduced a whole new spectrum of objective assessment to what had been a very subjective exercise. Peak expiratory flow (PEF) is a cheap and simple test and shows a strong correlation with other measures of airflow obstruction. PEF is quick to record, and serial measures also provide an indication of the variability of airflow. It is tempting to extrapolate all the above to COPD. However, the physiology and uses of the measurements are very different in the two conditions.

PEF measures the maximum expiratory flow a patient can achieve over a fraction of a second. The level of PEF is related to the airway calibre in asthma, and there is a reasonable correlation of falling PEF with increasing symptoms and vice versa. Asthma is very variable, and the PEF may vary by 200 L/min between periods of wellness and periods of illness. This may be from 50% of predicted to normal. This is greatly in excess of the variability of the measurement (single measurements can vary by ±60 L/min), and moreover the effect of variability of an individual reading is reduced by making serial readings over a day or week. The serial PEF chart is a measure of the variability of the airways and of the average levels of function being achieved. It provides a useful method for monitoring average levels of lung function and for documenting the improvement that should follow a successful change in asthma therapy.

In COPD, the situation is quite different. Symptomatic COPD patients have much less variability. The range of possible PEF variability is reduced, such that most COPD patients will not exceed the variation that might be expected from the measurement itself. If the airflow limitation is essentially fixed, it is not helpful to use change in lung function as a primary outcome variable, either when assessing treatment or as a marker of short-term decline. The prime reasons for a measurement in COPD are to make the diagnosis of airflow obstruction and to assess the severity of the abnormality. This requires a single-visit measure that is robust and repeatable.

Advantages of spirometry

- Spirometry records both FEV_1 and FVC and thus FEV_1/FVC, which is a measure of obstruction—PEF cannot differentiate between restrictive and obstructive impairments.
- Spirometry can be performed by patients at any level of severity of airway obstruction with similar reproducibility.
- There are well-defined normal ranges that allow for the effects of age, ethnicity and sex, against which the severity of the impairment can be calculated.
- The level of the FEV_1 predicts future mortality and to the severity of breathlessness.
- The variance of repeated measurements is lower than for PEF. In COPD, the variability of the FEV_1 between testing occasions is about 170 mL [19] Hence, if values change by more than an absolute value of 200 mL, it is unlikely that the difference is due to chance.
- Serial measurements (over several years) are evidence of the rate of progression.

Against these advantages must be set the disadvantage that the equipment is significantly more expensive, and good measurement depends on having a good technician operating the spirometer [20].

There is one more important reason for preferring spirometry in COPD. The physiological processes causing the airflow limitation differ between COPD and asthma. This leads to an altered relationship between FEV_1 and PEF. The airway narrowing of asthma is mostly from bronchospasm of major airways. During expiration in COPD, it is due to a combination of bronchospasm in larger to medium airways, small-airway narrowing and obliteration, and collapsibility of the segmental airway secondary to the loss of elastic tissue within the lungs. It is probably the latter feature that upsets the relationship. Fig. 3.1 shows the expiratory flow volume loop for a patient with severe COPD compared with that for a healthy person. The patient's FEV_1 is reduced to 0.8 L or 33% of the normal example, whereas the PEF is relatively preserved at 5.7 L/s (340 L/min) (80% of predicted).

As normal expiration begins (point 'a'), there is a rapid increase in expiratory flow until the flow becomes limited by the airway dimensions and peak flow is reached (point 'b'). As expiration continues in the healthy subject (upper trace), flow decreases slowly and progressively until the person reaches their residual volume when flow ceases (point 'd').

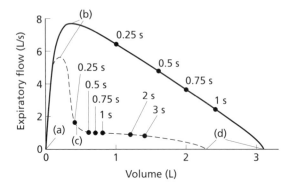

Fig. 3.1 Expiratory flow volume traces from a healthy person (solid line) and someone with emphysema (dashed line). Timings refer to the elapsed time from onset of the expiratory effort.

In the COPD patient, the initial rapid rise in expiratory flow is similar, but to a lower peak (point 'b'); then, as intrathoracic pressure increases in the early part of expiration, that pressure is transmitted to the segmental airways, which have lost the elastic attachments that enable normal airways to resist compression [21]. The airways therefore 'collapse' and obstruct the passage of air through those airways. This results in the rapid reduction in flow after the peak has been attained (point 'c'). Flow in the remainder of the expiration remains low, limited by the collapsed airways. A feature of severe COPD such as this is that airflow during tidal breathing (when the patient is generating less intrathoracic pressure) may be better than in the forced expiratory manoeuvre.

What differential diagnoses must be considered and how should other diagnoses be excluded?

* Heart failure
* Bronchiectasis
* Asthma.

The diagnostic overlap with asthma has already been described. Table 3.2 compares the symptoms, signs and test results typical in COPD, ischaemic heart disease and bronchiectasis.

In early to moderate disease, the symptomatic overlap between COPD and ischaemic heart disease (IHD) is almost complete and there are no reliable distinguishing features. The radiographic features are a guide, but are not absolute. COPD patients may have no evidence of hyperinflation and may have a large heart (without failure) on a radiograph, whereas cardiac patients do not necessarily exhibit cardiac enlargement. It is the FEV_1 that is most helpful, although even then chronic cardiac failure is often associated with mild reductions of FEV_1. However, a clue to a cardiac problem is that the level of dyspnoea is disproportionately more severe than the reduction in FEV_1. COPD patients with symptoms will always have a significant FEV_1 reduction.

Table 3.2 A comparison of clinical features in three overlapping conditions.

	COPD	Ischaemic heart disease	Bronchiectasis
History to childhood	No	No	Often
Smoking history	Always	Often	Sometimes
Breathlessness	+++	+++	+++
Wheeze	++	+	+
Sputum	+−	+−	+++
Early morning symptoms	+−	+−	
Nocturnal wakening	+	++	
Cyanosis	++	++	
Ankle swelling	++	++	
Auscultation for crackles	Variable, scanty coarse	Fine if failure present	Coarse
Abnormal FEV$_1$	Severe	Normal or mild	Usually
CXR	Overinflation	Large Ht/LVF	Increased markings
ECG	Variable	Variable	Often normal
CT scan	Emphysema	Normal lungs	Dilated bronchi

COPD, chronic obstructive pulmonary disease; CT, computed tomography; CXR, chest X-ray; ECG, electrocardiography; FEV$_1$, forced expiratory volume in 1 s; LVF, left ventricular failure.

The overlap with bronchiectasis is different, and here it is the long history and the volume and colour of sputum that usually will distinguish it from COPD. Some auscultatory but scanty crackles are common in COPD and are not always present in mild or focal bronchiectasis. Similarly, the FEV$_1$ can be abnormal in both, but the chest radiograph and particularly the computed tomography (CT) scan usually make the differentiation obvious.

The message from these examples is that sorting out a differential diagnosis in individual patients on the basis of history and clinical signs alone is often unreliable, so that the best management will almost always be dependent on further investigations. Once made, the diagnosis is likely to be unchanged for many years, and the costs of these investigations are therefore proportionately quite low compared with the benefits to the patient of getting the therapy correctly focused (Table 3.2).

Some diagnostic examples

Most books describe the typical features of each condition, and it is often difficult for the clinician to relate the rather dry descriptions to the particular individual in the consulting room. This section describes the diagnostic problems in five real patients as they presented to the author. They are by no means inclusive of all the situations that may arise, but are intended to illustrate the need for objective assessment in order to deliver appropriate therapy for conditions that will require the patient to continue attending for medical help over many years. The first three arrived in the clinic over a 2-week period, and show

how failure to measure lung function and to evaluate that information critically led to inappropriate management, which in one case had continued for many years.

• A 56-year-old man was referred because he wanted to be considered for early retirement on the grounds of 'emphysema', which had been treated with nebulized bronchodilators for the preceding 15 years. Unusually for a man requiring high-dose therapy, he had had little time off from work as a warehouseman during the 15 years. His occupational health physician was concerned because his FEV_1 was 79% of predicted and this did not 'fit'. The consultant agreed that despite a long smoking history, the almost normal spirometry meant that this man had little or no respiratory limitation and that his nebulizer was entirely inappropriate. There were no clues to suggest asthma, and he was not receiving steroids in any form. Further investigation included a cardiorespiratory exercise test, which showed he was capable of a normal maximum workload. The patient was pleased that he did not have severe emphysema, but was concerned as to whether he could claim back the 15 years of charges for the drugs that he had been prescribed unnecessarily!

• A 62-year-old woman was referred to the clinic as having COPD, with an FEV_1 of 60% of predicted, that had been unresponsive to inhalers or oral steroids over some months. She had ceased to smoke some 3 years before. She complained bitterly of a dry, ticklish cough and was breathless when climbing stairs at home or on going to the shops. The response to inhalers had been disappointing. On examination in the clinic, there was no wheeze on auscultation and the chest was clinically clear. On inspection of the spirometric traces, it was immediately obvious that the pattern of the trace was not obstructive; the FVC was also reduced to 60% of predicted and had been overlooked. The eventual diagnosis was a fibrosing alveolitis, possibly related to her (at that time) very mild rheumatoid disease. Inhalers were withdrawn.

• The third man was 67, had been a heavy smoker (45 pack-years), and was referred as having 'COPD that was responding poorly and should be assessed for a nebulizer prescription'. He had become progressively more limited in his ability to walk since his retirement 5 years earlier and had a productive cough, worst in the mornings. His FEV_1 was markedly reduced to 0.7 L. A single dose of nebulizer in the clinic caused an improvement to 1.3 L, and after a trial of oral steroids, his FEV_1 rose to 2.7 L and he described feeling 20 years younger. Although he had been symptomatic for many years, he and his doctors had ascribed the symptoms to his smoking and had never considered the diagnosis of asthma. Even on reflection in this case, there were no particular clues that could or should have made the general practitioner specifically consider asthma.

• A 60-year-old housewife complained of having experienced increased breathlessness for some years, especially when shopping and hoovering. She had become unable to join friends for bridge because she was too breathless to make the journey. She had smoked 15 cigarettes per day for 34 years and was intelligent enough to have linked this to her breathlessness, although not intelligent enough to have stopped smoking. Her FEV_1 was 0.8 L and her FVC 1.9 L. A peak flow chart over 2 weeks showed a low level of variability between 120 and 150 L/min. She was given a trial of oral prednisolone (30 mg/day) over 2 weeks and her FEV_1 increased to over 1.5 L with concomitant symptomatic benefit. She stopped smoking then and there and remained well and active on inhaled steroids.

• A man of 57 was referred with a 15-year history of cough and sputum and wheezing, which had at first responded 'well' to asthma inhalers but had become progressively less responsive. He was now struggling for breath after walking 100 m on level ground. His FEV_1 was just 0.6 L and his PEF flow chart was unvarying. In the previous 4 years, oral prednisolone had been added and in the previous 12 months he had begun using nebulized bronchodilators. In addition, osteoporosis had been diagnosed. He insisted that he had stopped smoking. No treatment helped and he died 6 months later. The post-mortem revealed gross centrilobular emphysema, and it also emerged from a relative that he had actually continued to be a 'secret smoker' despite his denial.

Accurate diagnosis does matter. In each of the above cases, a little more care initially and an objective measurement (i.e. spirometry) could have saved time and effort for the health services, as well as being better for the patient. COPD management can be quite logical.

References

1 Reid L. The pathology of chronic bronchitis. In: Reid L. *The Pathology of Emphysema*. London: Lloyd-Luke Medical Books, 1967.

2 Medical Research Council. Definition and classification of chronic bronchitis for clinical and epidemiological purposes. *Lancet* 1965; i: 775–9.

3 Report of the Government Chemist, London, 1973.

4 Rogan JM, Attfield MD, Jacobsen M *et al.* Role of dust in the working environment in development of chronic bronchitis in British coal miners. *Br J Ind Med* 1973; 30: 217–26.

5 Brinkman GL, Block DL, Cress C. The effects of bronchitis on occupational pulmonary ventilation over an 11-year period. *J Occup Med* 1972; 14: 615–20.

6 Hankinson JL, Reger RB, Morgan WKC. Maximal expiratory flows in coal miners. *Am Rev Respir Dis* 1977; 116: 175–80.

7 Cosio M, Glazio H, Hogg JC *et al.* Relations between structural change in small airways and pulmonary function tests. *N Engl J Med* 1977; 298: 1277–81.

8 Gould GA, Redpath AT, Ryan M *et al.* Parenchymal emphysema measured by CT lung density correlates with lung function in patients with bullous emphysema. *Eur Respir J* 1993; 6: 698–704.

9 Fletcher C, Peto R. The natural history of chronic airflow obstruction. *BMJ* 1977; i: 1645–8.

10 Vestbo J, Prescott E, Lange P. Association of chronic mucus hypersecretion with FEV_1 decline and chronic obstructive pulmonary disease morbidity. Copenhagen City Heart Study Group. *Am J Respir Crit Care Med* 1996; 153: 1530–5.

11 Hankinson JL, Reger RB, Morgan WKC. Maximal expiratory flows in coal miners. *Am Rev Respir Dis* 1977; **116**: 175–80.

12 Nisar M, Walshaw MJ, Earis JE, Pearson MG, Calverley PMA. Assessment of airway reversibility of airway obstruction in patients with chronic obstructive airways disease. *Thorax* 1990; **45**: 190–4.

13 Tager IB, Segal MR, Speizer FE, Weiss ST. The natural history of forced expiratory volumes, effect of cigarette smoking and respiratory symptoms. *Am Rev Respir Dis* 1988; **138**: 837–49.

14 Global Initiative for Chronic Obstructive Lung Disease. *NHLBI/WHO Workshop Report: Global Strategy for the Diagnosis, Management, and Prevention of COPD.* Bethesda, MD: National Heart, Lung and Blood Institute, 2001 (NIH Publication No. 2701).

15 Lung and Asthma Information Agency. *Prevalence of Asthma Treated in the General Population.* London: St George's Hospital Medical School, 1999 (Factsheet 99/1).

16 Confronting COPD in North America and Europe. www.gsk.com 2001.

17 Global Initiative for Chronic Obstructive Lung Disease National Institute for Health, NHLBI publication 2701 April 2001.

18 *BTS Guidelines for the Management of Chronic Obstructive Pulmonary Disease. Thorax* 1997; **52** (Suppl. 5): S1–28.

19 Tweedale PM, Alexander F, McHardy GJR. Short-term variability in FEV_1 and bronchodilator responsiveness in patients with chronic obstructive ventilatory defects. *Thorax* 1987; **42**: 487–90.

20 American Thoracic Society. Standardization of spirometry: 1994 update. *Am J Respir Crit Care Med* 1995; **152**: 1107–36.

21 Kelly CA, Gibson GJ. Relation between FEV_1 and peak expiratory flow in patients with chronic obstructive pulmonary disease. *Thorax* 1988; **43**: 335–6.

4: Is it possible for spirometry to become a universal measurement?

David Bellamy

Introduction

Spirometry is an essential tool for the diagnosis and long-term monitoring of chronic obstructive pulmonary disease (COPD). It is the only means to accurately assess the severity of airflow obstruction and is helpful in planning treatment and its response in COPD. Spirometry can separate obstructive lung conditions from restrictive diseases and is of great value in the investigation of breathlessness. In addition, abnormal spirometric tests can act as a marker for increased mortality and risk in coronary artery disease, stroke and lung cancer [1].

Basically, spirometry measures airflow from fully inflated lungs together with the total volume of air that can be exhaled. The three indices that are clinically important are:
- Forced vital capacity (FVC)—the volume of air that can be exhaled from fully inflated lungs
- Forced expiratory volume in 1 s (FEV_1)—the volume of air that can be expired with maximal effort from fully inflated lungs in one second.
- The ratio of FEV_1/FVC as a percentage. The normal range lies above 70%. FEV_1 tends to be an index of airflow and FVC of lung volume. The FEV_1/FVC ratio when reduced below 70% indicates airflow obstruction.

Historically, spirometry was expressed as a curve of exhaled volume versus time. With the development of flow transducers, many spirometers also produce a representation of the exhaled manoeuvre as a flow–volume curve. Normal volume–time and flow–volume curves are shown in Fig. 4.1.

Why is spirometry the measurement of choice in COPD?

The FEV_1 is accurate and reproducible. The variance of repeated measurements in the same individual is low and normally less than 200 mL.

There are well-defined tables of normal values for FEV_1 based on age, sex, height and ethnic origin.

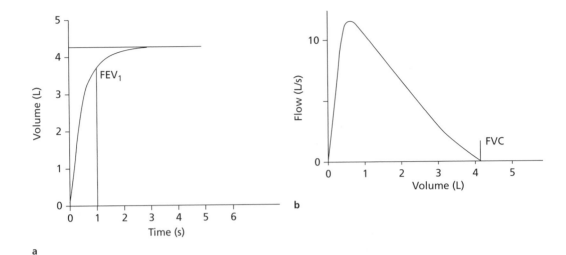

Fig. 4.1 Normal spirometry. (a) Normal volume–time curve. (b) Normal flow–volume curve.

FEV_1 is the best predictor of prognosis in COPD. Spirometry is relatively quick and easy to measure and is applicable for children over 6 years to old age. It is appropriate for all levels of severity of COPD.

The FVC, being more effort-dependent, is slightly less reproducible and more susceptible to errors such as poor effort and stopping blowing too early. In addition, some flow-dependent spirometers may underestimate FVC at the low flow rates found in severe COPD. If the FVC is underestimated, the FEV_1/FVC ratio may give a falsely high result.

Peak expiratory flow (PEF) is unreliable for airflow obstruction in COPD, often seriously underestimating the degree of airflow present [2]. This is related to COPD being a disease of smaller airways that is identified by FEV_1 but not by PEF, which measures flow mainly in the larger airways.

What equipment is needed?

There are many types of spirometer currently in use, and in general they perform measurements accurately. Spirometers broadly fall into two categories — those that measure volume directly, such as bellows-type spirometers; and those that measure flow and derive volume. The flow-based spirometers use a pneumotachograph or turbine, which records pressure change with time and integrates the flow–time signal to obtain volume. Computer enhancement has greatly improved the accuracy of these instruments.

Spirometers have an assortment of graphical displays, from paper printouts to digital real-time visual display of either flow–volume or volume–time curves. Hard copy can be obtained from the latter, or the signal can be passed through a computer for storage or printing. More expensive and accurate equipment tends to be used in lung function laboratories in hospitals, and simpler (less expensive) portable electronic units in primary care. The cheapest hand-held spirometers for primary care tend to provide only numerical values for FEV_1 and FVC, but no printout. This is undesirable, as it offers no way of assessing the accuracy and quality of the blows.

All spirometers require calibrating, preferably with a 3 L syringe. Calibration is carried out daily in lung function laboratories, but far less so in primary care. Some manufacturers of spirometers claim their equipment's calibration remains stable over 2–3 years without regular calibration.

It is important for reliable consecutive readings on a given patient that the same spirometer should be used. Some research from the UK [3,4] has compared pneumotachograph, turbine and wedge bellow spirometers. The FEV_1 volumes were similar, but measurements of FVC and vital capacity (VC) with the turbine machine were 400–500 mL less than with the other types of spirometer. The authors suggest this could be due to inadequate volume measurement at low flow rates, which is frequently found in patients with moderate to severe COPD. Since these studies, manufacturers of turbine spirometers have made modifications to correct the tendency to low readings of FVC.

The essential requirements for a spirometer are thus:
• The need for calibration.
• A hard copy or visual display of blows in real time, to assess accuracy and reproducibility.
• Ideally, the ability to superimpose traces with repeated blows.
• Some electronic spirometers calculate the percentage variation between blows, or give a bleep if blows are performed inadequately.

What constitutes an acceptable test?

The following criteria need to be satisfied:
• At least three technically satisfactory readings.
• The volume–time traces are smooth and free from irregularities suggesting a slow start, submaximal effort or coughing.
• At least two of the readings of FEV_1 should be within 100 mL or 5% of each other.
• The reading has been continued for long enough for a volume plateau to be achieved. This can take up to 15 s in patients with severe COPD.
• The best FEV_1 and FVC are reported and compared with predicted normal results.
• Temperature and atmospheric pressure measurement may be appropriate in hospital lung function laboratories, but not in primary care.

Training

The key to accurate and meaningful spirometry readings is through approved training in the techniques and interpretation of spirometry. The importance of training cannot be over-emphasized.

Respiratory technicians in hospitals will usually have a university degree and then undergo a year's specific training in respiratory physiological measurement and interpretation. In the UK, the Association for Respiratory Technology and Physiology (ARTP) set standards for training, examination and quality control. Criteria for the recommended performance of lung function measurement and equipment specification are set out by the American Thoracic Society [5,6] and European Respiratory Society [7].

In the UK, the ARTP, in conjunction with the British Thoracic Society (BTS), has developed a certificate in spirometry with accredited training, course work and examination, which is available to doctors and nurses in primary care or hospital staff. Training and knowledge in primary care are generally poor and inadequate.

What are normal and predicted values?

It is common practice for the results of spirometry to be interpreted in relation to reference values and in terms of whether or not they are considered to be within the 'normal' range [8,9]. Most equipment manufacturers follow these guidelines.

There may be potential causes for variation in clinical measurement, which include:
- Technical variation of the instrument.
- Performance of the test.
- Interpretation of the procedure by the operator.
- Position of patient during the procedure.

These variations must be evaluated and standardized as much as possible.

Clinically, the most important factors responsible for individual variations are: 1, gender; 2, height; 3, age; and 4, ethnic origin, together with the presence or absence of respiratory disease. Compared with a Caucasian population, black races tend to have predicted normal values approximately 13% less. Asians are intermediate.

The distribution of FEV_1 and FVC in population studies are near to Gaussian in the middle range but less so at the extremes. Reference values are most commonly calculated by a linear regression equation, but care should be taken in interpreting data outside the age range from which the population of normal individuals is sampled.

In clinical practice at hospitals and in primary care, values of FEV_1 and FVC are traditionally expressed as a percentage of the mean normal value for that individual. A value below 80% predicted is said to be abnormal. This has the major advantage that it immediately defines the level of severity of COPD present within a given patient. Many electronic spirometers provide results in this format. However, statistically, a more accurate representation of normal and abnormal values is by using the 95% confidence limits of the regression equation. An abnormal result is one which falls below the 5th percentile range. The figure can be calculated from: lower limit of normal = predicted value − 1.645 × SEE, where SEE is the standard error of the estimate (the average standard deviation, SD, of the data around the regression line). A recent review by Quadrelli et al. [10] has compared normal values using the two methods above for different prediction equations and found that, particularly in shorter and more elderly people, the lower normal range figure is often in the 60–80% predicted range. Thus, the percentile calculation provides a more accurate assessment of normal limits, where percentage predicted can provide a measure of the degree of deviation from the predicted value. Data for patients whose values lie close to lower limits should be interpreted with caution. It is also not acceptable to use a fixed FEV_1/FVC ratio as a lower limit of normal [8].

Predicted value reference equations

Reference values are derived by measuring lung function in a standardized way in a large group of non-smoking normal individuals. Many such reference ranges exist in the US [11–14]. In Europe, most lung function departments and equipment manufacturers use the European Community for Coal and Steel (ECCS) equation [15]. This was derived from a review of the European literature for lung function in normal Caucasian men and women age 25–70 years, and an overall mean of the reviewed data is represented. There are also reference ranges for different ethnic groups and children.

Quadrelli et al. [10] have compared the values of FEV_1 and FVC for a range of commonly used predictive ranges from the USA and Europe (Table 4.1). There are significant differences for both men and women, especially with increasing age. The differences may be explained to some extent on the basis of ethnic, social and geographical variations, as well as environmental exposure.

From a practical point of view, it is important to chose an appropriate predictive equation that is pertinent to the majority of patients being studied and to keep to it. Changing electronic equipment with different normal values will introduce unnecessary error.

Table 4.1 Predicted values for forced expiratory volume in 1 s (FEV$_1$) and forced vital capacity (FVC) in men 1.70 m in height and women 1.60 m in height, derived from different reference equations. Adapted from Quadrelli *et al.* [10].

Age (y)	FVC					FEV$_1$				
	Morris [11]	Cherniack [12]	Crapo [13]	Knudson [14]	ECCS [15]	Morris [11]	Cherniack [12]	Crapo [13]	Knudson [14]	ECCS [15]
Men										
20	5.17	4.63	5.11	4.96	4.93	4.25	4.13	4.35	4.20	4.14
30	4.92	4.49	4.90	4.66	4.67	3.92	3.90	4.11	3.91	3.83
40	4.67	4.35	4.69	4.36	4.41	3.60	3.67	3.87	3.62	3.52
50	4.42	4.21	4.48	4.06	4.15	3.29	3.44	3.63	3.33	3.21
60	4.17	4.07	4.27	3.76	3.89	2.97	3.21	3.39	3.04	2.90
70	3.92	3.93	4.06	3.46	3.63	2.65	2.98	3.15	2 75	2.59
80	3.67	3.79	3.85	3.16	3.37	2.33	2.75	2.91	2.48	2.28
Women										
20	3.91	3.58	3.84	3.57	3.83	3.17	3.23	3.40	3.44	3.64
30	3.67	3.43	3.625	3.40	3.56	2.92	3.04	3.14	3.24	3.33
40	3.43	3.28	3.405	3.23	3.29	2.67	2.85	2.88	3.04	3.02
50	3.19	3.13	3.18	3.06	3.02	2.42	2.66	2.62	2.84	2.71
60	2.95	2.98	2.96	2.89	2.75	2.17	2.46	2.36	2.64	2.40
70	2.71	2.83	2.74	2.72	2.48	1.92	2.28	2.10	2.44	2.09
80	2.47	2.68	2.52	2.55	2.21	1.67	2.00	1.84	2.24	1.78

ECCS, European Community for Coal and Steel; FEV$_1$, forced expiratory volume in 1 s; FVC, forced vital capacity.

What do the traces show?

A forced expired spirogram may show a number of characteristic patterns:
• Normal
• Obstructive pattern
• Restrictive pattern

Normal

The volume–time trace should have a rapid smooth initial rise in volume, with flattening of the trace to a plateau within 3–5 s. Greater than 70% of the total expired volume should be exhaled in the first second. The flow–volume trace also has a steep smooth initial phase leading to the maximal expiratory flow level and then flow rate decreases in a fairly linear way until the residual volume is reached. Following three satisfactory blows, values for FEV$_1$, FVC and the FEV$_1$/FVC ratio can be obtained and compared with predicted values for the individual.

Obstructive pattern

Airflow obstruction is seen most commonly in asthma and COPD. It repre-

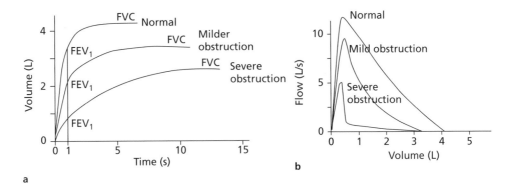

Fig. 4.2 Obstructive pattern.

sents narrowing of larger to peripheral airways. Spirometry provides the best means for assessing the degree of severity of airflow obstruction and also the response to bronchodilator or corticosteroid treatment.

With increasing levels of obstruction, the initial slope of the volume–time curve becomes progressively less steep and it frequently takes longer to empty the lungs and achieve an FVC plateau. In severe COPD, this may take 15–20 s. The absolute value of FEV_1 falls, as does the ratio of FEV_1/FVC. The FVC tends to be better maintained until severe levels of obstruction are observed, when it falls. The flow–volume trace continues to show a steep initial rise, but the maximal flow decreases as obstruction becomes worse. The characteristic part of the trace is a concavity of the second part of the curve, the depth of which increases with greater airflow obstruction. Patients with more advanced emphysema may show the diagnostic 'steeple' appearance, with a rapid fall of flow from the maximum levels and then a slow, long tail to residual volume (RV). Illustrative examples are shown in Fig. 4.2.

Restrictive pattern

This type of trace occurs in parenchymal lung disease such as fibrosing alveolitis, sarcoid and conditions that constrict the lungs or thoracic cage. The shape of both volume–trace and flow–volume curves is similar to that of normal individuals. On examining the absolute values for FEV_1 and FVC, they will be reduced in parallel, indicating small lungs. The FEV_1/FVC ratio, however, will be normal or even high (Fig. 4.3).

Combined obstruction and restriction

This is often difficult to interpret accurately. The traces will show evidence of airflow obstruction, with concavity of the second phase of the flow–volume

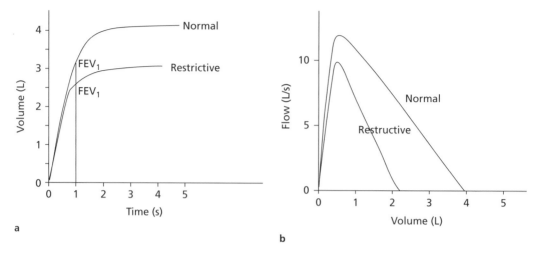

Fig. 4.3 Restrictive pattern.

trace. The value of FVC will be significantly reduced, but the ratio of FEV_1/FVC should still be below 70%. It is not easy to differentiate this from more severe obstruction with loss of FVC without more detailed lung function tests.

The choice of severity values in COPD guidelines

Over the last few years, national and international clinical guidelines have been produced for the management of COPD. Each set of guidelines has chosen values of FEV_1 percent predicted to categorize mild, moderate and severe levels of COPD.

Values of FEV_1 greater than 80% are within two standard residuals of the predicted mean and are thus considered to be within the normal range. The American thoracic Society (ATS), in assessing levels of respiratory disability [16], choose 60% and 40% FEV_1 as indicators for mild, moderate and severe disability. The same levels were used for the British Thoracic Society (BTS) guidelines [17].

The ATS COPD guidelines [18] decided on three levels of severity based on 80%, 50% and 35% predicted. The European Respiratory Society guidelines [19] opted for 90%, 70% and 50% predicted. There has been no scientific evidence quoted for justifying these values (Table 4.2).

How does FEV_1 correlate with various clinical parameters?

FEV_1 is the best predictor of progress and mortality in COPD. It also corre-

Table 4.2 Chronic obstructive pulmonary disease guidelines — severity levels of forced expiratory volume in 1 s (FEV_1) % of predicted.

	Mild	Moderate	Severe
ATS guidelines [18]	80%	50%	35%
ERS guidelines [19]	90%	70%	50%
BTS guidelines [17]	80%	60%	40%
GOLD global guidelines [30]	$FEV_1/FVC<70\%$ with $FEV_1 \geq 80\%$ with or without symptoms	30–80%	<30% predicted (or<50% plus respiratory failure or right heart failure)

ATS, American Thoracic Society; BTS, British Thoracic Society; COPD, chronic obstructive pulmonary disease; ERS, European Respiratory Society; GOLD, Global Initiative for Chronic Obstructive Lung Disease; FEV_1, forced expiratory volume in 1 s; FVC, forced vital capacity.

lates well with morbidity, those with lower functions having more respiratory symptoms.

Reduced FEV_1 is also associated with worse prognosis in lung cancer, cardiovascular diseases and diabetes. The Renfrew study [20] showed increased risk of death in cardiovascular disease in those with reduced FEV_1, even in lifelong non-smokers.

FEV_1 is useful in monitoring disease progression with serial readings, but these should be taken under conditions of clinical stability and not after exacerbation.

FEV_1 does not correlate well with symptomatic improvement after bronchodilator reversibility testing. The VC, if carried out properly, may be a better indicator here, as bronchodilators work mainly to reduce hyperinflation and the work of breathing.

Although decreasing FEV_1 is associated with greater respiratory symptoms, it does not correlate particularly well with quality of life questionnaires or with the Sickness Impact Profile [21]. The relationship with walking distance also shows only poor to moderate correlation [22].

How is spirometry used in primary care?

Perhaps the greatest challenge in COPD management is to encourage the widespread, accurate and appropriate use of spirometry in primary care, where the majority of COPD is diagnosed and managed.

Until the publication of the British Thoracic Society (BTS) COPD guidelines in 1997 [17], COPD management had been largely neglected and was very much considered a disease process for which little could or, indeed, needed to be done other than to suggest that patients should give up smoking. The use of spirometers on a regular basis to diagnose and assess the severity of COPD was minimal.

In 1996, a postal survey [23] of 2548 randomly selected general practitioners (GPs) in the UK revealed that, of the 931 who returned the questionnaire, 39% had a spirometer in their practice. Of those who owned or were intending to buy a spirometer, 86% said that the practice nurse would carry out the testing. Ninety percent agreed that the nurse needed appropriate training. At the time of the survey, 61% of the owned spirometers were of the simple hand-held electronic variety, with no graphical display. Disappointingly, only 11% of responders had access to open-access spirometry at the local hospital. The disadvantage of postal surveys is that the data obtained tend to be biased by the interests of those who return the questionnaire. It is therefore likely that the true figures for the proportion of practices with a spirometer was considerably less than 39%.

When the BTS COPD guidelines were produced, a considerable effort was put into disseminating an attractively presented four-page summary to a wide range of health professionals. All primary-care physicians received a copy, as well as approximately 15 000 practice nurses who were known to have an interest in asthma or run clinics in asthma. This mailing, coupled with postgraduate meetings and the setting up of training courses in COPD and spirometry for practice nurses, greatly increased the awareness of COPD, its effective treatment, and the measurement of FEV_1 to make a diagnosis and assessment of disease severity.

Primary-care practitioners are now systematically evaluating patients with chronic respiratory symptoms, many of whom have been diagnostically labelled as asthmatic, to determine the correct diagnosis and assess severity and reversibility. The most appropriate therapy can then be provided. An analysis by Pinnock et al. [24] of 100 consecutive patients with respiratory symptoms referred for spirometry in a large general practice in Kent has clearly outlined the value of spirometry. Sixty-five patients with airflow obstruction were identified, and with bronchodilator reversibility testing, COPD was differentiated from asthma. Twelve previously undiagnosed restrictive defects were identified, with the remainder of the patients being normal.

In the last few years, many practices have purchased spirometers, a high proportion of which have the preferred facility for graphical display and thus allow more effective evaluation of blowing technique and reproducibility. Hospital pulmonary function laboratories are also making access to lung function testing more readily available.

A face-to-face marketing survey of 209 general practitioners and 102 practice nurses carried out on behalf of the BTS COPD Consortium in 1999 [25] revealed that 50% of GPs and 69% of practice nurses had spirometers in their practices. Where there was no spirometer in the practice, over 75% sent patients to the local hospital for lung function testing. Spirometers are used in primary care twice as often by nurses than by GPs. Encouragingly, 93% of the nurses had received some training in spirometry, compared with 60% of GPs.

The survey is to be repeated after the circulation of a simple, practical booklet on the uses, technique and interpretation of spirometry in primary care.

A postal survey carried out by the author in Dorset in 2002 showed the number of practices with a spirometer has risen to 80%.

Should spirometric screening of asymptomatic smokers be organized?

Since some degree of impaired lung function is likely to be measurable by the age of 40–50 years in the 20% of smokers who are susceptible to tobacco smoke, there might appear to be some logic in screening this group of smokers to detect early disease. Symptomatic COPD may be totally prevented if patients can be persuaded to quit smoking at this early stage of mild airflow obstruction.

Attractive though this idea might initially seem, there are many questions that need to be asked about the efficacy, manpower implications and cost benefits of widespread screening before it can become routine practice in primary care. There are relatively few data on the prevalence of airflow obstruction in asymptomatic smokers over the age of 40 years, but as yet unpublished studies from Poland, the USA and the UK suggest figures between 15% and 25%. A study by Freeman [26] found 19 smokers with mild or moderate levels of COPD in the first 100 patients she screened.

As yet, there have been no studies to measure the effect on smoking quit rates if smokers are found to have abnormal lung function. It is always difficult to persuade symptomatic COPD suffers to stop smoking, but will the knowledge that their lungs are not normal encourage a greater proportion to quit smoking? This would surely be a primary goal of screening. A large controlled study is urgently needed.

A negative aspect of spirometric screening of smokers might be a reassurance that if their lung function is normal, it is perfectly all right to continue smoking.

Large-scale screening in primary care will have considerable time and cost implications, particularly for practice nurse involvement. Screening could be opportunistic, or more formalized in special clinics. However, formal evaluation needs to take account of the cost–benefit ratio of such screening.

Using a case finding approach, van Schayck et al. [27] found that when smokers were preselected on the basis of chronic cough the proportion with abnormal FEV_1 rose to 27%, making screening more time and cost efficient.

How can quality control of measurement be achieved in primary care?

Whereas respiratory technicians in hospital have at least one year's formal training in respiratory function testing, no such schemes exist in primary care. Training of practice nurses at best may run to 1–2-day courses, some of which will deal with affiliated topics other than pure spirometry. Courses for GPs are likely to be no more than a half-day session, which may provide the basics but contain little in-depth knowledge.

Hospital technicians will check and calibrate equipment daily, but depending on the type of spirometer, no such regular calibration is likely to occur in primary care. If spirometry occurs in designated clinics, equipment can be calibrated beforehand, but as much work in primary care is opportunistic and appointments are likely to be less than 10 min in duration, there is often no time. There is thus an attraction for GPs to purchase electronic spirometers, with which the manufacturers say no calibration is required except at an annual service. Being able to switch on a spirometer and type in height, age and sex details and immediately be able to perform the blows is much more compatible with the hectic pace of a general-practice surgery. The choice of spirometer for primary care should certainly be influenced by the way it is likely to be used. Opportunistic measurements definitely require a very quick and simple-to-use machine. Clinics can better utilize machines with which more calibration has to be performed initially.

Whichever spirometer is selected, it is essential that the doctor or nurse is fully aware of patient preparation, the technique for performing the blows, the problems that arise with poor blows and the criteria for good reproducibility. Knowledge is also needed to interpret traces and figures.

The following points constitute the basis of good spirometric technique.

Preparing the patient

1 Patients should be clinically stable over the previous 4 weeks.
2 The subject's age and height are obtained.
3 Ideally (particularly if performing a bronchodilator reversibility test), the patient should not have taken a bronchodilator for the previous 6 h, a long-acting β-agonist for 12 h and theophyllines for 24 h. This may not be feasible for opportunistic measurement.
4 Ensure that patients are comfortable. Invite them to empty their bladder, request that they loosen any tight-fitting clothing and remove loose dentures.
5 When prebooking the patient for a spirometry clinic, written instructions should ideally be provided.

Blowing technique

1 Patients should be relaxed and seated in an upright position (performing tests while standing may cause faintness and dizziness after repeated blows).

2 Explain and demonstrate the technique.

3 The subject should take a maximal breath in and place the lips around the mouthpiece to form an airtight seal. A nose clip is generally not required.

4 Exhale as hard, fast and completely as possible, with lots of encouragement from the operator. In a healthy subject, it usually takes 3–4 s to complete the blow. With airflow obstruction, it is more difficult for the patient to blow air out rapidly, and exhalation in more severe COPD may take 15–20 s.

5 Allow adequate time — including time for recovery — between blows, with a maximum of six forced manoeuvres in one session.

6 The operator should observe the patient during the manoeuvres to check for leaks around the mouthpiece and that the procedure is being performed correctly.

Technical standards

1 Three technically satisfactory manoeuvres should be made with good reproducibility. At least two readings of FEV_1 should be within 100 mL or 5% of each other. Some electronic spirometers calculate the variation between blows automatically.

2 Usually, the best readings of FEV_1 and FVC are accepted.

3 Common technique problems include:
- An incomplete blow — stopping too soon.
- Slow start to the blow.
- A cough in the middle of the blow.

4 It is very difficult to assess correct technique and reproducibility without a visual graphical display.

5 The best values of FEV_1, FVC and FEV_1/FVC are compared with the predicted values for the subject.

6 A hard copy of the tracings and results should be kept in the patient's records.

The limited published literature on quality assurance for spirometry in primary care paints a rather gloomy picture. A recent study [28] from New Zealand assessed the effect of a 2-h workshop for doctors and practice nurses where particular attention was paid to the practical aspects of spirometry and quality assurance. Over the following 12 weeks, 'trained' staff and a control group who did not attend the spirometry workshop performed tasks on an electronic hand-held Vitalograph device that had a capability for alerting operators when the quality of blows was poor (e.g. a slow start) and also gave the level of variance between blows. All blows were analysed for acceptability on the fairly strict ATS criteria. Only 18.9% of the trained group and 5.1% of the control group performed three acceptable blows. Two acceptable blows (which may be adequate for primary care) were achieved in 33.1% and 12.5%

of the trained and control groups, respectively. The main reason for non-acceptability was failure to satisfy a blow lasting at least 6 s. The study suggests that the majority of FEV_1 measurements may thus be acceptable.

The study also demonstrated a good learning effect from the workshop. However, in a random selection of 559 traces, only 55% were shown to have the correct interpretation when reviewed by expert pulmonologists.

A study from the Netherlands [29] examined the quality of instruction and subsequent patient use of the spirometer in a group of practice nurses or practice assistants who had been given several training sessions. Overall, about half the instructors and half the patient performance items were considered to have been carried out satisfactorily.

A review of primary-care spirometry has recently been published [30], which provides a good overview of some of the topics discussed in this chapter.

Conclusions

Spirometry is obviously in its infancy as a diagnostic tool in primary care. To establish reliable, accurate and reproducible spirometric readings together with the knowledge to interpret traces correctly, there needs to be:

- A large number of good-quality accredited teaching courses.
- Follow-up assessment of practical and theoretical knowledge.
- Encouragement for primary-care practitioners to become involved in performing spirometry.
- Support and teaching by local respiratory physicians and lung function laboratory staff.

It is unrealistic to assume that in the near future, primary care will achieve the high standards of accuracy demanded from an accredited hospital respiratory function unit. Primary care must be encouraged and nurtured to start performing spirometry. The essential training process involved must always emphasize quality and correct technique.

The types of spirometer used in primary care will need to be simple to use and access, provide real-time graphical displays and printouts and be fairly inexpensive. Most will be electronic devices, which have the added advantage of being small, portable and containing technology that will allow storage of multiple blows and provide instant feedback on reproducibility of blows. They also calculate predicted values, thus saving the busy practitioner valuable time. By hospital standards, such equipment may be thought inferior and possibly inaccurate, particularly when calibration is not regularly performed. However, the devices definitely fulfil the role and clinical needs of primary care in helping to screen, diagnose and assess severity of COPD, as well as giving valuable information about many other forms of respiratory disease.

References

1 Kannel WB, Lew EA. Vital capacity as a prediction of cardiovascular disease: the Framingham Study. *Am Heart J* 1983; **105**: 311–15.

2 Pearson MG. FEV_1 and PEF in COPD management. *Thorax* 1999; **54**: 468–9.

3 Marshall M, Jackson J, Cooper BG. Does it matter what type of spirometer is used to measure FEV_1, FVC and VC? *Thorax* 1999; **54** (Suppl. 3): A78.

4 Harrison J, Hancox L, Carter J, Hill SL. The influence of device on the measurement of spirometric indices. *Thorax* 1999; **54** (Suppl. 3): A78.

5 American Thoracic Society. Standardisation of spirometry; 1987 update. *Am Rev Respir Dis* 1987; **136**: 1285–98.

6 American Thoracic Society. Standardisation of spirometry: 1994 update. *Am J Respir Crit Care Med* 1995; **152**: 1107–36.

7 Quanjer PhH, Tammeling GJ, Coles JE *et al.* Standardisation of lung function tests. European Community for Steel and Coal. *Eur Respir J* 1993; **6** (Suppl. 16): 85–100.

8 American Thoracic Society. Lung function testing: selection of reference values and interpretative strategies. *Am Rev Respir Dis* 1991; **144**: 1202–18.

9 Miller MR, Pincock AC. Predicted values: how should we use them? *Thorax* 1988; **43**: 265–7.

10 Quadrelli S, Rancoroni A, Mantiel G. Assessment of respiratory function: influence of spirometry references values and normality criteria selection. *Respir Med* 1999; **93**: 523–35.

11 Morris JF, Koski A, Johnson LC. Spirometric standards for healthy non-smoking adults. *Am Rev Respir Dis* 1971; **103**: 57–67.

12 Cherniack RM, Raber MB. Normal standards for ventilatory function using an automated wedged spirometer. *Am Rev Respir Dis* 1972; **106**: 38–44.

13 Crapo RO, Morris AH, Gardiner RM. Reference spirometric values using techniques and equipment that meet ATS recommendations. *Am Rev Respir Dis* 1981; **123**: 659–64.

14 Knudson RJ, Lebowitz MD, Holberg CJ, Burrows B. Changes in the normal maximal expiratory flow volume curve with growth and ageing. *Am Rev Respir Dis* 1983; **127**: 725–34.

15 European Community for Coal and Steel. Standardisation of lung function tests. *Bull Eur Physiopathol Respir* 1983; **19** (Suppl.): 1–93.

16 American Thoracic Society. Evaluation of impairment/disability secondary to respiratory disorders. *Am Rev Respir Dis* 1986; **133**: 1205–9.

17 BTS Guidelines for the management of chronic obstructive pulmonary disease. *Thorax* 1997; **52** (Suppl. 5): S1–28.

18 American Thoracic Society. Standards for the diagnosis and care of patients with chronic obstructive pulmonary disease. *Am J Respir Crit Care Med* 1995; **152**: S77–121.

19 Siafakas NM, Vermeire P, Pride NB *et al.* Optimal assessment and management of chronic obstructive pulmonary disease (COPD). *Eur Respir J* 1995; **8**: 1398–420.

20 Hole DJ, Watt GCM, Davey-Smith G *et al.* Improved lung function and mortality risk in men and women: findings from the Renfrew and Paisley prospective population study. *BMJ* 1996; **313**: 711–15.

21 Mahler DA, Maekowiak JI. Evaluation of the short-form 36-item questionnaire to measure health-related quality of life in patients with COPD. *Chest* 1995; **107**: 1585–9.

22 Oren A, Sue DY, Hansen JE *et al.* The role of exercise testing in impairment evaluation. *Am Rev Respir Dis* 1987; **135**: 230–5.

23 Bellamy D, Hoskins G, Smith B *et al.* The use of spirometers in general practice. *Asthma Gen Pract* 1997; **5**: 8–9.

24 Pinnock H, Carley-Smith J, Kalideen D. Spirometry in primary care: an analysis of the first 100 patients referred in one general practice. *Asthma Gen Pract* 1999; **7**: 23–4.

25 Rudolf M. Making spirometry happen. *Thorax* 1999; **54** (Suppl. 3): A43.

26 Freeman D. Personal communication. 2000.

27 Van Schayck CP, Loozen JMC, Wagena E *et al.* Detecting patients at a high risk of developing chronic obstructive

pulmonary disease in general practice: cross-sectional case finding study. *BMJ* 2002; **324**: 1370–3.

28 Eaton T, Withy S, Garrett JE *et al.* Spirometry in primary care practice: the importance of quality assurance and the impact of spirometry workshops. *Chest* 1999; **116**: 416–23.

29 Den Otter JJ, Knitel M, Akkermans RPM *et al.* Spirometry in general practice: the performance of practice assistants scored by lung function technicians. *Br J Gen Pract* 1997; **47**: 41–2.

30 Schermer TRJ, Folgering HTM, Bottema BJAM *et al.* The value of spirometry for primary care: asthma and COPD. *Prim Care Respir J* 2000; **9**: 51–5.

31 Pauwels R, Buist AS, Calverley RMA *et al.* Global strategy for the diagnosis, management and prevention of COPD. *Am J Respir Crit Care Med* 2001; **163**: 1256–76.

5: Assessment of disability: what test, or combination of tests, should be used?

Denis O'Donnell and Michael Fitzpatrick

Assessment of disability

Disability is defined by the World Health Organization as 'any restriction or lack of ability to perform any activity within the range of normal for a human being' [1]. In COPD, structural and physiological impairment of the respiratory system is associated with varying degrees of disability. However, the clinical assessment of the COPD patient in the past has relied heavily on the quantification of physiological impairment with little attention given to the assessment of the consequent disability. The increasing realization that common spirometric measures of pulmonary impairment correlate only weakly with exercise intolerance, symptom intensity, and quality of life, has prompted a search for better evaluative methods. This review focuses on the interface between physiological impairment and disability in COPD and forms the basis for a more comprehensive clinical assessment of the symptomatic patient.

Why does decrement in FEV_1 not correlate precisely with disability?

The forced expiratory volume in 1 s (FEV_1) is the most common test of physiological impairment in COPD, and has stood the test of time. It is a simple reproducible test, it is of unquestionable diagnostic utility, it is useful in following the course of the disease, and is a valuable prognostic indicator. The term COPD, however, encompasses heterogeneous pathophysiological derangements of the small and large airways, lung parenchyma and capillary bed in highly variable combinations and these diverse structural abnormalities are unlikely to be reflected in one simple spirometric test. Therefore, it is not surprising that the FEV_1, which is a crude measurement of overall physiological impairment, has been shown repeatedly in research studies to correlate poorly with measures of disability such as symptom intensity and exercise capacity in COPD [2–4]. This poor statistical correlation is borne out by common clinical observation. Thus, patients with the same measured FEV$_1$ (expressed as percentage predicted) may vary greatly in their level of disability; patients may deteriorate clinically, either acutely (e.g. during infective exacerbations) or chronically, while preserving spirometric FEV$_1$. Moreover, patients may achieve considerable improvements in symptoms and exercise endurance as a result of interventions such as bronchodilators, oxygen therapy or exercise training, with little or no change in the FEV$_1$ [5–7]. These observations collectively attest to the fact that disability is multifactorial and often independent of the FEV$_1$. Factors that determine the level of disability (or its change over time) in a given individual include: the level of expiratory flow limitation, gas exchange abnormalities, ventilatory demand, extent of thoracic overinflation, extent of mechanical loading of the inspiratory muscles, degree of ventilatory muscle and peripheral muscle weakness/deconditioning, and cardiac factors. Moreover, the level of disability is also profoundly influenced by interactions among multiple physiological, psychological, social, and environmental factors.

Spirometric FEV$_1$ is prone to measurement artifact because a forced manoeuvre, initiated from total lung capacity, introduces gas compression effects, airway compression effects, and results in an altered pattern of lung emptying compared with that which occurs during normal tidal breathing over a range of operating lung volumes. Spirometric FEV$_1$ gives no information about the extent of prevailing expiratory flow limitation, the extent of dynamic lung hyperinflation (DH) required to maximize expiratory flow rates and therefore does not provide an assessment of the 'dynamic' expiratory flows available under conditions of increased ventilation such as exercise (Fig. 5.1). All of these factors can vary greatly for a given FEV$_1$ and contribute importantly, either singly or in combination, to symptom generation, ventilatory limitation and exercise capacity [4].

Despite the multifactorial nature of disability in COPD, it is reasonable to assume that the degree to which an individual is disabled ultimately reflects the extent of ventilatory mechanical abnormalities present. Given the limitations of the FEV$_1$ as a measure of mechanical impairment, additional physiological measurements such as dynamic lung volumes, together with direct measurements of symptom intensity and exercise impairment, are used increasingly to clinically evaluate patients and to determine the success of therapeutic interventions. A variety of parameters can be employed to comprehensively assess impairment, disability and handicap in the symptomatic COPD patient (Table 5.1).

What causes dyspnoea in COPD?

In a recent American Thoracic Society Consensus Statement [8], dyspnoea was defined as 'a term used to characterize a subjective experience of breath-

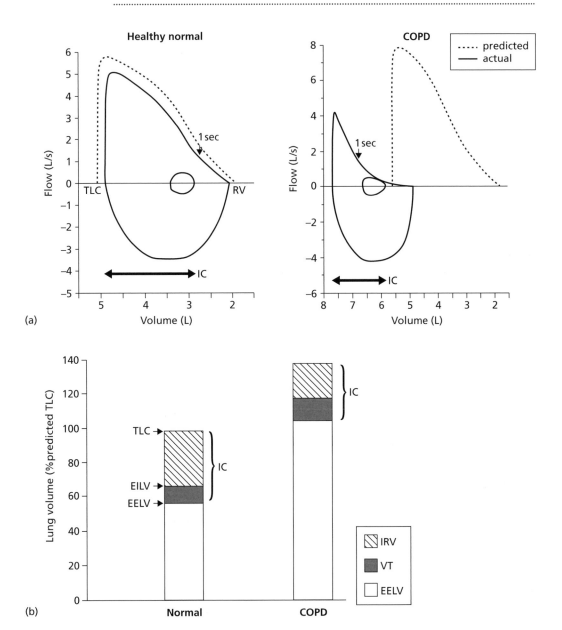

Fig. 5.1 (a) Maximal and tidal flow-volume loops in a healthy subject and in a patient with COPD. The patient exhibits markedly reduced FEV_1 (1 s), expiratory flow limitation and lung hyperinflation (i.e. reduced inspiratory capacity [IC]). (b) Lung volume compartments in the same patient. Note marked lung hyperinflation with reduced IC compared with normal. EELV, end-expiratory lung volume; EILV, end-inspiratory lung volume; TLC, total lung capacity; IRV, inspiratory reserve volume; V_T, tidal volume.

Table 5.1 Evaluation of the symptomatic COPD patient.

• Symptoms (BDI, MRC)	
• Body mass index (BMI)	
• Spirometry	Impairment
• Hyperinflation (IC, FRC)	
• D$_L$CO and CT scan	
• Exercise performance:	Disability
Peak V̇o$_2$	
Ventilatory reserve	
Gas exchange	
• Peripheral muscle strength	
• Health status	Handicap

ing discomfort that consists of qualitatively distinct sensations that vary in intensity'. Exertional dyspnoea in COPD consists of multiple qualitative dimensions: the majority of patients describe predominant inspiratory difficulty with only a minority describing significant expiratory difficulty at the peak of symptom-limited exercise [9]. The perception of inspiratory difficulty further encompasses an awareness of unsatisfied inspiration ('can't get enough air in', or 'my breath does not go in all the way'), which appears to be peculiar to the diseased state and not encountered in healthy subjects even at the breakpoint of exhaustive exercise [9]. Dyspnoea in COPD is provoked or aggravated by activity, so it is only fitting that mechanistic studies on symptom generation are carried out during exercise. Pathophysiological factors known to contribute to the quality and intensity of exertional dyspnoea and to exercise limitation in COPD include:

1 Intrinsic mechanical loading (elastic and resistive) of the inspiratory muscles.
2 Increased mechanical (volume) restriction during exercise.
3 Functional inspiratory muscle weakness.
4 Excessive ventilation.
5 Gas exchange abnormalities.
6 Dynamic airway compression in expiration.
7 Cardiovascular factors.
8 Any combination of the above [10].

These factors are highly interdependent and their relative contribution to dyspnoea intensity may vary considerably among different COPD patients. In general, as the disease advances, more of these factors become instrumental in dyspnoea causation [10].

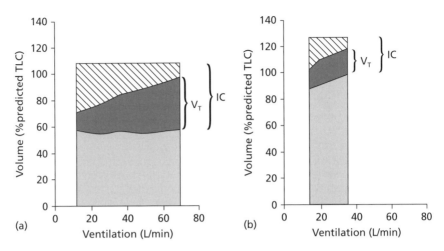

Fig. 5.2 Changes in operational lung volumes over ventilation during exercise (a) in health and (b) in COPD. Note, compared with normal, there is increased resting and dynamic hyperinflation as ventilation increases with the result that the tidal volume response is constrained and IC progressively diminishes.

Mechanical abnormalities in COPD—the importance of dynamic hyperinflation

The hallmark of COPD is expiratory flow limitation which results from a combination of reduced lung recoil and airway tethering, as well as intrinsic airway narrowing [11]. However, while the most obvious mechanical defect is obstructive, in expiration, the most important mechanical consequence is a 'restrictive' ventilatory deficit in inspiration due to the effects of dynamic lung hyperinflation (DH) (Figs 5.1 and 5.2). One of the earliest descriptions of DH was provided by William Stokes, an Irish physician, in his treatise, *Diseases of the Lung and Windpipe*, published in 1837 [12]. Stokes recounted the following lucid clinical observations of a patient with emphysema: 'I shall describe a sign which promises to be of the greatest importance in diagnosis. By making the patient perform a number of forced inspirations rapidly, the repetition of the inspiratory efforts caused such an accumulation of air in the diseased portion of the lung as ultimately to nearly prevent its further expansion. The results of this experiment are readily explained by referring to the difficulty in expiration which occurs in this disease' [12].

DH occurs in flow-limited patients when ventilation increases, either voluntarily or reflexly (as for example during exercise) in response to increased levels of arterial carbon dioxide (Fig. 5.2). Thus, at higher levels of ventilation, tidal lung emptying becomes incomplete and lung volume fails to decline to its equilibrium point (i.e. functional residual capacity), causing dynamic end-

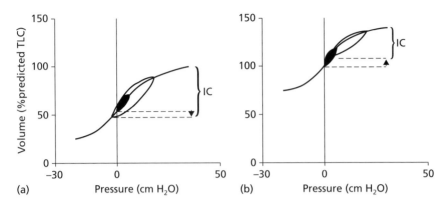

Fig. 5.3 Pressure-volume (P–V) curves of the respiratory system in (a) health and (b) COPD. Tidal loops at rest (enclosed area) and during exercise (open area) are constructed on each curve. In contrast to health, IC is reduced in COPD and tidal volume is positioned on the upper alinear extreme of the P–V relation where there is increased elastic loading.

expiratory lung volume ($EELV_{dyn}$) to progressively increase as a result of air trapping (Fig. 5.2) [11,13–15]. The extent of DH during exercise depends on:

1   The extent of expiratory flow limitation
2   The level of baseline lung hyperinflation
3   Ventilatory demand, and
4   The breathing pattern at any given ventilation.

The level and pattern of DH during exercise in COPD is highly variable: in a recent study, the average increase in $EELV_{dyn}$ during exercise in 105 patients with COPD was 0.37 ± 0.39 L or $14\pm15\%$ of predicted [15].

Although DH serves to optimize tidal expiratory flow rates, it adversely affects dynamic ventilatory mechanics in three major ways: (i) it causes patients to breathe at a high lung volume where further volume expansion during exercise is seriously restricted (Fig. 5.2); (ii) it burdens inspiratory muscles with additional elastic loading; and (iii) it causes functional inspiratory muscle weakness. Theoretically, DH would also be expected to impair cardiovascular function during exercise but this question remains to be studied.

The inability to expand V_T during exercise results in greater reliance on increasing breathing frequency to increase ventilation, but this tachypnoea results in further DH in a vicious cycle [11,15]. Tachypnoea also contributes to the reduced dynamic lung compliance which is known to have an exaggerated frequency dependence in COPD [11]. Because of DH, V_T encroaches more and more on the upper alinear extreme of the respiratory system's (combined lung and chest wall) pressure–volume relationship, where there is increased elastic loading of inspiratory muscles already overburdened with the work of overcoming increased airways resistance in COPD (Fig. 5.3) [11]. By

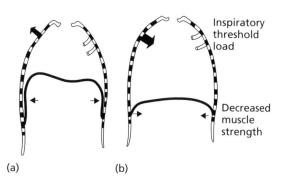

Inspiratory threshold load

Decreased muscle strength

Fig. 5.4 Illustration of the rib cage and diaphragm in (a) health and (b) COPD. In COPD the diaphragm is shortened and functionally weakened because of hyperinflation and the combined recoil of the lung and chest wall at end-expiration is inwardly rather outwardly directed as in normals, creating an inspiratory threshold load (see text for details).

(a)   (b)

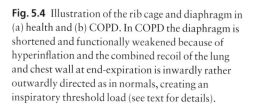

contrast, V_T remains within the linear portion of the pressure–volume (P–V) relationship in health, even at much higher levels of exercise (Fig. 5.3). Inspiratory threshold loading is another more recently recognized consequence of DH. In flow-limited patients with positive intrathoracic pressures at the end of expiration (the autoPEEP phenomenon) [11], the inspiratory muscles must first overcome the combined inward recoil of the lung and chest wall at end-expiration, before inspiratory flow is initiated (Fig. 5.4). This threshold load occurs throughout inspiration and the pressure required to overcome it can be substantial, particularly if DH is severe during higher levels of ventilation [9]. Lastly, DH alters the length–tension relationships of the inspiratory muscles, particularly the diaphragm (which becomes flattened), and compromises their ability to generate pressure (Fig. 5.4) [11]. Attendant tachypnoea during exercise, with increased velocity of inspiratory muscle shortening, results in further functional muscle weakness [11]. Moreover, DH may alter the pattern of ventilatory muscle recruitment to a more inefficient pattern with negative implications for muscle energetics and performance.

Due to the increased loading and functional inspiratory muscle weakness occasioned by DH, tidal inspiratory pressures represent a much higher fraction of their maximal force generating capacity than in health at similar work rates and ventilation (Fig. 5.5) [9]. Since, in exercising COPD patients, the ability to breathe enough air in is progressively curtailed despite mustering near maximal inspiratory efforts, the ratio of effort (tidal esophageal pressure swings relative to maximum) to tidal volume (V_T) is significantly higher than in health (Fig. 5.5) [9]. This may have important implications for respiratory sensation. It is reasonable to assume that some of the distinctive qualitative dimensions of dyspnoea in COPD, such as unsatisfied inspiration, may have their physiological basis in the marked disparity between inspiratory effort, which approaches the maximum, and the mechanical response of the system, which is greatly impaired because of breathing at high lung volumes and increased inspiratory airways resistance. The intensity of dyspnoea during exercise has been shown to correlate strongly with the extent of dynamic lung hyperinflation and with the

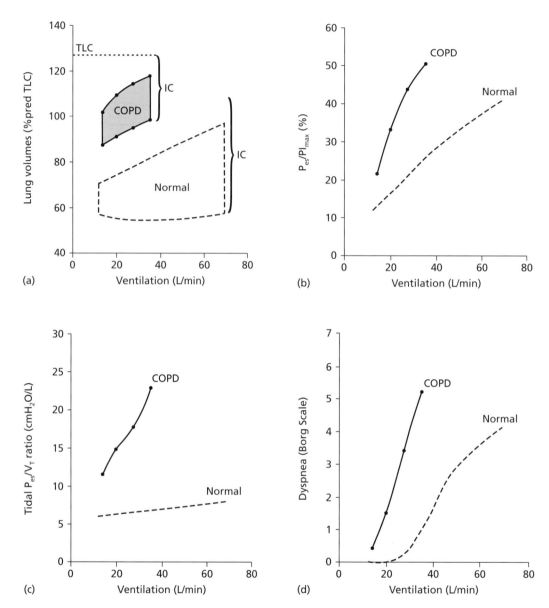

Fig. 5.5 Plots of (a) operational lung volumes, (b) inspiratory effort (esophageal pressure relative to maximal P_{es}/PI_{max}) and the (c) ratio of effort to tidal volume (P_{es}/V_T), and (d) Borg dyspnoea ratings, all expressed as a function of increasing ventilation during exercise. Compared with normals, in COPD inspiratory effort is greatly increased despite a reduced tidal volume response and this likely contributes to increased exertional dyspnoea. (Adapted from [9]).

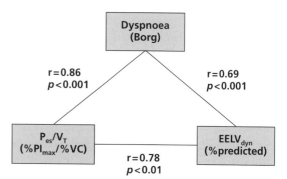

Fig. 5.6 Statistical correlations between Borg ratings of inspiratory difficulty, end-expiratory lung volume (reduced dynamic inspiratory capacity), and the ratio of inspiratory effort to tidal volume standardized for vital capacity (P_{es}/PI_{max}:V_T/% VC) at a standardized level of exercise in COPD patients [9].

increased ratio of inspiratory effort to thoracic displacement; the latter ultimately reflects severe neuromechanical uncoupling of the respiratory pump (Fig. 5.6) [6,9,14]. Further indirect evidence of the importance of DH in dyspnoea causation comes from a number of recent studies which have shown that dyspnoea can effectively be ameliorated by interventions that reduce operational lung volumes, either pharmacologically [5–7] or surgically [16,17]. We can conclude therefore, that measurements of resting and dynamic lung volumes in COPD may be more relevant to functional disability than traditional spirometric expiratory measurements. Further studies are required to determine if lung volume (or capacity) estimations such as inspiratory capacity (which reflects $EELV_{dyn}$), slow or timed vital capacity (which reflects residual volume), or direct plethysmographic measurements of thoracic gas volume, correlate better with disability in COPD than expiratory flow measurements per se, and whether such measurements are more sensitive when assessing responses to combination bronchodilator therapy.

Dyspnoea and excessive ventilation in COPD

The level of disability can be greatly influenced by the interaction of dynamic mechanics and ventilatory drive. An excessive ventilatory response, regardless of its cause (i.e. exercise, anxiety, infective exacerbations, acute metabolic alterations) will amplify the mechanical derangements outlined above. In other words, DH is increased at high ventilation levels and causes earlier limiting ventilatory constraints of flow and volume generation. Thus, for a given level of expiratory flow limitation, the extent of DH and its negative mechanical and sensory consequences will vary with ventilatory demand. Factors contributing to excessive ventilation in COPD during exercise include: high physiological deadspace, early lactate acidosis, hypoxemia, high O_2 cost of breathing, low arterial carbon dioxide (CO_2) set points, and other non-metabolic sources of ventilatory stimulation (i.e. anxiety, hyperventilation) [18–21]. Several studies have shown that dyspnoea during exercise in COPD correlated strongly with the change in ventilation expressed in absolute terms or as a fraction of the estimated maximal breathing capacity [14,22,23]. Studies have shown that for a given FEV_1, COPD patients with low diffusion capacity for carbon monoxide and with higher ventilatory demands during exercise (as a result of higher physiological deadspace) experience greater acute and chronic activity-related dyspnoea than those with normal ventilatory responses to exercise [15,22]. Indirect evidence of the importance of excessive ventilation in contributing to exertional dyspnoea and exercise limitation in COPD comes from a number of studies which have shown that exercise training, oxygen therapy and opiate medication relieve dyspnoea and improve exercise performance, in part, by reducing submaximal ventilation levels [24–27]. It has become clear that even modest reductions in ventilation (i.e. 3–6 L/min) can provide important symptomatic alleviation in severely mechanically compromised patients [24–27].

Does arterial oxygen desaturation cause dyspnoea in COPD?

In some patients, arterial hypoxemia during rest or exercise may contribute to dyspnoea through ventilatory stimulation secondary to an altered metabolic load (i.e. excessive acidosis during exercise secondary to reduced O_2 delivery or utilization), or directly via altered peripheral chemoreceptor activation, independent of the level of ventilation [25,26,28]. While large controlled studies have provided convincing evidence of the beneficial effects of continuous oxygen therapy on survival in severely hypoxemic patients with COPD, the effects of such therapy on chronic symptoms and disability is unknown. Case-controlled studies during exercise have shown that symptomatic responses to supplemental oxygen are entirely unpredictable in an individual patient with COPD, regardless of the level of baseline or exertional arterial oxygen desaturation [25,26,28]. Patients who do not improve their dyspnoea or exercise endurance during added oxygen (compared with placebo) likely have other predominant sources of symptom generation such as mechanical abnormalities. It must be remembered that hypoxia, increased ventilatory stimulation and dynamic lung hyperinflation are inextricably linked such that supplemental oxygen, by depressing ventilation, will reduce air trapping for a given level of expiratory flow limitation and improve symptoms and activity levels in those patients who respond (Fig. 5.7) [26]. Since responses to ambulatory oxygen therapy are unpredictable in COPD, a single blind, constant-load exercise study with measurements of symptoms and exercise endurance time is required to identify responders [26]. Even COPD patients, who are normoxic at rest and exercise, have been shown to benefit in a dose–response manner from incremental supplemental oxygen during exercise: Somfrey et al. [29] have shown progressive

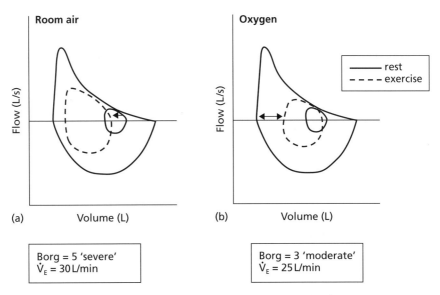

Room air

Oxygen

Flow (L/s)

Volume (L)

(a)

Flow (L/s)

Volume (L)

(b)

—— rest
- - - exercise

Borg = 5 'severe'
$\dot{V}_E$ = 30 L/min

Borg = 3 'moderate'
$\dot{V}_E$ = 25 L/min

Fig. 5.7 Comparison of maximal and tidal resting and exercise flow-volume loops at a standardized exercise level in a patient with COPD during exercise receiving either room air (a) or supplemental oxygen (b). Added oxygen resulted in reduced ventilation (by 5 L/min) with consequent reductions in dynamic hyperinflation and reduced exertional dyspnoea (Borg scale).

reduction in lung hyperinflation and increase in inspiratory reserve volumes during exercise, with a plateau effect at a fractional oxygen concentration of 0.5.

It is well established that patients with chronic hypoxemia can develop secondary pulmonary hypertension, which may be further aggravated acutely during activity. Such patients often experience severe activity-induced dyspnoea. In these patients, the relative contribution to dyspnoea generation of cardiovascular factors (i.e. activation of pulmonary and right sided cardiac receptors), mechanical factors and excessive ventilation has never been determined with precision. It is possible that direct afferent inputs from the right heart and vasculature may directly give rise to unpleasant respiratory sensations, but this remains speculative [30].

Dyspnoea and psychological factors

Patients with COPD are known to have a higher incidence of anxiety-depressive states than a healthy population, and these psychological factors undoubtedly contribute to perceptions of respiratory distress and general disability [31]. Anxiety may of itself, induce dyspnoea in mechanically compromised patients: for example, the accompanying tachypnoea may worsen lung hyperinflation. Alternatively, anxiety may represent the affective response to unpleasant respiratory sensations. There is anecdotal evidence that in some patients with COPD, treatment of morbid anxiety by psychological counselling and sedative medication can reduce dyspnoea and improve activity levels but, in general, responses to these interventions in the published literature are highly variable.

The importance of psychological factors in contributing to disability is borne out by the favourable responses achieved following supervised exercise training in such patients [24]. Many of the benefits of pulmonary rehabilitation programs are attributable to the patient's overcoming their anxiety or fear of breathlessness during activity.

Do exercise tests add anything to the assessment of disability?

Resting physiological measurements are poorly predictive of maximal exercise capacity (i.e. peak symptom-limited oxygen consumption) or exercise endurance in individual patients with COPD; therefore, direct assessment of exercise performance is required to assess functional disability. Exercise tests vary considerably in their level of sophistication. The simple observation of the patient as he/she walks along the corridor, or climbs a flight of stairs, provides useful qualitative information. Supervised timed walking distances, such as the 12-minute walk distance or the more convenient 6-minute walk distance (6MWD) tests have been used extensively as a measure of functional disability [32]. Concurrent measurements of dyspnoea intensity using validated scales enhance the value of this test.

Although the 6MWD is a useful clinical indicator of functional disability, and correlates with both quality of life and mortality, it has limitations. Such tests are highly motivationally dependent. It is impossible to control the pace of walking or power output during the test and this becomes important, particularly when comparisons of two tests are being made in the same individual over time. Because of a definite learning effect, it is recommended that two 'familiarization' tests be conducted and that the third test should be accepted as the baseline test [33]. If tests are to be compared over time, great care must be taken by the supervisor to standardize the instruction and encouragement of the patient [33]. These recommendations collectively increase the complexity of testing. In addition, access to adequate facilities to conduct the test (i.e. long unimpeded corridors) is also a definite practical consideration. Concomitant measurement of dyspnoea (using validated scales [34,35]) and arterial oxygen saturation enhance the value of the test. The inability to carry out pertinent physiological measurements during the 6MWD test is a potential disadvantage. Because of these limitations, modifications in timed walking distance tests have been made. For example, 6-minute testing using a treadmill, where the power output can be controlled and where physiological measurements can be more easily undertaken, may have advantages over the traditional hallway testing [36].

The shuttle test

The incremental shuttle test is designed to overcome some of the limitations of the 6MW test, and there is evidence of its reliability and responsiveness, at least to exercise training [36]. With this test the pace, or work rate, is progressively increased using an auditory cue, which allows observation of the patient over a range of activity levels. The patient walks fixed distances of 10 m between two cones [37,38]. The time available to complete each 10-metre distance is progressively decreased and the distance walked when the patient stops becomes the outcome measure of interest. The test is terminated when patients develop intolerable symptoms and heart rate reaches 85% of maximum. The endurance shuttle test at a fixed fraction of the pre-established peak power output during the incremental shuttle test is likely to be more responsive than the incremental test in evaluating the effects of therapeutic interventions, such as ambulatory O_2 [38–40]. However, its sensitivity in the evaluation of bronchodilator efficacy remains unknown. There is anecdotal evidence that, in patients with severe functional disability, the 6MWD is more sensitive in assessing bronchodilator efficacy. However, for less disabled patients, the shuttle test may prove superior.

Cardiopulmonary exercise testing

Increasingly, disability and dyspnoea assessment is conducted in the setting of formal exercise testing in the laboratory (Fig. 5.8). This more rigorous, integrative approach to the measurement of the physiological and perceptual responses to exercise has several advantages:

1   It provides an accurate assessment of the patient's exercise capacity;
2   It measures the perceptual responses to a quantifiable dyspneogenic stimulus (i.e. O_2 consumption (VO_2), ventilation, power output);
3   It provides insights into pathophysiological mechanisms of dyspnoea in a given patient (e.g. excessive ventilation, dynamic hyperinflation, arterial oxygen desaturation);
4   It can identify other coexisting conditions that contribute to dyspnoea and exercise limitation (i.e. cardiac disorders, intermittent claudication, musculoskeletal problems); and
5   Standardized comparisons of perceptual responses to measurable dyspnoea-provoking stimuli allow an accurate assessment of symptom responses to therapeutic interventions [41].

There is currently no consensus about which exercise testing protocol

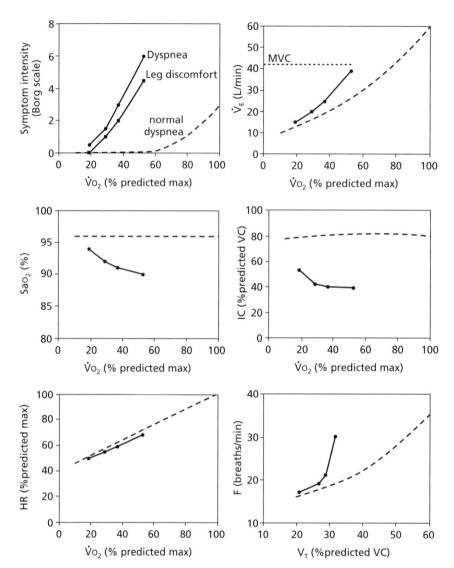

Fig. 5.8 An incremental exercise test in a patient with COPD (solid lines) compared with normal responses in health (dashed lines). Exertional symptoms, ventilation (V_E), oxygen saturation, inspiratory capacity (IC), and heart rate (HR) responses are plotted against oxygen consumption (V_{O_2}). Breathing patterns [frequency (F) vs. tidal volume (V_T)] are plotted on the lower left panel. This patient stopped exercise at 50% of V_{O_2} predicted maximum because of severe breathlessness and leg discomfort. Contributing factors to exercise limitation in this patient included excessive ventilation, arterial oxygen desaturation, progressive lung hyperinflation (i.e. reduced IC), and a rapid shallow breathing pattern. MVC, maximal ventilatory capacity.

should preferentially be used for disability assessment. Both incremental and constant load endurance testing, using cycle ergometry or treadmill, are used extensively and these different approaches have the potential to produce different, but complimentary, clinical information. Estimations of symptom-limited, maximal oxygen consumption (VO_{2max}) during incremental cycle exercise testing is frequently used in the assessment of disability in patients with occupational lung diseases, but is used less extensively in COPD, where endurance tests may be preferable. Knowledge of the VO_{2max} and of the MET equivalents (metabolic rates based on multiples of the resting VO_2) of various activities of daily living permit a crude estimation of the patient's functional capacity. Precise stratification of the VO_{2max} *vis-à-vis* overall functional disability in individual patients with COPD is not available. However, generally speaking, a VO_{2max} of <15 mL/kg/min in a patient with COPD represents severe functional disability. Standard cardiopulmonary exercise testing measures the following physiological responses: metabolic load (VO_2, VCO_2), ventilation, breathing pattern, arterial oxygen saturation, heart rate, oxygen pulse, and blood pressure. More recently, other ventilatory parameters relevant to dyspnoea assessment, such as the exercise tidal flow-volume loop analysis relative to the maximal resting loop, are being used (Fig. 5.7) [41]. This approach allows a more comprehensive evaluation of the ventilatory constraints that apply in a given individual compared with traditional estimates of ventilatory limitation such as the ventilatory index (i.e. estimated maximal ventilatory capacity minus peak ventilation). Repeated inspiratory capacity measurements during exercise allow an indirect assessment of the extent of dynamic hyperinflation which, as already mentioned, contributes importantly to both symptoms and exercise intolerance (Figs 5.6 and 5.8) [7,41].

Dyspnoea is measured during exercise using the Borg or visual analogue scales. Both scaling methods have been shown to be reliable (reproducible) and responsive (ability to detect change) in patient populations with COPD [34,35]. Constant load cycle ergometry at 50–80% of the patient's predetermined maximal work rate has been shown to have excellent reproducibility and to be responsive to interventions such as bronchodilators, oxygen therapy, opiates, and exercise training [7]. For the clinical assessment of bronchodilator efficacy, comparisons of the dyspnoea (Borg) scale—time slopes at a standardized constant load (e.g. 75% peak VO_2) has been shown to be highly responsive, and concomitant quantitative flow-volume loop analysis allows additional insights into the mechanisms of functional improvement [7].

Does CT assessment of the extent of emphysema predict disability?

High resolution computed tomography (HRCT) has made it possible to quantify, with considerable precision, the extent and pattern of emphysematous destruction of the lung *in vivo* [42,43]. Emphysema scores, based on the magnitude and distribution of low attenuation areas on HRCT, correlate well with morphometric measurements of microscopic emphysema in subsequently resected lungs. Several studies have shown reasonable correlations between HRCT derived emphysema scores and physiological indices such as the diffusion capacity for carbon monoxide (DLCO), lung volumes, and spirometric expiratory flow rates [42,43]. HRCT performed at end-inspiration correlates most closely with the extent of emphysema on pathological examination, whereas HRCT performed at end-expiration correlates best with measurements of airflow obstruction [44]. Intensive research is currently underway on the potential role of HRCT in differentiating the various pathological components of COPD (i.e. emphysema, chronic bronchitis and asthma). However, the classical findings in chronic bronchitis of bronchial wall thickening and gas trapping at low lung volumes are unreliable and often absent. Given the heterogeneity of pathological abnormality in COPD, it is unlikely that refinements in HRCT quantification and differentiation will enhance our ability to predict disability in a given patient. However, preliminary studies suggest that HRCT assessments, in combination with detailed physiological measurements, have the potential to elucidate mechanisms of disability in individual COPD patients [43]. For example, it has been shown that symptomatic patients with a history of cigarette smoking, who have only minor spirometric abnormalities, but with disproportionately reduced DLCO, may have a localized upper zone centrilobular emphysema on HRCT [43]. Such patients may have significant ventilation/perfusion inhomogeneity and extensive small-airways dysfunction, not reflected by the FEV_1. In these patients, the combination of excessive ventilatory stimulation (due to high physiological deadspace) can aggravate expiratory flow limitation and DH, with consequent premature ventilatory limitation, heightened dyspnoea and exercise intolerance [15].

Patients with both interstitial lung disease and emphysema may have normal expiratory flow rates and lung volumes. HRCT is useful in such patients to determine the relative extent of each disease and the likely contribution of each condition to the clinical and functional abnormality [45].

Advances in nuclear medicine and magnetic resonance imaging in COPD hold promise for the future. Single photon emission computed tomography (SPECT) ventilation images can be used to provide quantitative volumetric mapping of regional gas trapping [46]. In this technique, equilibrium phase images with xenon-133 are used to generate 3D views of the total lung volume, while washout images provide 3 dimensional views of regional gas trapping. Static magnetic resonance imaging (MRI) allows three dimensional reconstructions of the chest wall and diaphragm, which may improve evaluation of structure-function relationships in COPD, and also provide reliable measurements of lung volumes in these patients (for example, pre and post surgical intervention) [47]. Dynamic MRI during the breathing cycle has been used to depict asynchronous movement of the chest wall and diaphragm in severe emphysema, and improvement in respiratory mechanics with surgical intervention (lung volume reduction surgery) [47]. Magnetic resonance ventilation imaging with hyperpolarized He-3 gas has shown potential to allow volumetric mapping of enlarged airspaces in COPD that are below the resolution capability of HRCT [48]. High resolution volumetric MR imaging of regional pulmonary perfusion has also become possible.

Hence, there is reason for considerable optimism that highly accurate quantitative imaging of both structural and functional abnormalities in patients with COPD will be available in the future. How much this imaging will add to the clinical and functional assessment of disability in the patient with COPD remains to be seen.

Will it be possible to measure small-airway function in future?

It has long been recognized that small-airways disease may precede the overt clinical manifestations of chronic bronchitis and emphysema in smokers. Chronic bronchiolitis of small airways is an integral component of established COPD. There is little doubt that small-airways disease contributes importantly to both impairment and disability in COPD. However, the small airways have been termed the 'silent zone' because extensive narrowing of these peripheral airways contributes little change to measurements of overall airways resistance. A reliable test of small-airways dysfunction is therefore desirable. Moreover, given our increased understanding of the nature of the inflammatory process in small airways in COPD, and the development of new, non-steroidal anti-inflammatory (mediator antagonists) and bronchodilator therapies (tiotropium and long-acting beta agonists), the assessment of small-airway function is of obvious importance in ascertaining the eventual clinical utility of these agents.

The development of a simple reproducible test of small-airway function has remained an elusive goal, as witnessed by the plethora of physiological tests that are currently available in clinical practice or in the research setting [49]. Examples include:

1 Expiratory flow-volume loops derived by variable-volume plethysmography;

2 Partial and maximal flow–volume loop isovolume comparisons;

3 Flow volume loops during helium breathing;

4 Tests of expiratory flow limitation such as negative expiratory pressure (NEP) application;

5 Tests of ventilation distribution (i.e. frequency dependence of compliance and closing volume);

6 Measurement of thoracic gas volumes (i.e. residual volume); and

7   Measurements of dynamic hyperinflation and dynamic elastance during exercise [7,41].

All of the above listed tests have limitations; many are technically demanding or are unavailable and, in particular, the responsiveness of these tests to various therapeutic interventions has not been established. To the extent that air trapping and lung hyperinflation fundamentally reflect small-airway dysfunction in COPD, then bronchodilator induced reduction in lung hyperinflation serves as an indirect measure of improved dynamic small-airway function [41]. Recent innovations in HRCT permit precise morphometric assessments of higher generations of peripheral small airways than were, hitherto, possible [36,37]. Classical HRCT imaging features of smoking-related bronchiolitis—areas of ground glass opacity, centrilobular nodules and bronchial wall thickening—have been described. Unfortunately, however, HRCT is usually normal in this early stage of disease. It is conceivable that in the future, combined structural and functional assessments of small-airway disease, such as those alluded to above will increase our understanding of the mechanisms of disability in COPD.

Summary

Disability in COPD is complex and multifactorial, and this makes clinical evaluation a challenging task. However, recent advances in our understanding of the interface between pathophysiological impairment and functional disability in COPD has set the stage for the development of better evaluative methods. More research and dialogue is required to devise an acceptable staging system for disability in COPD, akin to that which is already available for other chronic diseases such as congestive heart failure. The comprehensive assessment of disability might incorporate the following elements:

1   Measurement of impairment: FEV_1, inspiratory capacity, and D_LCO, each expressed as percentage predicted;

2   Measurement of body mass index;

3   Measurement of exercise performance, together with exertional symptoms and ventilatory reserves;

4   Assessment of chronic activity-related dyspnoea using validated self-rated scales or multidimensional instruments; and

5   Measurement of disease-specific quality of life using validated questionnaires.

A composite score derived from the above listed components would permit stratification of patients with respect to disability level, and could also be used to facilitate the evaluation of the overall clinical impact of therapeutic interventions in patients with symptomatic COPD.

References

1   World Health Organization. *International Classification of Iimpairments, Disabilities and Handicaps*. Geneva: World Health Organization, 1980; 10–11 (26–31): 86–7.

2   Wolkove N, Dajczman E, Colacone A, Kreisman H. The relationship between pulmonary function and dyspnoea in obstructive lung disease. *Chest* 1989; 96: 1247–51.

3   Hay JG, Stone P, Carter J, Church S *et al*. Bronchodilator reversibility, exercise performance and breathlessness in stable chronic obstructive pulmonary disease. *Eur Respir J* 1992; 5: 659–64.

4   Bauerle O, Chrusch CA, Younes M. Mechanisms by which COPD affects exercise tolerance. *Am J Respir Crit Care Med* 1998; 157: 57–68.

5   Chrystyn H, Mulley BA, Peake MD. Dose–response relation to oral theophylline in severe chronic obstructive airways disease. *Br Med J* 1988; 297: 1506–10.

6   Belman MJ, Botnick WC, Shin JW. Inhaled bronchodilators reduce dynamic hyperinflation during exercise in patients with chronic obstructive pulmonary disease. *Am J Respir Crit Care Med* 1996; 153: 967–75.

7   O'Donnell DE, Lam M, Webb KA. Measurement of symptoms, lung hyperinflation and endurance during exercise in chronic obstructive pulmonary disease. *Am J Respir Crit Care Med* 1998; 158: 1557–65.

8   Meek PM, Schwartzstein RMS, Adams L *et al*. Dyspnoea mechanisms, assessment and management: a consensus statement (American Thoracic Society). *Am J Respir Crit Care Med* 1999; 159: 321–40.

9   O'Donnell DE, Bertley JC, Chau LL, Webb KA. Qualitative aspects of exertional breathlessness in chronic airflow limitation: pathophysiologic mechanisms. *Am J Respir Crit Care Med* 1997; 155: 109–15.

10 O'Donnell DE. Exertional breathlessness in chronic respiratory disease. In Mahler DA, ed. *Lung Biology in Health and Disease*, Vol. III: Dyspnoea. New York: Marcel Dekker Inc, 1998; 97–147.

11 Pride NB, Macklem PT. Lung Mechanics in Disease. In: AP Fishman., eds. *Handbook of Physiology*, Section 3, Vol. III Part 2: The Respiratory System. Bethesda MD: American Physiological Society, 1986; 659–92.

12 Stokes WA. A treatise on the diagnosis and treatment of diseases of the chest. *Part 1: Diseases of the Lung and Windpipe*. London: The New Sydenham Society 1937: 168–9.

13 Dodd DS, Brancatisano T, Engel LA. Chest wall mechanics during exercise in patients with severe chronic airflow obstruction. *Am Rev Respir Dis* 1984; 129: 33–8.

14 O'Donnell DE, Webb KA. Exertional breathlessness in patients with chronic airflow limitation: the role of hyperinflation. *Am Rev Respir Dis* 1993; 148: 1351–7.

15 O'Donnell DE, Revill S, Webb KA. Dynamic hyperinflation in exercise intolerance in chronic obstructive pulmonary disease. *Am J Respir Crit Care Med* 2001; 164: 770–7.

16 Martinez FJ, Montes de Oca M, Whyte RI, Stetz J, Gay SE, Celli BR. Lung-Volume reduction improves dyspnoea, dynamic hyperinflation and respiratory muscle function. *Am J Respir Crit Care Med* 1997; 155: 1984–90.

17 Laghi F, Jurban A, Topeli A *et al*. Effect of lung Volume reduction surgery on neuromechanical coupling of the diaphragm. *Am J Respir Crit Care Med* 1998; 157: 475–83.

18 Dillard TA, Piantadosi S, Rajogopal KR. Prediction of ventilation at maximal exercise in chronic airflow obstruction. *Am Rev Respir Dis* 1985; 132: 230–5.

19 Jones NL, Jones G, Edwards RHT. Exercise tolerance in chronic airway obstruction. *Am Rev Respir Dis* 1971; 103: 477–91.

20 Levison H, Cherniack RM. Ventilatory cost of exercise in chronic obstructive pulmonary disease. *J Appl Physiol* 1968; 25: 21–7.

21 Jones NL. Pulmonary gas-exchange during exercise in patients with chronic airway obstruction. Clin Sci 1966: 3139–50.

22 O'Donnell DE, Webb KA. Breathlessness in patients with severe chronic airflow limitation: physiologic correlates. *Chest* 1992; 102: 824–31.

23 Leblanc P, Bowie DM, Summers E, Jones NL, Killian KJ. Breathlessness and exercise in patients with cardio-respiratory disease. *Am Rev Respir Dis* 1986; 133: 21–5.

24 O'Donnell DE, McGuire M, Samis L, Webb KA. The impact of exercise reconditioning on breathlessness in severe chronic airflow limitation. *Am J Respir Crit Care Med* 1995; 152: 2005–13.

25 Swinburn CR, Wakefield JM, Jones PW. Relationship between ventilation and breathlessness during exercise in chronic obstructive airways disease is not altered by prevention of hypoxemia. *Clin Sci* 1984; 67: 515–9.

26 O'Donnell DE, Bain DJ, Webb KA. Factors contributing to relief of exertional breathlessness during hyperoxia in chronic airflow limitation. *Am J Respir Crit Care Med* 1997; 155: 530–5.

27 Light RW, Muro JR, Sato RI, Stansbury DW, Fischer CE, Brown SE. Effects of oral morphine on breathlessness and exercise tolerance in patients with chronic obstructive pulmonary disease. *Am Rev Respir Dis* 1989; 139: 126–33.

28 Lane R, Cockcroft A, Adams L, Guz A. Arterial oxygen saturation and breathlessness in patients with chronic obstructive airways disease. *Clin Sci* 1987; 72: 693–8.

29 Somfay A, Porszasz J, Lee SM, Casaburi R. Dose–response effect of oxygen on hyperinflation and exercise endurance in non-hypoxemic COPD patients. *Eur Resp J* 2001; 18: 77–84.

30 Jones PW, Huszczuk A, Wasserman K. Cardiac output as a contributor of ventilation through changes in right ventricular load. *J Appl Physiol* 1982; 53: 218–24.

31 Gift AG, Cahill CA. Psychophysiologic aspects of dyspnoea in chronic obstructive pulmonary disease: a pilot study. *Heart Lung* 1990; 19: 252–7.

32 McGavin CR, Artvinli M, Naoe H, McHardy GJ. Dyspnoea, disability and distance walked: comparison of estimates of exercise performance in respiratory disease. *Br Med J* 1978; 2: 241–3.

33 Guyatt GH, Puglsey SO, Sullivan MJ *et al.* Effect of encouragement on walking test performance. *Thorax* 1984; 39: 818–22.

34 Borg G, Simple rating methods for estimation of perceived exertion. *Wenner-Gren Center Int Symp Series* 1976; 28: 39–47.

35 Gift AG. Validation of a vertical visual analogue scale as a measure of clinical dyspnoea. *Rehab Nurs* 1989; 14: 313–25.

36 Stevens D, Elpern E, Sharma K, Szidow D, Ankin M, Kesten S. Comparison of hallway and treadmill six minute walk tests. *Am J Respir Crit Care Med* 1999; 160: 1540–3.

37 Singh SJ, Morgan MD, Scott S, Walters D, Hardman AE. Development of a shuttle walking test of disability in patients with chronic airways obstruction. *Thorax* 1992; 47: 1019–24.

38 Singh SJ, Morgan MD, Hardman AE, Rowe C, Bardsley PA. Comparison of oxygen uptake during a conventional treadmill test and the shuttle walking test in chronic airflow limitation. *Eur Resp J* 1994; 7: 2016–20.

39 Revill SM, Morgan MD, Singh SJ, Williams J, Hardman AE. The endurance shuttle test. A new field test for the assessment of endurance capacity in chronic obstructive pulmonary disease. *Thorax* 1999; 54: 213–22.

40 Revill SM, Singh SJ, Morgan MD. Randomized controlled trial of ambulatory oxygen and an ambulatory ventilator on endurance exercise in COPD. *Respir Med* 2000; 94: 778–83.

41 O'Donnell DE. Exercise Limitation and Clinical Exercise Testing in Chronic Obstructive Pulmonary Disease. In: Wiseman IM, Zebellos RJ, eds. *Clinical Exercise Testing*. Prog Respir Res: Karger, 2002: 32, 138–58.

42 Nakano Y, Sakai H, Muro S *et al.* Comparison of low attenuation areas on computed tomographic scans between inner and outer segments of the lung in patients with chronic obstructive pulmonary disease: incidence and contribution to lung function. *Thorax* 1999; 54: 384–9.

43 Klein JS, Gamsu G, Webb WR, Golden JA, Muller NL. High resolution CT diagnosis of emphysema in symptomatic patients with normal chest radiographs and isolated low diffusion capacities. *Radiology* 1992; 182: 817–21.

44 Genevois PA, de Vuyst P, Sy M, Scillia P *et al.* Pulmonary emphysema: Quantitative CT during expiration. *Radiology* 1996; 199: 825–9.

45 Wiggins J, Strickland B, Turner-Warwick M. Combined cryptogenic fibrosing alveolitis and emphysema: The value of high-resolution computed tomography in assessment. *Respir Med* 1990; 84: 365–9.

46 Suga K, Kume N, Nishigauchi K *et al*. Three-dimensional surface display of dynamic pulmonary xenon-133 SPECT in patients with obstructive lung disease. *J Nucl Med* 1998; 39: 889–93.

47 Gierada DS, Hakimian S, Slone RM, Yusen RD. MR analysis of lung Volume and thoracic dimensions in patients with emphysema before and after lung Volume reduction surgery. *Am J Roentgenol* 1998; 170: 707–14.

48 de Lange EE, Mugler JP, Brookeman JR *et al*. Lung air spaces: MR imaging evaluation with hyperpolarized 3He gas. *Radiology* 1999; 210: 851–7.

49 Anthonison NR. Tests of mechanical function. In: AP Fishman, ed. *Handbook of Physiology* Vol. III *Part 2: The Respiratory System. Mechanics of Breathing*, American Physioloical Society. Baltimore, Maryland: Williams & Wilkins Co, 1986, 753–84.

6: Do older patients with COPD need a different approach?

Martin Connolly

Introduction

Respiratory disease is the second commonest cause of disability in old age [1], and chronic obstructive pulmonary disease (COPD) in turn is the commonest disabling respiratory condition in this age group. Estimates of the overall prevalence of COPD in the elderly population vary widely, from around 16% to nearly 30% [2–6]. These differences are likely to be largely dependent on differences in smoking prevalence, pollution levels, and poverty levels between subpopulations examined. Most epidemiological surveys, however, agree on the point that a large proportion of chronic obstructive pulmonary disease in old age remains undetected and untreated. A further complicating factor in epidemiological assessment is the accuracy of diagnostic labelling. Many elderly patients with chronic asthma and limited treatment responsiveness could equally well be (and often interchangeably are) labelled as either asthmatics or COPD sufferers. For the purpose of this chapter, chronic poorly responsive asthma in old age will be included under the COPD umbrella [7]. However, the historical lack of agreement in terminology has meant that medical practitioners often vary in diagnostic labelling, with a tendency to overdiagnose COPD in elderly men and overdiagnose asthma in young women [8].

There are several potent questions that should challenge physicians dealing with elderly COPD patients. This chapter does not claim to answer these questions comprehensively, merely to pose them and attempt an analysis.

Is COPD a different condition in old age?

This question has perhaps two main aspects: (i) is the disease aetiologically different?; and (ii) is the disease clinically different?

The answer to the first question must be in the widest sense a resounding 'no'. There is no evidence to suggest that cigarette smoking is not the major cause of COPD in the elderly. Indeed, smoking uptake reached its maximum in Britain in men born within 10 years of the turn of the 20th century and in women born 20 years later [9]. It is these populations that have COPD and will continue for 20 years or more to supply physicians with the majority of their (elderly) COPD patients. Whether the 'Dutch hypothesis' that an interaction between smoking and atopy may have a differential effect with ageing is an interesting question. Many studies have shown associations between lung function and measures of atopy in smokers and non-smokers [10–17], and have also shown that smokers have elevated atopic markers, particularly IgE levels [10–17]. Renwick and Connolly [18] have tentatively suggested that measures of atopy may be *more strongly* associated with both airways obstruction and bronchial hyperresponsiveness in older rather than younger adults. This is a surprising finding and contradictory to accepted wisdom concerning the decline of the atopic tendency with ageing.

More conventionally, however (as discussed above), the overlap between asthma and COPD is wider in the elderly than in the young, in large part because of the reduced treatment response [19] particularly to bronchodilators seen in elderly asthmatics, whether due to long duration of disease or even short duration of disease in more elderly individuals [8]. Whilst this may have limited practical import at present, with the clinical management of elderly subjects with stable 'COPD-like chronic asthma', these patients (and perhaps all elderly COPD patients, in view of the atopy–smoking interaction) should not be ignored as potential beneficiaries of new anti-asthma developments, such as leukotriene antagonists. This area, however, has no evidence base and needs research endeavour.

In terms of the clinical presentation of the condition, there is very good reason to argue that COPD may, for many elderly subjects at least, be a different condition to that seen in young sufferers. Whilst the insidious onset of the disease is well-recognized in all age groups, this is particularly so in old age. Predictive factors for various obstructive symptoms of cough, wheeze, sputum production and breathlessness are particularly low in old age [20]. Whether this reflects merely reduced expectation and activity level in the elderly, compounded by a reduced index of suspicion among carers and physicians, is unclear. There is evidence to suggest that the subjective perception of bronchoconstriction is impaired with increasing age [21,22]. The association of COPD with other disabling conditions (see below) is in many elderly patients a further confounding factor. Whatever the reasons, COPD is often not clinically detected at all in the elderly [6,23] or may be detected late, resulting in more likely progression to end-stage disease, with less opportunity for life-prolonging intervention. There is no justification in this regard for any therapeutic nihilism in terms of, for example, smoking cessation in old age—the motivated elderly smoker being just as likely to quit as a motivated young smoker [24,25], and with no age-related decline in the beneficial effects of nicotine replacement therapy [25,26].

The elderly patient with moderate or severe COPD will often present with a kaleidoscope of symptomatic, diagnostic and therapeutic characteristics, with impairments and disabilities influenced by a wide variety of factors both directly related and unrelated to COPD. In particular, the high incidence of depressive symptoms in COPD patients, including the elderly [27,28], and its effect on performance is a matter of great concern, particularly as depression is usually under-recognized in the elderly patient group [28]. The above argues for a specialist multidisciplinary team approach to the assessment of such patients, as it is only by use of the skills and facilities available to such a team that a full diagnostic and therapeutic package can be assembled.

How can perceived disabilities due to COPD be distinguished from those due to other age-related conditions?

The large number of septuagenarians and octogenarians completing marathon events across the world each year is striking evidence that ageing itself is not a cause of disability. Despite age-related reductions in performance of the cardiorespiratory and musculoskeletal system, the reserve of the human body is such that the mere addition of years in the span given to humans is not a major concern in terms of performance of normal activities of daily living. Impairment and disability at all ages has a clinical and pathological cause. As mentioned above, however, many elderly people may be affected by more than one age-associated condition. This is particularly true when there is a major aetiological factor (cigarette smoking) at play, often resulting in multiple-system disorder.

Clinicians and researchers attempt to quantify disability using scales that measure activities of daily living (ADL). In the context of COPD, some hospital-based ADL scales, particularly the Barthel Index [29], have ceiling effects that make them of little value [30]. ADL scales that measure more 'extended' community-based activity, such as the Nottingham Extended ADL Scale [31], are of more use. However, most ADL scales currently in use in geriatrics practice do not attempt to distinguish between respiratory-related disability and disability due to other conditions, and indeed most were designed to measure stroke-related disability. The Nottingham Extended ADL Scale, for example, though distinguishing well between elderly COPD sufferers and normals, is not responsive to COPD interventions [32]. Our own group has modified the Nottingham Extended ADL Scale to produce the Manchester Respiratory ADL Scale, which in addition to distinguishing elderly COPD subjects from normals is responsive to intervention by respiratory rehabilitation [32]. In clinical practice, however, the physician faced with a patient with multiple-system problems rarely has the luxury of treating each one in temporal isolation, and it may thus be individually difficult to estimate which element of any alleviation of disability is explained by treatments for separate conditions. There is some evidence to support the routine use of ADL scales in elderly COPD outpatients (see below). Furthermore, in the context of rehabilitation following acute admission for exacerbation of COPD, extrapolation of data on other conditions (particularly stroke) suggests that they have an important place. More research is needed in this general area.

What is the value of FEV_1 in the elderly?

There are three separate questions here:
- Is forced expiratory volume in 1 s (FEV_1) in itself 'accurate' in old age?
- Is FEV_1 useful for diagnosis?
- Is FEV_1 useful for staging of disease?

In terms of the first question, it is clear that both FEV_1 and FEV_1/forced vital capacity (FVC) ratio are strongly related to gender and to age. Use of FEV_1 expressed as percentage of predicted values does not remove the age bias completely because, as there is a positive relationship between FEV_1 and height and a negative relationship between FEV_1 and age, the use of predictive FEV_1 increases the number of short and elderly individuals appearing to have abnormal results [33]. The use of FEV_1 expressed as standardized residual (SR) has been advocated to remove such bias [33]. SRs should probably be employed in all research studies (particularly epidemiological studies) involving lung function measurements in old age, particularly when comparing elderly subjects to younger subjects.

However, this is almost certainly impractical in the clinical setting. Unfortunately, even after accepting the above, age-adjusted percentage predicted levels may be unreliable, as many of the normal populations employed to ascertain these values have not included elderly subjects and have mistakenly extrapolated above the age of 65, usually overestimating age-related decline in lung function. True age-related data up to the age of 85 have been supplied by the studies by Enright *et al.* [34], and these are probably the most suitable for clinical studies, at least in elderly Caucasian patients. In practice, many elderly patients with COPD find it difficult to complete an FVC manoeuvre, and thus although the FEV_1/FVC ratio is in theory less affected by normal ageing, it is probably of less clinical value. In contrast to popular opinion, most elderly subjects *are* able to perform FEV_1 manoeuvres satisfactorily.

In terms of diagnosis, formal lung function tests are if anything even more valuable in old age than in the relatively young. The multiplicity of system disorder and subsequent disability, together with the impaired perception of bronchoconstriction in old age [21,22], argues strongly for the use of objective lung function measures. Although peak flow may seem easier for many elderly patients to perform, its limited value in COPD is well recognized, and this is no less true in old age. There is increasing recognition that the use of FEV_1 in epidemiological surveys both in the community and in hospital sub-populations detects previously undiscovered cases of COPD [6,35,36]. However, there is as yet no evidence to advocate the widespread use of lung function screening in populations or subpopulations of the elderly.

In terms of staging of disease in old age, the value of FEV_1 is less clear. The British Thoracic Society Guidelines employ FEV_1 in large part because of its prediction of mortality and its ability to at least roughly correlate with level of symptoms and intervention needed. It is however, well recognized even in younger subjects that the relationship between FEV_1 and disability is poor, and this is if anything even more so in old age. Our own studies [30,37,38] have shown that FEV_1 is not an independent predictor of quality of life in COPD, does not predict exercise capacity and predicts only 3% of the variance in disability as measured by an extended ADL scale.

Given that simple lung function tests are a poor measure of treatment response, how then is the latter to be assessed? Interest in recent years has focused on the use of quality of life (QoL) scales, both in terms of giving a holistic, patient-centred approach to treatment response and also (recognized more recently) a potentially more sensitive index of response. Any QoL scales contain a very large element of disability assessment, and thus in addition it would seem sensible and logical to have valid and responsive disability scales (ADL measures). This area has been discussed above; ADL scales, which have been widespread in geriatrics practice generally for many years, should perhaps be extended to COPD assessment, at least for elderly patients.

In our own studies [37], we have found the Breathing Problems Questionnaire [39] to be a particularly valid quality of life scale in old age and a better discriminatory tool than the Chronic Respiratory Disease Questionnaire [40]. Our studies were carried out in patients with a mean age of 78 years and a maximum age of 90 years. Another QoL scale, The St George's Respiratory Questionnaire [41], has been shown to be valid (independent of age) in subjects up to the age of 75, and thus for research studies comparing elderly populations (particularly the young elderly) to younger populations, this is perhaps the best-validated tool.

In a clinical setting however, perhaps the main factors to consider when choosing a QoL questionnaire are: how long it takes to complete; what percentage of the variance in quality of life score can be explained by variance in other measurable parameters; and how responsive it is to intervention. In our hands, in elderly COPD subjects, 70% of the variance in Breathing Problems Questionnaire scores were explained by other measurable parameters, most importantly disability measure and a depression screening tool [30]. It is unclear, however, whether in a purely clinical setting both a disability measure (ADL scale) *and* a QoL tool need to be assessed. Disability measures have a greater track record in elderly patients generally, and this author would therefore advocate using ADL scales in clinical practice.

Are the same treatment algorithms applicable to the elderly?

The British Thoracic Society guidelines on the management of COPD [7] are a valuable tool, not least because they specifically addressed many of the problems that elderly patients with COPD face. The cornerstone of COPD management is smoking cessation, and the fact that the ability (or otherwise) of the elderly to quit is no less than that of younger smokers has already been addressed. On the more fundamental issue of whether it is worthwhile for an elderly subject to stop smoking, there are fewer data, but the benefits of quitting on the rate of decline in lung function, though lower in the elderly, are probably worthwhile up until about 80 years, especially in women [42]. Almost all data (in all age groups) on quit rates have been acquired in smokers motivated to quit, however. Though anecdotal evidence would suggest that such motivation falls with increasing age, there is no true evidence base here, and this area is worthy of study.

The only other currently proven life-prolonging treatment, long-term oxygen therapy (LTOT), has not been critically assessed in the very elderly, and indeed one of the major trials, the MRC LTOT trial, specifically excluded patients over the age of 70 years [43]. However, clinical experience suggests that the elderly patient with incipient or current cor pulmonale is no less likely to benefit from LTOT than his or her younger counterpart. Though it is self-evident that the very elderly patient is unlikely to achieve the absolute prolongation in survival of a younger subject when using LTOT, there is need for research examining the other potential benefits, particularly the effect of adequate oxygenation on cognitive function and mood in old age.

The British Thoracic Society guidelines [7] specifically acknowledge that elderly patients may prefer to take inhaled β-adrenergic agonists on a regular basis rather than 'on demand'. This is at least in part in deference to the impaired perception of bronchoconstriction in old age [21]. In addition, although the bronchodilator response to both beta-agonists and ipratropium falls with age, the fall is less for ipratropium, emphasizing the potential added benefit of the use of muscarinic antagonist inhalers.

There is a wealth of literature on inhaler devices, and it is not with the scope of this chapter to discuss this topic further. Suffice it to say that there is good evidence in the elderly for the use of large-volume spacer devices (without the disadvantage seen in younger patients of poor patient acceptability), the Turbuhaler and the Autohaler.

Whilst theophyllines (and occasionally oral beta-agonist preparations) may be particularly useful in cognitively impaired elderly patients who are unable to use any form of inhaled bronchodilator, the side effects of theophylline are often prohibitive in the elderly, particularly as significant therapeutic benefit is only obtained at the upper end of the previously accepted 'therapeutic range' [44]. In practice, however, many elderly patients are taking regular theophyllines, and it is important to maintain a high index of clinical suspicion regarding side effects (particularly related to drug interactions) and to monitor serum levels regularly.

The prescription of nebulized bronchodilator therapy to the elderly should be made in accordance with published guidelines [45]. UK national guidelines currently caution against the use of high-dose beta-agonists in elderly patients with ischaemic heart disease and also suggest the use of mouthpieces rather than face masks in elderly patients with known or suspected glaucoma when using high doses of anticholinergic drugs. Particular emphasis should also be placed on whether the elderly patient can technically manage the nebulizer, and the help of carers may need to be recruited in this regard. The need for adequate follow-up and servicing cannot be overstressed. There may be a lower threshold for the use of nebulizers in elderly patients unable to manage standard inhalers. The use of oral corticosteroids should once again adhere to the British Thoracic Society guidelines on COPD management [7]. There is a particular concern about steroid-induced osteoporosis (or perhaps more accurately, steroid-exacerbated osteoporosis) in elderly patients, especially women. There is no indication for bone densitometry assessment prior to the use of oral corticosteroids in old age, as the vast majority of elderly persons will show osteoporotic indices in any case. However, the use of 'bone prophylaxis' is advisable, and the current recommendations of the British Osteoporosis Society are that calcium and vitamin D supplementation is acceptable in elderly patients receiving corticosteroids. This has the advantage of convenience and minimal side effects.

Particular attention in old age should be given to non-drug management. The uptake of influenza and pneumococcal vaccination is poor and as well as the standard methods of recruiting for this (in the community) an opportunistic policy should perhaps be pursued in hospital outpatients and even ward discharges. The dietary intake of frail and elderly patients in general is often limited whether or not they suffer COPD, often as a result of impaired ADL abilities. This clearly merits attention. Elderly patients as well as the young are able to benefit from pulmonary rehabilitation programmes [38] and should be included in them.

The high incidence of depression in elderly patients with COPD has already been mentioned [27,28], as has its under-recognition [28]. In these respects, COPD is little different from many other chronic disabling illnesses in the elderly, where the need for screening tests for depression is well recognized, the symptoms of the underlying disease often mimicking those of depression. Less well understood, however, are appropriate treatment strategies, and there is some evidence that elderly patients with depression associated with organic conditions will fail to accept a diagnosis of depression and decline antidepressant therapy when offered [46,47].

Management of acute exacerbations should once again follow the British Thoracic Society guidelines [7]. Perhaps the most important time in the hospital management of acute exacerbation in an elderly patient is the day or two prior to discharge, where particular emphasis should be given to discharge medication (particularly including inhaler technique) and a multidisciplinary assessment (sometimes requiring a home visit) of the patient's abilities to manage at home. The skills of the occupational therapist have so far been underused in the management of elderly patients with COPD.

References

1 Hunt A. *The Elderly at Home: a Study of People Aged Sixty-Five and Over Living in the Community in England in 1976*. London: HMSO, 1976.

2 Dow L, Coggon D, Holgate ST. Respiratory symptoms as predictors of airways lability in an elderly population. *Respir Med* 1992; **86**: 27–32.

3 Lundback B, Nystrom L, Rosenhall L, Stjernberg N. Obstructive lung disease in northern Sweden: respiratory symptoms assessed in a postal survey. *Eur Respir J* 1991; **4**: 257–62.

4 Banerjee DK, Lee GS, Malik SK, Daly S. Under-diagnosis of asthma in the elderly. *Br J Dis Chest* 1987; **81**: 23–9.

5 Biegi G, Paoletti P, Carrozzi L et al. Prevalence rates of respiratory symptoms in Italian general population samples exposed to different levels of air pollution. *Environ Health Perspect* 1991; **94**: 95–9.

6 Renwick DS, Connolly MJ. Prevalence and treatment of chronic airways obstruction in adults over the age of 45. *Thorax* 1996; **51**: 164–8.

7 COPD Guidelines Group of the Standards of Care Committee of the BTS. BTS guidelines for the management of chronic obstructive pulmonary disease. *Thorax* 1997; **52** (Suppl. 5): S1–28.

8 Dodge R, Cline MG, Burrows B. Comparisons of asthma, emphysema, and chronic bronchitis diagnoses in a general

population sample. *Am Rev Respir Dis* 1986; **133**: 981–6.

9 Lee PN, Fry JS, Forey BA. Trends in lung cancer, chronic obstructive lung disease, and emphysema death rates for England and Wales 1941–85 and their relation to trends in cigarette smoking. *Thorax* 1990; **45**: 657–65.

10 Burrows B, Hasan FM, Barbee RA, Halonen M, Lebowitz M. Epidemiological observations on eosinophilia and its relation to respiratory disorders. *Am Rev Respir Dis* 1980; **122**: 709–19.

11 Van der Lende R, De Kroon JPM, Van der Meulen GG et al. Possible indicators of host factors in CNSLD. In: Orie NGM, Van der Lende R, eds. *Bronchitis III. Third International Symposium*. Assen, Netherlands: Royal Van Gorcum/Springfield, IL: Thomas, 1969: 52–79.

12 Burrows B, Lebowitz MD, Barbee RA, Knudson RJ, Halonen M. Interactions of smoking and immunologic factors in relation to airways obstruction. *Chest* 1983; **84**: 657–61.

13 Burrows B, Knudson RJ, Cline MG, Lebowitz MD. A re-examination of risk factors for ventilatory impairment. *Am Rev Respir Dis* 1988; **138**: 829–36.

14 Kauffman F, Neukirch F, Korobaeff M *et al*. Eosinophils, smoking and lung

function: an epidemiologic survey among 912 working men. *Am Rev Respir Dis* 1986; **134**: 1172–5.

15 Annesi I, Oryszczyn MP, Frette C *et al.* Total circulating IgE and FEV$_1$ in adult men: an epidemiologic longitudinal study. *Chest* 1992; **101**: 642–8.

16 Frette C, Annesi I, Korobaeff M *et al.* Blood eosinophilia and FEV$_1$: cross-sectional and longitudinal analyses. *Am Rev Respir Dis* 1991; **143**: 987–92.

17 Vollmer WM, Buist AS, Johnson LR, McCamant LE, Halonen M. Relationship between serum IgE and cross-sectional and longitudinal FEV$_1$ in two cohort studies. *Chest* 1986; **90**: 416–23.

18 Renwick DS, Connolly MJ. Persistence of atopic effects on airway calibre and bronchial responsiveness in older adults. *Age Ageing* 1997; **26**: 435–40.

19 Brown PJ, Greville HW, Finucane KE. Asthma and irreversible airflow obstruction. *Thorax* 1984; **39**: 131–9.

20 Renwick DS, Connolly MJ. Do respiratory symptoms predict chronic airflow obstruction and bronchial hyperresponsiveness in older adults? *J Gerontol Med Sci* 1999; **54A**: M136–M139.

21 Connolly MJ, Crowley JJ, Charan NB, Nielson CP, Vestal RE. Reduced subjective awareness of bronchoconstriction provoked by methacholine in elderly asthmatic and normal subjects as measured on a simple awareness scale. *Thorax* 1992; **47**: 410–13.

22 Marks GB, Yates DH, Sist M *et al.* Respiratory sensation during bronchial challenge testing with methacholine, sodium metabisulphite, and adenosine monophosphate. *Thorax* 1996; **51**: 793–8.

23 Roberts SJ, Bateman DN. Which patients are prescribed inhaled anti-asthma drugs? *Thorax* 1994; **49**: 1090–5.

24 Vetter NJ, Ford D. Smoking prevention among people aged 60 and over: a randomized controlled trial. *Age Ageing* 1990; **19**: 164–8.

25 Campbell IA, Prescott RJ, Tjeder-Burton SM. Transdermal nicotine plus support in patients attending hospital with smoking-related diseases: a placebo-controlled study. *Respir Med* 1996; **90**: 47–51.

26 Russel MAH, Stapleton JA, Feyerbend C *et al.* Targetting heavy smokers in general

practice: randomised controlled trial of transdermal nicotine patches. *BMJ* 1993; **306**: 1308–12.

27 Craig TJ, Van Nutta PA. Disability and depressive symptoms in two communities. *Am J Psychiatry* 1983; **140**: 598–601.

28 Yohannes AM, Roomi J, Baldwin RC, Connolly MJ. Depression in elderly outpatients with disabling chronic obstructive pulmonary disease. *Age Ageing* 1998; **27**: 155–60.

29 Collin C, Wade DT, Davies S, Horne V. The Barthel ADL Index: a reliability study. *Int Disabil Stud* 1988; **10**: 61–3.

30 Yohannes AM, Roomi J, Waters K, Connolly MJ. A comparison of the Barthel index and Nottingham Extended Activities of Daily Living Scale in the assessment of disability in chronic airflow limitation in old age. *Age Ageing* 1997; **27**: 369–74.

31 Nouri F, Lincoln NB. An extended activities of daily living scale for stroke patients. *Clin Rehab* 1987; **1**: 233–8.

32 Yohannes AM, Roomi J, Connolly MJ. The Manchester Respiratory ADL (MRADL) questionnaire: validation and responsiveness. *Age Ageing* 1998; **27** (Suppl. 2): 41.

33 Miller MR, Pincock AC. Predictive values: how should we use them? *Thorax* 1988; **43**: 265–7.

34 Enright PL, Kronmal RA, Higgins M, Schenker M, Haponik EF. Spirometry reference values for women and men 65 to 85 years of age. Cardiovascular health study. *Am Rev Respir Dis* 1993; **147**: 125–33.

35 Pulford EC, Connolly MJ. Prevalence of airways obstruction in elderly hospital admissions. *Age Ageing* 1998; **27** (Suppl. 1): P62.

36 Patterson CJ, Dow L, Teale C. Prevalence of undiagnosed airflow limitation in acute elderly admissions. *Age Ageing* 1996; **25** (Suppl. 1): P27.

37 Yohannes AM, Roomi J, Waters K, Connolly MJ. Quality of life in elderly patients with COPD: measurement and predictive factors. *Respir Med* 1998; **92**: 123–6.

38 Roomi J, Johnson MM, Waters K *et al.* Respiratory rehabilitation, exercise capacity and quality of life in chronic airways disease in old age. *Age Ageing* 1996; **25**: 12–16.

39 Hyland ME, Bott J, Singh S, Kenyon CAP. Domains, constructs and the development of the Breathing Problems Questionnaire. *Qual Life Res* 1994; **3**: 245–56.

40 Guyatt GH, Townsend M, Berman LB, Pugsley SO. Quality of life in patients with chronic airflow limitation. *Br J Dis Chest* 1987; **81**: 45–54.

41 Jones PW, Quirk FH, Baveystock CM, Littlejohns P. A self-complete measure of health status for chronic airflow limitation: the St George's Respiratory Questionnaire. *Am Rev Respir Dis* 1992; **145**: 1321–7.

42 Burchfiel CM, Marcus EB, Curb D *et al.* Effects of smoking and smoking cessation on longitudinal decline in pulmonary function. *Am J Respir Crit Care Med* 1995; **151**: 1778–85.

43 Report of the Medical Research Council Oxygen Working Party. Long-term domiciliary oxygen therapy in chronic hypoxic cor pulmonale complicating chronic bronchitis and emphysema. *Lancet* 1981; i: 681–5.

44 McKay SE, Howie CA, Thomson AH *et al.* Value of theophylline treatment in patients handicapped by chronic obstructive lung disease. *Thorax* 1993; **48**: 227–32.

45 British Thoracic Society Nebuliser Project Group. Current best practice for nebuliser treatment. *Thorax* 1997: **52** (Suppl. 2): S1–3.

46 Koenig HG, Goli V, Shelp F *et al.* Antidepressant use in elderly medical inpatients: lessons from an attempted clinical trial. *J Gen Intern Med* 1989; **4**: 498–505.

47 Kaplan EM. Antidepressant noncompliance as a factor in the discontinuation syndrome. *J Clin Psych* 1997; **58** (Suppl. 7): 31–5.

7: Do COPD patients develop particular problems in sleep?

Walter McNicholas

Introduction

Sleep has well-recognized effects on breathing, which in normal individuals have no adverse impact. These effects include a mild degree of hypoventilation with consequent hypoxaemia and hypercapnia, and a diminished responsiveness to respiratory stimuli. However, in patients with chronic lung disease such as chronic obstructive pulmonary disease (COPD), these physiological changes during sleep may have a profound effect on gas exchange, and episodes of profound hypoxaemia may develop, particularly during rapid-eye-movement (REM) sleep [1], which may predispose to death at night [2]. Furthermore, COPD has an adverse impact on sleep quality itself [3], which may contribute to the complaints of fatigue and lethargy that are well-recognized features of the condition [4] (Table 7.1).

How does COPD affect sleep quality?

Sleep tends to be fragmented in COPD, with frequent arousals and diminished amounts of slow-wave and REM sleep [3]. The mechanism of sleep impairment in COPD is unclear, but probably relates at least in part to the disordered gas exchange. Although there have been many studies of breathing and gas exchange disturbances during sleep in COPD, few studies have focused on sleep quality. Furthermore, sleep impairment is an aspect of COPD that is frequently ignored by many physicians, even in research protocols designed to assess the impact of COPD on quality of life [5–8]. This aspect assumes particular importance in the context of assessing the impact of pharmacological therapy on quality of life in patients with COPD [9], since pharmacological agents that improve sleep quality in COPD [10] are likely to have a beneficial clinical impact over and above that simply associated with improvements in lung mechanics and gas exchange, particularly in terms of fatigue and overall energy levels.

Table 7.1 Impact of chronic obstructive pulmonary disease (COPD) on sleep.

- Disturbed sleep quality
- Diminished slow-wave and rapid-eye-movement (REM) sleep
- Frequent arousals
- Impaired gas exchange
- Hypoxaemia — may be severe in REM sleep
- Hypercapnia — usually mild

Table 7.2 Mechanisms of sleep-related hypoxaemia in chronic obstructive pulmonary disease (COPD).

- Hypoventilation — most important
- Impact of oxyhaemoglobin dissociation curve — amplifies the impact of hypoventilation
- Ventilation–perfusion mismatching
- Coexisting sleep apnoea — present in only 10–15% of patients

When should COPD patients have sleep studies?

The serious and potentially life-threatening disturbances of ventilation and gas exchange that may develop during sleep in patients with COPD raise the question of appropriate investigation of these patients. However, it is widely accepted that sleep studies are not routinely indicated in patients with COPD associated with respiratory insufficiency, particularly since the awake PaO_2 level provides a good indicator of the likelihood of nocturnal oxygen desaturation [11]. Sleep studies are only indicated where there is a clinical suspicion of an associated sleep apnoea syndrome or manifestations of hypoxaemia not explained by the awake PaO_2 level, such as cor pulmonale or polycythaemia. In most situations in which sleep studies are indicated, a limited study focusing on respiration and gas exchange should be sufficient, and full polysomnography with sleep staging is rarely required (Table 7.2).

What are the mechanisms of sleep-related breathing disturbances in COPD?

Sleep-related hypoxaemia and hypercapnia are well recognized in COPD, particularly during REM sleep, and may contribute to the development of cor pulmonale [1,12] and nocturnal death [2]. These abnormalities are most common in the 'blue bloater' type of patient, who also have a greater degree of awake hypoxaemia and hypercapnia than the 'pink puffer' type of patient [13]. However, many patients with awake arterial PO_2 (PaO_2) levels in the mildly hypoxaemic range can also develop substantial nocturnal oxygen desaturation, which appears to predispose to the development of pulmonary hypertension [12]. Furthermore, COPD patients develop levels of oxygen desaturation during sleep that are greater than those seen during maximum treadmill exercise testing [14]. There are a number of potential mechanisms for the development of these abnormalities.

Hypoventilation

Studies using non-invasive methods of quantifying respiration have shown clear evidence of hypoventilation, particularly during REM sleep, associated with periods of hypoxaemia in patients with COPD [15,16], but the semi-quantitative nature of these measurements makes it difficult to determine if this is the sole mechanism of oxygen desaturation, or whether other factors are involved. A recent report [14] in which ventilation, SaO_2, and transcutaneous PCO_2 ($PtcCO_2$) were continuously recorded during sleep in a group of patients with severe but stable COPD demonstrated that falls in SaO_2 were accompanied by a rise in $PtcCO_2$, and REM sleep, in particular, was frequently characterized by irregular, low tidal volume respiration and a high $PtcCO_2$. These observations support hypoventilation as the major cause of nocturnal desaturation in COPD, particularly during REM sleep.

Impact of the oxyhaemoglobin dissociation curve

There is a close relationship between awake PaO_2 and nocturnal oxygen saturation (SaO_2) levels, and it has been proposed that nocturnal oxygen desaturation in patients with COPD is largely the consequence of the combined effects of physiologic hypoventilation during sleep and the fact that hypoxaemic patients show a proportionately greater fall in SaO_2 with hypoventilation than normoxaemic, because of the effects of the oxyhaemoglobin dissociation curve [14–16]. However, PaO_2 has also been shown to fall more during sleep in major desaturators as compared with minor desaturators [14], which indicates that other factors must also play a part in nocturnal oxygen desaturation in patients with COPD.

Altered ventilation–perfusion relationships

The reduction in accessory muscle contribution to breathing particularly during REM sleep result in a decreased functional residual capacity (FRC), and contribute to worsening ventilation–perfusion relationships during sleep, which also aggravate hypoxaemia in COPD [15,16]. We have found that transcutaneous PCO_2 ($PtcCO_2$) levels rise to a similar extent in patients who develop major nocturnal oxygen desaturation to that in patients who develop only a minor degree of desaturation [14], which suggests a similar degree

Table 7.3 Management options for chronic obstructive pulmonary disease (COPD) patients with sleep-related respiratory failure.

General measures
Optimize therapy of underlying condition
Prompt therapy of infective exacerbations

Supplemental oxygen
Controlled flow to minimize risk of CO_2 retention

Pharmacologic therapy
Bronchodilators, particularly anticholinergics
Theophylline
Almitrine
Non-invasive positive pressure ventilation (NIPPV)

of hypoventilation in both groups, despite the different degrees of nocturnal oxygen desaturation. The much larger fall in PaO_2 among the major desaturators as compared with the minor desaturators, in conjunction with the similar rise in $PtcCO_2$ in both patient groups, suggests that in addition to a degree of hypoventilation operating in all patients, other factors such as ventilation–perfusion mismatching must also play a part in the excess desaturation of some COPD patients.

Coexisting sleep apnoea syndrome

The incidence of sleep apnoea in patients with COPD is about 10–15% [17], which is little higher than would be expected in a normal population of similar age. Factors that may predispose to sleep apnoea in patients with COPD include impaired respiratory drive, particularly in the 'blue bloater' type of COPD patient. Patients with coexisting COPD and sleep apnoea typically develop more severe hypoxaemia during sleep, because such patients may be hypoxaemic at the commencement of each apnoea, whereas patients with pure sleep apnoea tend to resaturate to normal SaO_2 levels in between apnoeas. Therefore, they are particularly prone to the complications of chronic hypoxaemia, such as cor pulmonale and polycythaemia [17] (Table 7.3).

Can sleep-related breathing abnormalities in COPD be treated?

General principles

The first principle of management of sleep-related breathing disturbance in COPD should be to optimize the underlying condition, since this will almost invariably have beneficial effects on breathing. For example, optimizing bronchodilator therapy has been shown to improve gas exchange during sleep

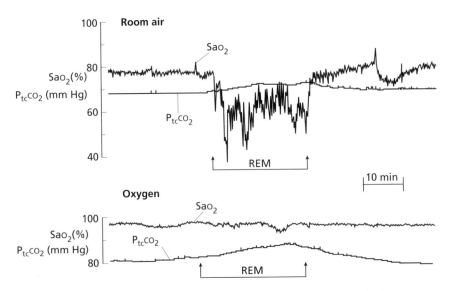

Fig. 7.1 SaO_2 and transcutaneous CO_2 levels in non-REM and REM sleep on and off supplemental oxygen. Adapted from [19] with permission.

[10,18] Respiratory infections in these patients should be treated promptly and vigorously.

Oxygen therapy

The role of oxygen therapy in COPD is covered in another chapter, but it is important to summarize the impact of oxygen supplementation in COPD during sleep. Oxygen therapy effectively corrects sleep-related hypoxaemia in COPD [19], but at the cost of some degree of CO_2 retention. However, this retention is usually modest (approximately 1 kPa) and non-progressive during the night. Oxygen therapy can also improve sleep quality (Fig. 7.1).

Pharmacologic therapy

Anticholinergics. Cholinergic tone is increased at night, and it has been proposed that this contributes to airflow obstruction and deterioration in gas exchange during sleep in patients with obstructive airways disease. There is recent evidence that ipratropium improves arterial SaO_2 in addition to sleep quality in patients with COPD [10].

Theophylline. Theophylline improves gas exchange during sleep in COPD [18], which may reflect the fact that in addition to being a bronchodilator, theophylline has important effects on respiration, including central respiratory stimulation and improved diaphragmatic contractility [20]. However, theophyllines have an adverse effect on sleep quality, and also have a relatively high incidence of gastrointestinal intolerance, which limits their usefulness in this setting.

β_2-agonists. There are only limited data on the efficacy of β_2-agonists on the management of sleep-related breathing abnormalities in COPD. One report found that a long-acting theophylline was superior to salbutamol in terms of nocturnal gas exchange and overnight fall in spirometry [21]. However, there are no studies of the impact of long-acting β_2-agonists on sleep and breathing in COPD.

Almitrine. Almitrine lessens hypoxaemia both awake and asleep, by means of carotid body stimulation and improved ventilation–perfusion matching within the lung [22], and it is beneficial in hypoxaemic patients with COPD [23]. Important side effects include pulmonary hypertension, dyspnoea and peripheral neuropathy [24].

Non-invasive ventilation

The role of non-invasive ventilation in acute exacerbations of COPD is covered in Chapter 16. However, in the past decade, increasing attention has been directed towards non-invasive methods of ventilatory support of COPD patients with chronic respiratory insufficiency, particularly during sleep [25,26]. Beneficial effects on gas exchange during wakefulness have been widely reported in patients treated with nocturnal ventilatory support in addition to improvements in respiratory muscle strength and endurance [27,28]. The mechanism by which non-invasive positive-pressure ventilation (NIPPV) produces improvements in daytime blood gases likely involve a number of factors, which include resting of the respiratory muscles, resetting of respiratory drive, particularly at the chemoreceptor level and a reduction in residual volume and in the degree of gas trapping.

The findings from studies of NIPPV during sleep in COPD offer exciting new prospects for the management of such patients with advanced disease who are in chronic respiratory failure. However, the health-care resource implications of this therapy are potentially very great, because of the high prevalence of COPD. While it is clear from the literature that NIPPV will play an increasing role in the management of patients with advanced COPD over coming years, it is likely that only a subset of patients with advanced COPD will benefit from this therapy. These considerations emphasize the importance of outcome studies that evaluate the efficacy of this therapy in different patient populations.

References

1 Douglas NJ, Calverley PMA, Leggett RJE *et al*. Transient hypoxaemia during sleep in chronic bronchitis and emphysema. *Lancet* 1979; i: 1–4.

2 McNicholas WT, FitzGerald MX. Nocturnal death among patients with chronic bronchitis and emphysema. *BMJ* 1984; **289**: 878.

3 Cormick W, Olson LG, Hensley MJ, Saunders NA. Nocturnal hypoxaemia and quality of sleep in patients with chronic obstructive lung disease. *Thorax* 1986; **41**: 846–54.

4 Breslin E, Van der Schans C, Breubink S *et al*. Perception of fatigue and quality of life in patients with COPD. *Chest* 1998; **114**: 958–64.

5 Ping-Shin T, McDonnell M, Spertus JA *et al*. A new self-administered questionnaire to monitor health-related quality of life in patients with COPD. *Chest* 1997; **112**: 614–22.

6 Jones PW, Quirk FH, Baveystock CM *et al*. A self-complete measure of health status for chronic airflow limitation. *Am Rev Respir Dis* 1992; **145**: 1321–7.

7 Tsukino M, Nishimura K, Ikeda A *et al*. Physiological factors that determine the health-related quality of life in patients with COPD. *Chest* 1996; **110**: 896–903.

8 Ketelaars CAJ, Schlosser MAG, Mostert R *et al*. Determinants of health-related quality of life in patients with chronic obstructive pulmonary disease. *Thorax* 1996; **51**: 29–43.

9 Jones PW, Bosh TK. Quality of life changes in COPD patients treated with salmeterol. *Am J Respir Crit Care Med* 1997; **155**: 1283–9.

10 Martin RJ, Bucher BL, Smith P *et al*. Effect of ipratropium bromide treatment on oxygen saturation and sleep quality in COPD. *Chest* 1999; **115**: 1338–45.

11 Connaughton JJ, Caterall JR, Elton RA, Stradling JR, Douglas NJ. Do sleep studies contribute to the management of patients with severe chronic obstructive pulmonary disease? *Am Rev Respir Dis* 1988; **138**: 341–4.

12 Fletcher EC, Luckett RA, Miller T *et al*. Pulmonary vascular hemodynamics in chronic lung disease patients with and without oxyhemoglobin desaturation during sleep. *Chest* 1989; **95**: 757–66.

13 DeMarco FJ Jr, Wynne JW, Block AJ *et al*. Oxygen desaturation during sleep as a determinant of the 'blue and bloated' syndrome. *Chest* 1981; **79**: 621–5.

14 Mulloy E, McNicholas WT. Ventilation and gas exchange during sleep and exercise in patients with severe COPD. *Chest* 1996; **109**: 387–94.

15 Caterall JR, Calverley PMA, McNee W *et al*. Mechanism of transient nocturnal hypoxemia in hypoxic chronic bronchitis and emphysema. *J Appl Physiol* 1985; **59**: 1698–703.

16 Fletcher EC, Gray BA, Levin DC. Nonapneic mechanisms of arterial oxygen desaturation during rapid-eye-movement sleep. *J Appl Physiol* 1983; **54**: 632–9.

17 Chaouat A, Weitzenbum E, Krieger J *et al*. Association of chronic obstructive pulmonary disease and sleep apnea syndrome. *Am J Respir Crit Care Med* 1995; **151**: 82–6.

18 Mulloy E, McNicholas WT. Theophylline improves gas exchange during rest, exercise and sleep in severe chronic obstructive pulmonary disease. *Am Rev Respir Dis* 1993; **148**: 1030–6.

19 Goldstein RS, Ramcharan V, Bowes G *et al*. Effects of supplemental oxygen on gas exchange during sleep in patients with severe obstructive lung disease. *N Engl J Med* 1984; **310**: 425–9.

20 Murciano D, Aubier M, Lecocguic Y *et al*. Effects of theophylline on diaphragmatic strength and fatigue in patients with chronic obstructive pulmonary disease. *N Engl J Med* 1984; **311**: 349–53.

21 Man GC, Chapman KR, Ali SH *et al*. Sleep quality and nocturnal respiratory function with once-daily theophylline (Uniphil) and inhaled salbutamol in patients with COPD. *Chest* 1996; **110**: 648–53.

22 Reyes A, Roca J, Rodriguez-Roisin R *et al*. Effect of almitrine on ventilation–perfusion distribution in adult respiratory distress syndrome. *Am Rev Respir Dis* 1988; **137**: 1062–7.

23 Bell RC, Mullins RC, West LG *et al*. The effect of almitrine bismesylate on hypoxaemia in chronic obstructive

pulmonary disease. *Ann Intern Med* 1986;
105: 342–6.

24 Howard P. Hypoxia, almitrine, and
peripheral neuropathy. *Thorax* 1989; **44**:
247–50.

25 Elliott MW, Simonds AK, Carroll MP *et al*.
Domiciliary nocturnal nasal intermittent
positive pressure ventilation in
hypercapnic respiratory failure due to
chronic obstructive lung disease: effects on
sleep and quality of life. *Thorax* 1992; **47**:
342–8.

26 Strumpf DA, Millman RP, Carlisle CC
et al. Nocturnal positive pressure
ventilation by nasal mask in patients with
severe chronic obstructive pulmonary
disease. *Am Rev Respir Dis* 1991; **144**:
1234–9.

27 Goldstein RS, De Rosie JA, Avendano MA
et al. Influence of noninvasive positive
pressure ventilation on inspiratory
muscles. *Chest* 1991; **99**: 408–15.

28 Elliott MW, Mulvey DA, Moxham J *et al*.
Domiciliary nocturnal nasal intermittent
positive pressure ventilation in COPD:
mechanisms underlying changes in arterial
blood gas tensions. *Eur Respir J* 1991; **4**:
1044–52.

8: Is it possible to help people stop smoking?

James Friend

Tobacco smoking is the single most important cause of chronic obstructive pulmonary disease (COPD), and smoking cessation is the most important measure in improving the long-term outlook for people with COPD.

What good does stopping smoking do?

The damage that smoking does to health is well known. It is estimated that someone who smokes 20 cigarettes a day during adult life has a 50% likelihood of dying of a smoker's disease, with an average loss of life expectancy of 8 years, or up to 11 min of life lost per cigarette smoked. The three major smokers' diseases include lung cancer, now the commonest cause of cancer deaths in the UK in both men and women; ischaemic heart disease; and COPD. On top of all this, a range of other malignancies and vascular diseases are commoner in smokers, and together all these diseases account for about 120 000 UK deaths per year in a population of 55 million—the biggest preventable cause of ill-health and death.

Most people know and accept that smoking does some harm to health, but the level of risk is not usually known or acknowledged. There is a tendency for smokers to feel that the risks of smoking may not be very large, and that the consequences are likely to be far in the future, and in any case, 'the damage has probably been done'. Health advisers have a responsibility to explain to smokers that the risks are considerable, that many of the diseases are often prolonged, disabling and miserable (and here COPD is pre-eminent) and that the benefits of stopping smoking are quick and important.

In the case of COPD, the average loss of forced expiratory volume in one second is 50–80 mL per year. However, people with COPD who stopped smoking in the Lung Health Study [1] showed an average *increase* of forced expiratory volume in 1 s (FEV_1) of 57 mL in the first year. Over 5 years, a person with COPD who stopped smoking had an average decline in FEV_1 of 34 mL per year, which is very similar to the 'normal' decline in FEV_1 in lifelong non-smokers as a result of ageing. In other words, there is good evidence to be able to say to smokers with COPD, 'If you stop smoking now, not only will your lung function stop getting rapidly worse, but there may be a small improvement in your lungs; and there is a good chance that you will live longer.'

Within 1–2 years of stopping smoking, the excess risk of death from heart disease is halved, and after 15 years, reaches almost the level of lifelong non-smokers. On top of this, smokers who stop smoking reduce their risk of developing lung cancer to 30–50% of that of continuing smokers within 10 years of stopping. Similar benefits accrue in terms of the risks of many of the other smokers' diseases. The health benefits of stopping smoking are not in doubt, and the financial benefits can be substantial—for example, in the UK in 2001, the average 20-a-day smoker spends over £1500 every year on cigarettes.

Finding out about smokers and their smoking—*ask!*

A careful smoking history is essential to a full understanding of smokers in deciding which approach is most likely to help them to stop smoking. The smoking history is as important a part of the history as the patient's name and age, or the presenting symptoms, or the recording of vital signs. After the first question, 'Do you smoke?' it is also essential to add, for those who say 'No', 'Have you ever been a smoker?' We have all come across clinical records which record 'non-smoker' for a patient who stopped smoking only weeks or days ago.

The next part of the smoking history is to gauge the lifetime dose of tobacco smoke and some idea of smoking behaviour. The following questions may also give an idea of lifetime habits and 'dose':
- 'How old were you when you started smoking?'
- 'How many cigarettes do you smoke now?'
- 'How many cigarettes a day have you smoked on average over the years?'

In the USA, it is common to estimate cigarette smoke consumption in 'pack-years', assuming a pack to contain 20 cigarettes. The calculation is simply made by multiplying the number of packs smoked per day by the number of years smoked; so to smoke a pack a day for 10 years makes for a 10 pack-year smoker, and 30 cigarettes (one and a half packs) a day for 30 years would be a 45 pack-year smoker.

Another area of enquiry relates to how well the smoker manages without nicotine doses, to gain some idea of the level of dependence on nicotine. Various measures have been developed for this, including the Fagerström Test for Nicotine Dependence (FTND) [2], in which the subject is asked the series of questions shown in Table 8.1). Many other scales and questionnaires have also been developed. However, in practice, asking about the number of cigarettes smoked each day and the time to the first cigarette probably give a simple idea of the level of dependence.

Table 8.1 The Fagerström Test for Nicotine Dependence (FTND) [2], in which the subject is asked a series of questions. A score of 6 or more on this scale is usually considered to represent high nicotine dependency.

Question	Answer	Score
How soon after you wake up do you have your first cigarette?	Within 5 min	3
	6–30 min	2
	31–60 min	1
	Over 60 min	0
Do you find it difficult to refrain from smoking in places where it is forbidden?	Yes	1
	No	0
Which cigarette would you hate giving up most?	The first in the morning	1
	Others	0
How many cigarettes per day do you smoke?	Less than 10	0
	11–20	1
	21–30	2
	More than 30	3
Do you smoke more frequently during the first hours after waking than during the rest of the day?	Yes	1
	No	0
Do you smoke if you are so ill that you are in bed most of the day?	Yes	1
	No	0

Further questions will be needed before the questioner can move forward towards helping the smoker to stop; these will be discussed later, but should include:

- 'Have you ever thought about giving up smoking?'
- 'Have you ever tried to stop smoking?'
- If 'Yes', an inquiry about previous attempts and relapses.

What are the barriers to stopping smoking?

Barriers in the smoker

Smokers will not stop smoking unless they want to stop, and also if they believe that they can stop. To want to stop, smokers must acknowledge the advantages of stopping, which will include improved health, saving money, and other individual factors; these may include benefits to their families, feelings of being in control, smelling nicer, and so on. It is valuable to explore these with the smoker, and to record them. Smokers also find it hard to believe that they could stop, because a number of barriers may exist to successful stopping. It is the job of the stop-smoking advisor to understand and look for these barriers, and to help the smoker overcome them.

Addiction

There has always been debate as to whether smoking is a pastime, habit, or a true addiction, and the reality is that different people may be more or less dependent on nicotine. However, for many people, nicotine use does fulfil many of the criteria for substance dependence listed by the World Health Organization International Classification of Diseases (ICD-10). Withdrawal of nicotine is for many smokers extremely stressful, and for a few, virtually impossible. It is clearly easier for less addicted smokers to stop.

Social disadvantage and psychiatric problems

Smoking rates are highest among the poorest social groups, and cessation often poses particular difficulties for socially deprived people for whom daily survival against the odds is the major preoccupation. For many people, smoking is a (relatively) cheap, immediately available pleasure, which may take precedence over other needs and long-term goals. Others who have particular difficulty in stopping include those with psychiatric disorders, including anxiety states, affective disorders, and other psychoses.

Concerns about weight gain

Cigarette smoking has sometimes been promoted as an aid to keeping slim, and smoking may reduce appetite and impair the taste of food. During smoking cessation efforts, weight gain often occurs, perhaps because appetite improves along with an improved sense of taste. Snacking may also be a replacement activity for smoking. On average, weight gain of 4–5 kg can occur in the first year of smoking cessation, and for a few, much greater weight gains may occur. The fear of weight gain can deter the figure-conscious smoker from attempting to stop smoking, particularly among women. Although a lean body image is a high priority, encouraged by the fashion press and often highlighted in tobacco advertising, particularly aimed at women, the risks of mild weight gain are far outweighed by the health risks of smoking. Any weight gain from smoking cessation need only be temporary, and need not occur at all with supportive advice and forewarnings. The use of nicotine replacement therapy and bupropion may reduce the tendency to weight gain.

Physical disease

In studies involving patients with diseases strongly linked to smoking, the occurrence of an acute and often dramatic episode, such as a recent acute myocardial infarction, often resulted in improved cessation rates. On the other hand, those with long-term disabling chronic respiratory disease, in-cluding COPD, demonstrated lower success rates in smoking cessation than unaffected people of similar age and sex. Perhaps the people with these chronically progressive diseases who were most likely to stop smoking did so in the earlier stages of their disease, when symptoms first started to have an im-pact on their lives—while on the other hand, those who did not stop earlier were the more addicted ones, who continued to smoke despite the develop-ment of increasingly obvious disability.

Advertising, social pressures

Tobacco manufacturers claim that advertising seeks only to inform smokers of brands, and attempts to switch brand loyalty among smokers. They also claim that advertising plays no part in recruiting new smokers. Despite this, there is good evidence that advertising encourages young people to try smoking, rein-forces the social acceptability of smoking, and makes the whole product more attractive. Smokers also find it harder not to smoke if their parents, siblings, work mates or friends smoke, and where smoking forms a part of normal so-cial activities at social gatherings, in pubs, and at work breaks. Such smokers may suffer some degree of social loss by giving up smoking.

Barriers to smoking cessation created by the counsellor

Smokers are more likely to succeed in stopping smoking with the help of an empathetic person who creates a good rapport and shows genuine, uncritical understanding of the smoker's needs and difficulties. The smoking cessation counsellor has to be able to retain enthusiasm for the task despite many fail-ures—and doctors, particularly, are not good at seeing the value of spending time on smoking cessation. Even if they achieve a cessation rate of 10%, the nine out of 10 failures loom large in proportion to the single success, and enthusiasm can evaporate.

What can I do in a few minutes to help COPD patients stop smoking?—the brief intervention

If the average medical consultation in primary care lasts 8 min, and hospital doctors are often rushed for time too, the intervention on smoking must be very focused if it is to have any impact. Despite this, studies suggest that even very brief advice to stop, taking 3 min of a clinician's time, can increase 6-month cessation rates by about 2%. This means that in the average UK general practice of about 9000 patients cared for by five partners, with 2600 smokers, brief advice could help 50 patients per year to stop smoking. Over the United Kingdom, such simple measures could achieve 300 000 ex-smokers per year in a country with around 12 million smokers. There is no reason why other health professionals, including practice nurses, ward nurses, and health visitors, and also members of the paramedical professions such as physiotherapists, dietitians, pharmacists and others could not have an equal or greater impact. So far there is no evidence as to how effective professionals other than doctors are in giving opportunistic advice and assisting smoking cessation. It seems likely that 'brief intervention' is most likely to be successful with light smokers, smoking 10 cigarettes a day or less. For heavier smokers, additional help or pharmacotherapy (nicotine replacement therapy or bupropion) is likely to be required.

How to undertake the brief intervention

The 'five As':
- Ask about smoking habits and history, as detailed above.
- Advise all smokers to consider stopping or stop.
- Assess their smoking habit and how best to:
- Assist the smoker to consider stopping, to prepare to stop, or to take action.
- Arrange follow-up for further support, or referral to specialist cessation service.

When asking about smoking habits, a good early question is, 'Have you ever thought about stopping smoking? If the answer is 'No', then it opens an opportunity to ask what the smoker likes about smoking, what they may dislike about smoking, and whether they see any advantage to not smoking. This may be a good moment to give factual information about the advantages of stopping, with improvements in health and money savings, good example to young people, depending on the individual. Some advisors may find the measurement of exhaled carbon monoxide a useful educational tool at this point. It may be a good moment to assess dependence by asking about the time to first cigarette, as one of the major indicators in the Fagerström Test for Nicotine Dependence (FTND) mentioned above. Supportive literature may be provided at this point. The intention is to encourage the smoker to consider the benefits of stopping, with a statement such as 'I'd really like to help you to stop smoking at some point, not too far away, so perhaps we can talk about this again soon, once you have thought about it.'

For the smoker who answers 'Yes' to the question, 'Have you ever thought about stopping?', the next question is, 'Have you ever tried to give up?' If yes, one needs to know about previous attempts to stop, how long the smoker managed to stop, and what happened to start them smoking again. If the smoker has thought of stopping but never actually tried, perhaps because they thought they wouldn't succeed, then it is helpful for the smoker to know that:

1   There are 12 million successful ex-smokers in the UK in a population of 55 million.

2   Most of them report that once they had decided to try to stop smoking, it proved less difficult than they had expected.

3   Most successful ex-smokers have made one or more attempts to stop before they finally succeed in stopping.

The counsellor should express every willingness to help the smoker stop smoking if he or she wants to, in an open, supportive way without criticism or derision.

Having identified a smoker as wishing to give up, the counsellor can assist the smoker by stressing one or more of the 'five Rs':

- Relevant benefits for the smoker
- Risks of continuing to smoke
- Rewards from stopping
- Roadblocks to stopping
- Repeat attempts are more successful.

Finally, it is always good practice to arrange a follow-up visit to discuss progress and give further support. For some patients, much more intensive support and more specialized advice may be needed, and referral to one of the many more specialized smoking cessation support services should always be considered as an addition to brief advice.

How can I understand more and improve success rates?

The majority of successful cessation strategies either result from the smoker's own decision and strategy, often with help from friends or family, or from brief interventions by committed health professionals. Success is encouraged by a supportive environment, which should include the absence of advertising and promotion, and restrictions on smoking in public places and at work, which most smokers support. In addition, there is a place for more specialized smoking advice from trained counsellors who are able to devote more time and expertise to the more addicted smokers. There is strong evidence that experts, spending more time, with regular follow-up and access to the full range of pharmacotherapeutic aids, can achieve the highest success rates. 'Smoking Advice Services' have been established throughout England and in many other areas of the UK to provide easily accessible advice, and try to ensure that the services are available to less affluent groups, who have the highest smoking rates. Telephone support is a further valuable option, together with self-help materials.

Which treatments will increase success rates — nicotine replacement, bupropion, and the rest?

Nicotine replacement therapy

Nicotine replacement therapy (NRT) first became widely available in the form of nicotine chewing gum. Since then, further nicotine delivery methods have become available, including transdermal patches, a nicotine inhaler, nicotine nasal spray, nicotine sublingual tablets and nicotine lozenges (both for buccal absorption). The British smoking cessation guidelines [3,4] offer detailed evidence on the effectiveness of nicotine replacement therapy as an aid to smoking cessation, indicating that use of nicotine replacement therapy doubles the chance of success in smokers who wish to stop.

Available delivery systems currently include:

- Nicotine chewing gum, 2 mg and 4 mg strengths.
- Nicotine transdermal patches — delivery over 16 h: 5 mg, 10 mg and 15 mg strengths; delivery over 24 h: 7 mg, 14 mg, and 21 mg strengths.
- Nicotine sublingual tablets, 2 mg.
- Nicotine lozenges, 1 mg.
- Nicotine inhalator, 10-mg doses for inhalation.
- Nicotine nasal spray, metered dose inhaler, 0.5 mg per puff.

Currently, nicotine replacement therapy is not recommended in pregnancy or in severe cardiovascular disease, and some products are not recommended for people under the age of 18. However, trials of safety and efficacy in such groups are needed, as it is unlikely that nicotine replacement will be more dangerous than the continued smoking it is intended to replace. Indeed, the benefits of stopping smoking may well outweigh the risks of using NRT.

Choosing the best form of NRT for a smoker who wants to stop

There is no clear information as to which type of NRT is most effective, and much depends on patient preference. In medium to heavy smokers, results are best when the higher dose formulations are used initially, such as the 4-mg gum, or the 15-mg, 16-h patch, or the 21-mg, 24-h patch. Many smokers prefer nicotine patches, and do not like chewing gum. It is best to discuss the options with smokers to find their preferences. The theory is that the 24-h patches, applied in the morning, will provide 'cover' until the next morning. Some smokers find that the continued release of nicotine through the night causes side effects such as vivid dreams, insomnia, and other side effects, and such people are likely to tolerate the 16-h preparations better.

It can be argued that the oral or inhaled varieties of NRT, having the quickest delivery after use, may have value in rapidly assuaging cravings in highly addicted smokers. In pregnancy, if cessation seems unlikely with advice alone, one of the oral or sublingual forms of NRT may be considered more appropriate than one of the more persistent dosing systems such as the transdermal patches.

Concurrent use of two or more different types of NRT is not at present recommended, as there have been no studies suggesting whether combined NRT therapies could be helpful. However, the use of different types of NRT together does have some logic, and there are anecdotal accounts of this being helpful to some individual smokers, using a patch for day-long nicotine levels and an oral tablet or lozenge to treat a particular short-term need.

Bupropion

This drug is an atypical antidepressant with both adrenergic and dopaminergic actions. Trials of the drug as a smoking cessation aid suggest that if bupropion is started 1 week before cessation, and continued for 7–12 weeks along with intensive support, smoking cessation rates are doubled when compared with placebo. As with other antidepressants, there is a one in 1000 risk of seizures, and epilepsy is regarded as a contraindication to its use. It is also not advised in pregnancy, in people with severe hepatic cirrhosis, with bipolar disorders, anorexia nervosa or people who have had a monoamine oxidase inhibitor (MAOI) within the previous 2 weeks. From trials conducted to date, it is not yet clear whether bupropion is more effective than NRT, whether it is effective without behavioural support, and whether, when used together, bupropion and NRT might be more effective than either treatment alone.

In COPD, there has been one published trial of bupropion; in subjects with relatively mild COPD who volunteered for the study, smoking cessation rates were approximately doubled. However, it may be harder to achieve success in patients with severe COPD.

Other interventions

In addition to NRT and bupropion, clonidine has been shown to have value in smoking cessation treatment, but tends to have more side effects than NRT or bupropion. A variety of antidepressants have also been tried, but without the success rates of NRT/bupropion. There is no good evidence for the value of hypnosis, acupuncture, or any other complementary therapy in smoking cessation.

Table 8.2 Interventions to assist smoking cessation (data from [4]).

Intervention	Group studied	Increase in success rates (%)
Simple brief advice by physician	Smokers attending GP surgeries	2
Specialist adviser, face to face, intensive	Moderate to heavy smokers seeking advice	7
Specialist adviser, face to face, intensive	Hospital admissions	4
Nicotine gum, intensive support,	Moderate to heavy smokers	8
Nicotine patches, intensive support	Moderate to heavy smokers	6
Nicotine nasal spray, intensive support	Moderate to heavy smokers	12
Nicotine sublingual tablet, intensive support	Moderate to heavy smokers	8
Intensive support, plus NRT or bupropion	Moderate or heavy smokers seeking help	13–19

GP, general practitioner; NRT, nicotine replacement therapy.

Is smoking cessation work worthwhile?

Various interventions to assist smoking cessation have been assessed as shown in Table 8.2, with success in each case being defined as 6 months or more of tobacco abstinence. It will seen from the Table that in properly validated studies, success rates increase with the amount of support given. Success also increases (roughly doubles) with NRT or bupropion, and with the motivation of the smoker—those who seek help are more likely to succeed than those who come to a doctor for another reason, or who are admitted to hospital. Bearing in mind the number of smokers (in the UK, perhaps 13 million out of a population of 55 million), even these apparently small success rates can represent large numbers of people.

A further way of looking at the issue of smoking cessation is by the benefit achieved in terms of life-years saved by successful smoking interventions. This issue is examined extensively in the British smoking cessation guidelines [3,4] but it has been calculated that an intervention based on an integrated area service and including brief advice, self-help, nicotine replacement therapy and a specialist service costs about £873 per quality-adjusted life year (QALY) saved. The cost of brief advice only is just over £2000 per QALY. Although this may sound expensive, many other forms of therapy are very much more expensive; for instance, the use of lipid-lowering agents (statins) has been estimated to cost around £9000 per QALY. It is estimated that £275 million will be spent on statins in the year 2001—about 10 times as much as is likely to be spent on smoking cessation drugs, with less than a tenth of the cost-effectiveness.

References

1 Anthonisen NR, Connet JE, Kiley JP *et al.* Effects of smoking intervention and the use of an inhaled anticholinergic bronchodilator on the rate of decline of FEV$_1$. *JAMA* 1994; **272**: 1497–505.
2 Heatherton TF, Kozlowski LT, Frecker RC, Fagerström KO. The Fagerström Test for Nicotine Dependence: a revision of the Fagerström Tolerance Questionnaire. *Br J Addict* 1991; **86**: 1119–27.
3 Raw M, McNeill A, West R. Smoking cessation guidelines for health professionals. *Thorax* 1998; **53**: S1–38.
4 West R, McNeill A, Raw M. Smoking cessation guidelines for health professionals: an update. *Thorax* 2000; **55**: 987–99.

Further reading

- Cochrane Tobacco Addiction Group. *Cochrane Library,* Issue 4, 2001.
- Royal College of Physicians of London. *Nicotine Addiction in Britain.* London: Royal College of Physicians, 2000.
- Royal College of Nursing. *Clearing the air: a nurse's guide to smoking and tobacco control.* London: Royal College of Nursing, 1999.
- US Department of Health and Human Services. *Treating Tobacco Use and dependence Clinical Practice Guideline,* 2000.

Valuable Internet sites

- Ash UK: http:/www.ash.org.uk
- Ash Scotland: http://www.ashscotland.org.uk
- Society for Research on Nicotine and Tobacco (SRNT): http://www.treatobacco.net
- The Quit Guide to Stopping Smoking: http:/healthnet.org.uk/quit/guide.htm

Telephone quit lines (UK telephone numbers)

- Quit: 0800-002200 (also has other lines for Asian languages and Turkish and Kurdish speakers)
- Scottish Smokeline: 0800-848484.

9: Bronchodilators in stable COPD — which one when?

Ronan O'Driscoll

Why use a bronchodilator in stable COPD?

Bronchodilator treatment provides symptomatic relief for patients with COPD. The main indication for the use of bronchodilator drugs is the relief of breathlessness or wheeze. For many patients with mild COPD, bronchodilator therapy (to be used as required) might be their only requirement.

Bronchodilator medication has no effect on prognosis in COPD [1]. Therefore, there is no need to insist on regular medication. The patient can be advised to take their bronchodilator therapy as required. Patients with troublesome symptoms are likely to use a short-acting bronchodilator several times per day. Many such patients may benefit from the introduction of a long-acting β-agonist bronchodilator.

For patients with more advanced COPD, bronchodilator therapy should be used as an adjunct to other therapy such as oxygen (if hypoxic), pulmonary rehabilitation (if disabled by breathlessness) and smoking cessation (if still smoking).

It is important to emphasize that bronchodilators will have no benefit in an asymptomatic patient in whom COPD is identified at routine screening tests. Such patients should be given smoking cessation advice (if still smoking) but bronchodilator therapy should not be started until the patient becomes symptomatic.

The aim of bronchodilator treatment is to provide relief of symptoms and, if possible, to extend exercise tolerance. Long-acting bronchodilators may reduce exacerbation rates in COPD as discussed below. For some patients with COPD, bronchodilator therapy may facilitate mucus expectoration. For a minority of patients with advanced COPD and problems with mucus clearance, this might best be achieved with nebulized bronchodilator therapy or with the use of nebulized saline as an adjunct to bronchodilator therapy from a metered dose inhaler.

When should bronchodilator therapy be commenced and how often should it be used?

The prescriber should begin bronchodilator therapy when patients with COPD report breathlessness or wheeze. Many patients with COPD are unaware of gradual loss of lung function over several decades. It is common for the first symptoms of breathlessness to occur during chest infections. At this stage, the patient may require bronchodilator therapy only during exacerbations but, as the FEV_1 declines over a period of years, the patient is likely to require bronchodilator therapy on many or most days.

Short-acting bronchodilator drugs are usually prescribed for use 'as required' to relieve breathlessness. Bronchodilators are also used to relieve breathlessness or chest tightness during exercise or they may be used before exercise to increase the patient's exercise capacity or to reduce breathlessness during the planned activity.

Bronchodilator drugs may also assist mucus clearance for some patients with COPD (especially in the morning). Mucus clearance is assisted by dilatation of narrowed airways [2]. It is possible that β-agonists may also assist muco-ciliary clearance although this remains controversial. This use of bronchodilator therapy is likely to be of greatest benefit to patients with copious sputum (for example those with coexisting bronchiectasis) or if the sputum is difficult to expectorate. Anticholinergic bronchodilators could theoretically cause some drying of bronchial secretions and could therefore make sputum more viscous in some cases although this would appear to be a rare problem in clinical practice.

Some patients prefer to use bronchodilator drugs on a regular basis to obtain a constant level of symptom relief throughout the day. There is no evidence to suggest that a prescription for regular bronchodilator therapy is better or worse than a prescription for bronchodilator therapy to be used 'as required'. In these circumstances, it is reasonable to let the patient choose whether the drug is to be used on an intermittent or regular basis. In practice, most patients with symptomatic COPD use their bronchodilator inhalers three or more times per day.

Patients requiring frequent short-acting bronchodilator therapy or patients with more severe symptoms should be considered for a trial of a long-acting bronchodilator.

What are the criteria of success to justify continuing treatment?

There has been much debate as to whether subjective criteria or objective criteria should be used to determine the outcome of a trial of bronchodilator treatment. There is relatively little correlation between symptoms and lung function in individual cases of COPD [3]. It is also possible that some patients may have physiological benefits such as reduced residual volume or reduced gas trapping that may not be detected by simple lung function tests [4]. Therefore, it is reasonable to aim at maximal symptom relief rather than maximum lung function as the main objective of bronchodilator therapy in COPD.

Many clinicians find it helpful to monitor FEV_1 or peak flow improvement during bronchodilator therapy, especially as a large change in FEV_1 or PEF may suggest that the diagnosis is asthma rather than COPD. Measurement of exercise capacity such as 6-minute walks, shuttle walks or step tests are helpful in research studies but they are of little value in assessing individual responses to treatment because improvements tend to be small (and variable). The main subjective criteria which are used are the patients' sensation of breathlessness and wheeze and their ability to undertake everyday activities. Patients should be specifically asked about these issues following a trial of bronchodilator therapy.

Sophisticated quality-of-life measures such as the St George's Respiratory Questionnaire are useful in trials involving large numbers of patients but they are insensitive (and inconvenient) for use in the management of individual cases. Additional benefits might include enhanced mucus clearance or reduced exacerbation rates. The presence or absence of side-effects is another important factor in determining whether or not to continue an inhaled treatment.

In summary, it is helpful to make objective measurements of lung function but bronchodilator therapy is given for symptomatic relief so most emphasis should be put on subjective benefit (and side-effects) when deciding whether or not to continue an individual bronchodilator agent.

When should a second drug be added and does the combination of β-agonist and anticholinergic really work better than higher doses of single drugs?

There is evidence that combined bronchodilator therapy (β-agonist with anticholingeric) produces greater bronchodilation than either drug given alone. This is true whether the agents are given in moderate dose (from hand-held inhalers) or in high doses (from small-volume nebulizers) [5,6].

If patients remains symptomatic despite treatment with a single bronchodilator agent, it is reasonable to initiate a trial of combined therapy. However, combined therapy should be continued only if the patient reports a definite improvement from the addition of the second agent. A combination metered dose inhaler (MDI) containing β-agonist and anticholinergic agent may be convenient for such patients. For some patients, higher doses of a single agent may give better symptomatic relief. However, combined therapy may deliver similar symptomatic relief with less side-effects (e.g. tremor from high doses of β-agonist).

It is suggested that the prescriber should start either a β-agonist or an anticholinergic on an 'as required' basis. In some clinical studies, anticholinergics have produced greater overall bronchodilation but the β-agonist agents have a quicker onset of action. It is reasonable to allow patients to assess their response to each agent and select the medication that gives them optimal symptom relief.

If the patient needs to use their 'as required' treatment with increasing frequency, they should be advised to try taking the medication on a regular basis (e.g. qid) to see if this diminishes symptoms. If symptoms remain troublesome, the prescriber may increase the bronchodilator dose or consider adding a second agent or a long-acting β_2-agonist (see next section).

Role of long-acting β-agnoists—do they act mainly on quality of life rather than on lung function variables?

There is increasing evidence that long-acting β_2-agonist treatment is effective for patients with COPD. This treatment has been shown to increase FEV_1 and peak flow, improve symptom control and improve quality of life compared with 'prn' use of short-acting β-agonist therapy [7,8]. Treatment with a long-acting β-agonist bronchodilator is likely to be of greatest benefit if prescribed for patients with persistent symptoms despite the use of short-acting β-agonists on a 'prn' basis. Some trials have shown a reduction in exacerbation rates or delay in the time to first exacerbation during treatment with long-acting β_2-agonists [9].

Long-acting β-agonists have been shown to be more effective than short acting anticholinergic agents in some studies [9]. Recently published evidence suggests that a long-acting anticholinergic agent (tiotropium bromide) is at least as effective as salmeterol and possible more effective for patients with COPD (see Chapter 11 on future treatments for COPD) [20].

If a patient with COPD is prescribed a long-acting β-agonist, they should continue to use their short-acting bronchodilator inhaler on a 'prn' basis for episodes of breathlessness. There is some evidence that combined treatment with salmeterol and anticholinergic treatment (ipratropium bromide) or with oral theophylline treatment is more effective than treatment with salmeterol alone [10,11].

Is the choice of inhaler device important?

Most patients with COPD are best treated with a hand-held device such as a metered dose inhaler or dry powder inhaler. There is not much clinical difference between the bronchodilator response achieved by different devices. The most important factor is to choose a device that the patient is able to use. For many COPD patients (especially the elderly), a breath-activated MDI or an MDI with spacer may be the easiest device for the patient to use.

Dry powder devices such as Diskhaler, Accuhaler, Clickhaler or Turbuhaler have all been used in COPD patients but there are few trials comparing the advantages and disadvantages of different hand-held inhaler devices in patients with COPD. For patients with extremely low inspiratory flow, an MDI with large volume spacer may achieve better lung delivery than a dry powder device or a breath-activated inhaler. For most patients, the key factor is the patient's ability to use the inhaler device.

A recent meta-analysis of trials of bronchodilator therapy using different hand-held inhaler devices showed that here was no important difference in clinical outcomes between metered dose inhalers, breath-activated inhalers or dry powder devices [12]. This meta-analysis involved patients with asthma but it is likely that these findings would apply equally to COPD patients (provided they can use the device which is prescribed for them).

Most bronchodilator studies with spacer devices have used large (750 mL) spacer devices such as the Volumatic or Nebuhaler device. However, these devices are rather large and many patients prefer a smaller device such as 'Aerochamber' although its use has not been as well validated in COPD as the larger devices. The smaller devices may not deliver as much aerosol to the lung, especially if used with the older CFC-containing inhalers which have a high spray velocity.

How should inhaler devices be selected for individual patients with COPD?

In theory, each patient would use the smallest and cheapest device that they could use effectively. In practice, some patients may achieve greater bronchodilation with specific devices as discussed in the previous section.

It is essential that each patient should have their inhaled therapy planned by a health-care professional who is familiar with the benefits and mode of use of all available devices. This could be a respiratory physician, a respiratory nurse specialist, a physiotherapist or a GP with a special interest in chest diseases.

This health-care professional should work with the patient to select the device which best suits the patient's needs. When possible, one type of device should be used for each patient. However, a patient who uses long- and short-acting inhaled β-agonist therapy together with anticholinergic agent an inhaled steroid may require two or more devices. The important issue is that the patient should understand how to use each device and demonstrate that they can use it effectively.

For patients on high doses of inhaled therapy or for patients requiring multiple inhaler devices, a spacer device may be the best solution. However, this may involve the use of some inhalers with spacer devices which are not licensed or tested for use with that inhaler. Patients with arthritis or weak hands may benefit from a Haler-Aid device used with an MDI and spacer. A gripping device is also available for the Turbohaler. If the patient cannot use an MDI, the prescriber should consider a spacer device, breath-activated inhaler or dry powder inhaler depending on what drugs are required and the reason why the patient cannot use a MDI. Whatever device is chosen, it is essential to recheck the patient's inhaler technique on a regular basis. Some patients will master the technique when supervised, but revert to a faulty technique during months or years of unsupervised use.

Is there a role for nebulized bronchodilators in severe but stable COPD?

A small minority of COPD patients may derive additional benefit from the very high dose of bronchodilator therapy that can be delivered from a nebulizer [13,14]. Most patients can derive equal benefit from treatment using hand-held inhalers or spacer devices. Nebulized treatment should only be prescribed after a formal trial comparing the response to nebulized treatment with the response to high-dose treatment using hand-held inhalers as recommended in British Thoracic Society and European Respiratory Society Guidelines for nebulizer use [13,14].

Hand-held inhalers and nebulizers each achieve about 10% lung deposition of the prescribed dose (depending on which individual device is used). However, a nebulizer will usually deliver a higher dose (e.g. 2.5 mg of nebulized salbutamol is the same dose as would be delivered by 25 puffs from a salbutamol inhaler). Most patients will derive no additional benefit from the higher dose of nebulized treatment (but side-effects may be increased).

However, for patients who do require high-dose treatment, a nebulizer may be more convenient than multiple puffs from an MDI spacer. The European Nebulizer Guidelines suggest that patients who require 10 or more puffs from hand-held inhalers to achieve symptomatic relief may find a nebulizer more convenient [14].

For some patients, especially with coexisting bronchiectasis, a nebulized β-agonist may assist mucus clearance [15]. Benefit of this sort can only be identified by a trial of nebulized treatment in the patient's home, ideally using loaned equipment. Some patients use nebulized saline between doses of bronchodilator treatment to assist mucus expectoration and relieve breathlessness [16].

Is there a role for oral bronchodilators in COPD?

Oral β-agonists such as salbutamol, terbutaline or bambuterol have been shown to have bronchodilator activity in COPD. However, oral β-agonists tend to cause side-effects such as tremor. Inhaled β-agonists can produce equivalent or superior bronchodilation for most patients with less side-effects.

Oral theophylline has been shown to have a modest bronchodilator effect in COPD. However, inhaled β-agonists, especially long-acting β-agonists, achieve greater bronchodilation with less risk of toxicity. In patients with severe symptoms, there may be some benefit from the combination of inhaled salmeterol supplemented by oral theophylline (but side-effects were also increased) [11].

It has been suggested that the best way to decide on optimal therapy for COPD patients is to conduct 'n or one' trials where additional drugs such as theophylline are introduced and withdrawn under careful medical scrutiny. However, conventional practice may be just as effective in identifying the subset of patients who respond to theophylline (about 20%) [17]. Each additional agent should be continued long-term only if the patient and the clinician are convinced that the additional agent has added worthwhile benefit for the patient.

Are bronchodilators cost effective in COPD?

Inhaled bronchodilator therapy is relatively inexpensive. For example, eight puffs of salbutamol per day from a metered dose inhaler costs approximately £70 per annum in the UK. This is clearly cost effective if a patient reports significant benefit. Breath-activated inhalers and dry powder inhalers are more expensive than MDIs. Therefore, for patients who can use an MDI effectively, it is the most cost-effective device. However, for patients who cannot use an MDI after careful instruction, these devices may be cost effective if the patient can use them more effectively.

Large volume spacers are a cheap means to enhance the clinical effectiveness of MDI therapy. They are useful and cost-effective for patients with poor inhaler technique. These devices may deliver more aerosol to the lungs than the use of a MDI alone. This is especially useful for patients who require high doses of bronchodilator drugs, thus achieving greater clinical benefit combined with cost-effectiveness. (However, it is important to instruct the patient that only one actuation at a time should be delivered via the large volume spacer, multiple actuations would result in reduced drug delivery to the lungs). For patients who spend most of the day outside their house, these devices are rather large and may be left at home. In these circumstances, a breath-activated device or dry powder device may become more cost-effective if it achieves better symptom control.

Long-acting β_2-agonists are considerably more expensive than short-acting β-agonists. However, there is some evidence that the long-acting β-agonists may reduce or delay COPD exacerbations which could make this treatment cost effective [9].

Nebulized bronchodilator therapy may help some patients with severe COPD to avoid hospital admissions but the effect on admission rates in clinical trials has been inconsistent and may apply to a subgroup of COPD patients that has not yet been defined clearly. If admission rates were reduced for some patients, this would make home nebulizer therapy cost-effective for some COPD patients. Some patients have been given nebulizers in the past without adequate assessment of their inhaled therapy using a range of devices. Such management was clearly not cost effective.

Are there any chronic side-effects from bronchodilator therapy?

The short-term side-effects of β-agonists are well known (mostly tremor and palpitations). The main side-effect of anticholinergic therapy is a dry mouth. Some patients find that inhaled medication makes them cough. Theophylline treatment carries dangers of theophylline toxicity if high doses are given or if the patient is given other drugs which interact with theophyllines. β-Agonists and anticholinergic treatment have been used for decades without any reports of significant cumulative side-effects. Long-acting β-agonists have also been evaluated in COPD without any major concerns about patient safety.

What developments are likely in the near future?

Tiotropium bromide is a once-daily long-acting anticholingeric medication which has been shown to be effective in clinical trials in COPD [18]. Tiotropium is probably more effective than short-acting anticholinergic treatment and it has been shown to reduce exacerbations and to improve health-related quality of life [19]. A recent trial has suggested that tiotropium bromide may achieve higher FEV_1 values than salmeterol for COPD patients [20]. Tiotropium bromide was licensed for clinical use in the UK just prior to publication of this chapter so clinical experience with this medication at the time of publication is confined to clinical trials. See Chapter 11.

New phosphodiesterase inhibitors such as Cilomilast are being developed. Cilomilast has been shown to improve FEV_1 compared with placebo in a study of 424 patients but there was no difference in quality of life between the groups. Further studies involving newer phosphodiesterase inhibitors are awaited [21]. See Chapter 11.

References

1 Anthonisen NR, Connett JE, Kiley JP *et al.* Effects of smoking intervention and the use of an inhaled anticholinergic bronchodilator on the rate of decline in FEV$_1$: the lung health study. *JAMA* 1994; 272: 1497–505.

2 Moretti M, Lopez-Vidriero MT, Pavia D, Clarke SW. Relationship between bronchial reversibility and tracheobronchial clearance in patients with chronic bronchitis. *Thorax* 1997; 52: 176–80.

3 Wijnhoven HA, Kriegsman DM, Hesslink AE *et al.* Determinants of different dimensions of disease severity in asthma and COPD. pulmonary function and health-related quality of life. *Chest* 2001; 119: 1034–42.

4 O'Donnell DE. Assessment of bronchodilator efficacy in sypmtpmatic COPD. is spirometry useful? *Chest* 2000; 117 (Suppl. 2): 42s–47s.

5 Friedman M, Serby C, Menjoge S *et al.* Pharmoeconomic evaluation of a combination of ipratropium plus albuterol compared with ipratropium alone and albuterol alone in COPD. *Chest* 1999; 115: 635–41.

6 Combivent Inhalation Solution Study Group. Routine nebulized ipratropium and albuterol together are better than either alone in COPD. *Chest* 1997; 112: 1514–21.

7 Boyd G, Morice AH, Poundsford JC *et al.* An evaluation of salmeterol in the treatment of chronic obstructive pulmonary disease (COPD). *Eur Respir J* 1997; 10: 815–21.

8 Jones PW, Bosch TK. Quality of life changes in COPD patients treated with salmeterol. *Am J Respir Crit Care Med* 1997; 155: 1283–9.

9 Mahler DA, Donohue JF, Barbee RA *et al.* Efficacy of salmeterol xinafoate in the treatment of COPD. *Chest* 1999; 115: 957–65.

10 Jarvis B, Markham A. Inhaled salmeterol: a review of its efficacy in chronic obstructive pulmonary disease. *Drugs Aging* 2001; 18 (6): 441–72.

11 Zu Wallack RL, Mahler DA, Reilly D *et al.* Salmeterol plus theophylline combination therapy in the treatment of COPD. *Chest* 2001; 119: 1661–70.

12 Ram FS, Wright J, Brocklebank D, White JES. Systematic review of the clinical effectiveness of pressurized metered dose inhalers versus other hand held inhaler devices for delivering B2 agonist bronchodilators in asthma. *BMJ* 2001; 323: 901–5.

13 ODriscoll BR. Nebulisers in chronic obstructive pulmonary disease. *Thorax* 1997; 152 (Suppl. 2): S49–S52 (Part of BTS guidelines on nebuliser use).

14 Boe J, Dennis JH, O'Driscoll BR. European Respiratory Society Guidelines on the use of nebulizers. *European Respiratory J* 2001; 18: 228–42.

15 Sutton PP, Gemmell HG, Innes N, Davidson J, Smith FW, Legge JS, Friend JAR. Use of nebulised saline and nebulised terbutaline as an adjunct to chest physiotherapy. *Thorax* 1988; 43: 57–60.

16 Poole PJ, Brodie SM, Stewart JM, Black PN. The effects of nebulised isotonic saline and terbutaline on breathlessness in severe chronic obstructive pulmonary disease (COPD). *Aust N Z J Medical* 1998; 28: 322–6.

17 Mahon JL. Laupacis A, Hodder RV *et al.* Theophylline for irreversible chronic airflow limitation: a randomized study comparing n of 1 trials to standard practice. *Chest* 1999; 115: 38–48.

18 Casaburi R, Briggs DD, Donojue JF *et al.* The spirometric efficacy of once-daily dosing with tiotropium in stable COPD. a 13-week multicenter trial. *Chest* 2000; 118: 1294–302.

19 Vincken W, van Noord JA, Greefhorst AP *et al.* Dutch/Belgian Tiotropium Study Group. Improved health outcomes in patients with COPD during 1 year's treatment with tiotropium. *Eur Respir J* 2002; **19**: 209–16.

20 Donohue JF, van Noord JA, Bateman ED *et al.* A 6-month, placebo-controlled study comparing lung function and health status changes in COPD patients treated with tiotropium or salmeterol. *Chest* 2002; **122**: 47–55.

21 Compton CH, Gubb J, Nieman R *et al.* Cilomilast, a selective phosphodiesterase-4 inhibitor for treatment of patients with chronic obstructive pulmonary disease: a randomized dose-ranging study. *Lancet* 2001; 358: 265–70.

10: Inhaled steroids — do they still have a role?

Jørgen Vestbo

It will come as no surprise to practicing clinicians that inhaled corticosteroids (ICS) are widely used in the management of chronic obstructive pulmonary disease (COPD). It is the general impression that as many COPD patients as asthma patients are treated with ICS; treatment often includes high-dose ICS, is continued for years without much thought of monitoring the effect, and little is done to evaluate potential systemic side effects. The widespread use of ICS was recently documented in a Canadian survey [1], in which 43% of hospitalized patients using ICS were suffering from COPD and not asthma, which is the registered indication in Canada as well as in most other countries.

There are no good studies on why inhaled corticosteroids became so popular in COPD in spite of their lack of official recognition and at a time when few data on long-term effects were available. It is my belief that they were used for several reasons — many doctors believed that COPD differed very little from asthma, where inhaled corticosteroids are the front-line drug; since systemic corticosteroids have been shown to be effective in the acute exacerbation of COPD, it seemed rational to use local steroids as maintenance treatment; and finally, what else could you use once you have tested all the available bronchodilators?

Today, however, we have more data available to determine the choice of whether or not to include ICS in the treatment for COPD.

The evidence

Early studies

Treatment of COPD with ICS has until recently not been evidence-based, no matter how that term is defined. This is reflected in findings from literature searches on the topic, with more editorials and comments being published than original papers. It is worth bearing in mind that there can be several reasons for choosing to treat COPD with ICS. Crudely, one can simply aim to relieve symptoms in COPD, or one can have the more ambitious goal of altering the future course of the disease. This may seem too simplistic, but the aim of treatment must be made clear. Whereas ICS, by diminishing acute inflammatory changes in the airways, can reduce cough, mucus hypersecretion, and perhaps even dyspnoea, the more ambitious long-term aim would be to alter the course of the disease, and most often this would imply reducing the excess decline in forced expiratory volume in 1 s (FEV_1), which is the hallmark of COPD. It would be fair, however, to state that a marked effect on other aspects of the disease—e.g. the number of exacerbations requiring medical treatment—would be beneficial and could be said to affect the course of the disease, although exacerbations are not traditionally considered significant in the natural history of the disease [2]. Recent analyses in the Lung Health Study [3] have shown that exacerbations result in an excess decline in FEV_1 that is not recovered later, and similar findings have been reported in abstract form by a British group [4].

Regarding the relief of symptoms, the data are not impressive. Data on the effect of ICS on FEV_1 decline are also limited, and leave much room for different interpretations. The most important studies will be briefly mentioned below.

Very often the early findings of Postma et al. [5,6] are quoted. These were uncontrolled studies of long-term treatment with low/moderate doses of systemic corticosteroids. The studies were not trials of medication, but observational studies from an ongoing epidemiological panel study in the towns of Vlagtwedde and Vlaardingen in the Netherlands, and no placebo-controlled long-term studies of oral corticosteroids exist. Few controlled long-term studies of inhaled corticosteroids in COPD have been conducted until recently. Kerstjens et al. [7] showed an effect on both FEV_1 and exacerbations. From today's point of view, the study is limited, because the Dutch at the time when the study was initiated seemed to make less distinction between asthma and COPD than is generally considered correct, judging from recent guidelines on asthma and COPD. This distinction between asthma and COPD was more obvious in the smaller study by Renkema et al. [8] from 1996. Their study showed some effect of inhaled corticosteroids on FEV_1, but the power of the study was limited. Recently, a meta-analysis [9] of the studies by Kerstjens et al. [7] and Renkema et al. [8], together with a study published as an abstract only [10] has appeared. The meta-analysis, by van Grunsven et al., showed an estimated 2-year difference in prebronchodilator FEV_1 between subjects treated with inhaled corticosteroids and placebo of 34 mL/year; this was statistically significant, in spite of the fact that approximately one-third of the patients originally included were excluded from the meta-analysis. The effect on postbronchodilator FEV_1 was less impressive, and the time course of FEV_1 did not fit in with our general understanding of the time course of the decline of FEV_1 in COPD. In a smaller Canadian study of 77 COPD patients irreversible

Table 10.1 Recent controlled trials of inhaled corticosteroids in chronic obstructive pulmonary disease.

Study	Ref.	Total number	Disease severity	ICS daily dose	Effect on FEV$_1$	Symptoms	Exacerbations
Paggiaro et al.	12	281	Moderate	Fluticasone 1000 μg	Yes (6 months)	Yes	Yes (severity)
Vestbo et al. (CCLS)	13	290	Mild/ moderate	Budesonide 1200/800 μg	None	None	None
Pauwels et al. (EUROSCOP)	14	1277	Mild/ moderate	Budesonide 800 μg	Initial rise; no effect on decline	None *	None *
Burge et al. (ISOLDE)	15	751	Moderate/ severe	Fluticasone 1000 μg	Initial rise; no effect on decline	None	Reduction 23%
Lung Health Study II	19	1116	Moderate	Triamcinolone 1200 μg	None	Yes	Reduction ≈ 40–50%

CCLS, Copenhagen City Lung Study; EUROSCOP, European Respiratory Society Study on Chronic Obstructive Pulmonary Disease; FEV$_1$ forced expiratory volume in 1 s; ICS, inhaled corticosteroids; ISOLDE, Inhaled Steroids in Obstructive Lung Disease in Europe. * reported in oral presentations only.

to systemic corticosteroids, Bourbeau et al. [11] found no effect of inhaled budesonide 1600 μg daily on FEV$_1$, dyspnoea and exercise capacity.

Recent studies

Five large placebo-controlled trials have recently been conducted—one 6-month study and four studies lasting 3 years. Crude results are shown in Table 10.1.

Paggiaro et al. [12] showed an effect of inhaled fluticasone on FEV$_1$, respiratory symptoms, and severity of exacerbations in patients with well-defined COPD; however, the study only lasted 6 months, which limits its value for assessing long-term effects.

The Copenhagen City Lung Study (CCLS) [13] included 290 subjects with predominantly mild COPD from an ongoing epidemiological study in which almost 10 000 subjects were screened using spirometry. Patients were recruited as non-asthmatic subjects with a decreased ratio between FEV$_1$ and vital capacity (VC); i.e. FEV$_1$/VC ≤ 0.7. Eligible patients had to be irreversible to oral prednisolone and inhaled terbutaline—i.e. have an increase in FEV$_1$ less than 15% of baseline; only 5% were reversible to prednisolone. A total of 290 patients were randomized to receive either budesonide, 800 + 400 μg daily for 6 months followed by 400 μg twice daily for 30 months, or placebo for 36 months. The study drug and placebo were given in a multidose powder inhaler, the Turbuhaler. The mean age of the patients was 59 years, 40% were women, and 77% were present smokers. The mean FEV$_1$ was 2.37 L or 86%

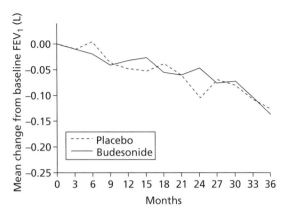

Fig. 10.1 Crude mean change from baseline forced expiratory volume in 1 s (FEV_1) in the Copenhagen City Lung Study. Reprinted with permission from [13].

of predicted. The main outcome parameter was FEV_1 decline, and crude FEV_1 declines turned out to be slightly smaller than expected—41.8 mL/year in the placebo group and 45.1 mL/year in the budesonide group. Post-bronchodilator FEV_1 over the course of the study is shown in Fig. 10.1. Using a regression model in the intention-to-treat population, patients in the placebo group had an FEV_1 decline of 49.1 mL/year, in contrast to 46.0 mL/year in the budesonide group; the estimated difference was 3.1 mL/year (95% confidence interval, 12.8 to 19.0) was both statistically and clinically insignificant ($P=0.70$). There was no initial rise in FEV_1 in the budesonide group. Before the study, the minimal relevant difference was decided as 20 mL/year; this difference was outside the two-sided 95% confidence interval. Secondary effect parameters were respiratory symptoms and number of exacerbations, and no effect of inhaled budesonide was seen on either of these outcomes.

The European Respiratory Society Study on Chronic Obstructive Pulmonary Disease (EUROSCOP) study [14] was a European multicentre study in which 39 study centres in nine countries participated. EUROSCOP included patients with mild COPD who continued to smoke in spite of a 3-month smoking cessation program including nicotine gum. A total of 1277 current smokers were randomized to either budesonide 400 µg b.i.d. or placebo, both given in the Turbuhaler. The patients' mean age was 52.5 years, 73% were men, and the mean postbronchodilator FEV_1 was 79.7% of predicted. There was a significant initial effect of inhaled budesonide on lung function; in the first 6 months, the placebo group experienced a rapid decline in FEV_1, 81 mL/year, whereas the budesonide group had an increase in FEV_1 of 17 mL/year. From 9 to 36 months, both groups declined in FEV_1, 69 m/year in the placebo group and 57 mL/year in the budesonide group. The difference was not statistically significant ($P=0.39$). After substratification according to pack-years of smoking, there was a tendency towards an effect of budesonide in subjects with ≤36 pack-years, but the difference in decline from 9 to 36 months did still not reach statistical significance. No information on symptoms or exacerbations is given in the report [14], but from early presentations of the study it seemed that no differences in the number of exacerbations were found. Side effects and safety were well documented. There was a statistically significant difference in the occurrence of skin bruises larger than 50 mm in diameter on the volar side of the forearms—10% in the budesonide group and 4% in the placebo group ($P < 0.001$). Apart from this, treatment was well tolerated.

The third study is the Inhaled Steroids in Obstructive Lung Disease in Europe (ISOLDE) study [15]. ISOLDE is the only study that has included patients with severe COPD, the mean FEV_1 being 50% of predicted. A total of 751 patients were included and randomized to either fluticasone 500 μg in metered-dose inhaler (MDI) via a Volumatic spacer twice daily, or placebo MDI via Volumatic spacer. All patients were immediately after randomization offered 2 weeks of treatment with oral prednisolone, 0.6 mg/kg once daily. The main effect parameter was FEV_1 decline; secondary effect parameters were exacerbations, symptoms, and health status, the latter evaluated using the St George's Respiratory Health Questionnaire. Only 219 patients in the fluticasone group and 182 in the placebo group completed the study; patients with more than three exacerbations within a 3-month period were excluded throughout the study, and this led to significantly more patients being excluded from the placebo arm than the fluticasone arm of the study. The course of lung function over the 3-year study is shown in Fig. 10.2 and was almost similar to that seen in the EUROSCOP study, except for the short effect of the oral prednisolone. There was an overall reduction in the number of exacerbations from 1.32 to 0.99 per year ($P = 0.03$). Most significantly, the gradual loss in health status was slowed down in the fluticasone group, from 3.2 units per year in the placebo group to 2.0 units per year in the fluticasone group ($P = 0.004$). These findings may be linked, as exacerbations are associated with loss of health status [16]. From preliminary reporting, it seems that the effect of fluticasone on exacerbations was mainly seen in those with low FEV_1, which in the ISOLDE study was the tertile with $FEV_1 < 1.25$ L and virtually ab-

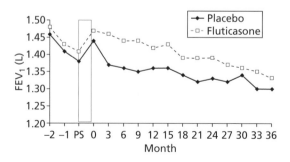

Fig. 10.2 Crude change from forced expiratory volume in 1 s (FEV_1) at randomization in the Inhaled Steroids in Obstructive Lung Disease in Europe (ISOLDE) study. The box illustrates the time of prednisolone. Modified from [15].

sent in the tertile with the best FEV_1. In the recruitment phase, a number of subjects were taken off ICS when entering the run-in period of the ISOLDE study, an 8-week wash-out period in which eligible subjects were followed without ICS. Thirty-eight percent of those taken off ICS experienced an exacerbation during the run-in, in contrast to only 6% of those entering run-in without previous treatment with ICS [17]. These findings have subsequently been confirmed in an American study in which withdrawal of inhaled steroids was associated with worsening of dyspnoea and a drop in FEV_1 [18].

Finally, the results of the Lung Health Study II have been published, to some extent confirming the findings of the previous studies [19]. Whereas Lung Health Study I [20] included both smoking cessation and usual care with or without an inhaled anticholinergic, Lung Health Study II (LHSII) was a pure controlled trial of inhaled triamcinolone. A total of 1116 patients with mild to moderate COPD were randomized in this multicentre trial, including 10 clinical centres in the USA and Canada. As in the previous studies, no effect of inhaled steroids was seen on FEV_1 decline; FEV_1 decline was 47 ± 3 mL/year in the placebo group and 44 ± 3 mL/year in the triamcinolone group. Exacerbations were not a predefined end-point, but as in the ISOLDE study, an effect was seen on effect parameters associated with exacerbations. Both hospitalizations and unscheduled outpatient visits for respiratory causes were reduced by approximately 50% in the triamcinolone group.

What else do we know?

If we look at studies using other outcomes than long-term change in lung function and exacerbations, a somewhat mixed picture emerges, and it is not obvious whether it helps us to clarify the position of ICS. Several short-term studies have been published looking at the effect of ICS on various surrogate markers, supposedly reflecting ongoing inflammation. Importantly, studies of cell types and mediators from bronchoalveolar lavage fluid have shown clear differences between asthma and COPD [21,22], and the choice of inflammatory markers is therefore crucial. It would be outside the scope of this chapter to summarize findings in this area; some studies have been interpreted as showing an effect of ICS on relevant measures, whereas others have been interpreted as negative.

Perhaps the most interesting findings come from a recent non-controlled study from Canada. Sin and Tu [23] used a pharmacoepidemiological set-up to study the effects of inhaled corticosteroids in elderly patients discharged from hospital with a diagnosis of COPD. Their register linkage study included more than 22 000 patients, and they were able to show a statistically significant 10% reduction in the 1-year risk of readmission or death. After controlling for markers of disease severity, the beneficial effect may be even larger, up to 25%. This study, which will inevitably be criticized for being uncontrolled, may show the true impact of the reduction in exacerbations shown in ISOLDE and LHSII. Its approach of looking at patients immediately after a hospitalization for COPD may provide us with an insight into a more optimal time for study inclusion than the one usually chosen [24].

Is there any point in reversibility testing?

Probably not. Data from the ISOLDE study presented at the 1999 American Thoracic Society meeting did not indicate any predictive value of the response to oral corticosteroids with regard to subsequent benefit from ICS. No other studies have convincingly shown any predictive value from reversibility testing [25], and in general 'reversibility' is not a discriminatory feature, but rather a characteristic with no obvious cut-off point, varying independently of reversibility, e.g. bronchodilator reversibility [26].

Is there a subgroup who should be treated as having 'asthma', and if so, what end points indicate success?

It seems that patients with 'asthma-like' features are more likely to show some response to a short course of systemic corticosteroids [27]; corticosteroid response was associated with eosinophilia and higher levels of eosinophil cationic protein (ECP) in bronchoalveolar lavage (BAL) fluid and thicker basement membrane in bronchial biopsies. As mentioned above, however, there is no evidence that this subgroup benefits from long-term treatment with inhaled or oral corticosteroids.

Should steroids be restricted to current smokers only?

The EUROSCOP study has been the only study so far that exclusively recruited smokers. However, all other studies have included fair proportions of smokers, and from subgroup analyses presented at meetings and informal discussions, the effect of inhaled steroids did not appear to differ between smokers and ex-smokers. If we draw on findings in asthma, it seems likely that current smokers will actually respond less favourably to ICS than ex-smokers [28].

What dose of inhaled steroids is justified in COPD, and with which device?

It is obvious from the above that far too few data exist for a satisfactory answer to be given to this important question. In the studies described above, doses were high in comparison with the doses generally used to treat asthma.

No dosing studies exist, and it therefore seems reasonable to treat patients with doses similar to those tested in the published trials if treatment with ICS is found to be indicated. Doses should therefore approximate to 1 mg of fluticasone per day, or equipotent doses of other inhaled corticosteroids. In the two most positive studies [12,15], the ICS were administered in MDIs using a spacer device. There are comparative studies with dry powder inhalers in asthma, but this is not the case in COPD. If a device other than an MDI plus spacer is used, it therefore seems crucial that a minimum inhalation technique should be taught properly to ensure maximal effectiveness of the device chosen.

What are the risks of long-term inhaled steroid use?

In asthma, there is general agreement that the benefits of ICS clearly outweigh the side effects and possible risks associated with long-term use [29]. As this may not be the case in COPD, it is worthwhile to consider both side effects and the potential risks associated with including ICS in the armamentarium of drugs for COPD.

Local side effects such as oral candidiasis and hoarseness are quite frequent, and systemic side effects are perhaps not as infrequent as is often believed in asthma. In EUROSCOP, an excess 6% developed bruises on the forearms > 5 cm in diameter at least once during the trial [14], and although it was firmly stated that no other systemic side effects were seen, bruises are markers of systemic effects and it is likely that the study was underpowered to detect more deleterious effects. In a subsample in EUROSCOP, no effects of treatment with ICS were seen on bone mineral density, but as long-term treatment will often be offered to patients with an unfavourable osteoporosis profile (smoking, minimal physical activity and inappropriate nutrition), this potential problem has not been solved. In fact, in LHSII an increased loss of bone mineral density was found in the femoral neck, but not in the lumbar spine, and this should indicate a need for caution. Wisniewski et al. [30] showed an association between the cumulative dose of ICS and loss of bone density, and two other studies have also increased awareness of the risk of cataracts developing in elderly patients taking ICS [31,32].

Can it be cost-effective to give inhaled steroids in COPD?

First, treatment with ICS is costly. Treatment such as that used in ISOLDE would in Denmark cost €760 (£480) per year. Based on the crude effects in ISOLDE, it thus costs approximately £1440 to avoid one exacerbation. In a subsequent analysis of data from the 6-month study by Paggiaro et al. [12], it was claimed that inhaled fluticasone was cost-effective, and the differences

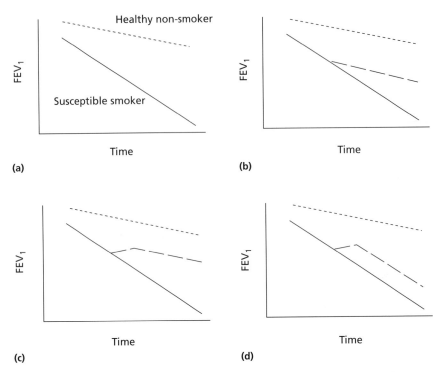

Fig. 10.3 The excessive decline in forced expiratory volume in 1 s (FEV₁) in COPD (a), the theoretical benefit of an effective intervention (b), the effect of smoking cessation (c), and the effect of inhaled corticosteroids in the European Respiratory Society Study on Chronic Obstructive Pulmonary Disease (EUROSCOP) and Inhaled Steroids in Obstructive Lung Disease in Europe (ISOLDE) studies (d).

were substantial with regard to costs per symptom-free day [33]. The results have, however, only been presented in abstract form and are based on the very positive 6-month study. With the lack of effect in the long-term studies in patients with mild to moderate COPD, it seems highly unlikely that ICS can be cost-effective without proper selection of patients. More data are, nevertheless, clearly needed.

There is no doubt that exacerbations are costly, especially when requiring hospitalization in patients with severe disease [34], but inferences from the ISOLDE study are difficult to make at present, as no data on the frequency of hospitalization in the ISOLDE study are available.

How then should inhaled corticosteroids be used in COPD?

First of all, it seems clear that not all COPD patients should be given ICS. As illustrated in Fig. 10.3, there is no evidence of any disease-modifying effect; that is, no effect on FEV₁ decline has been observed. From the studies reported, patients with mild COPD have no benefit whatsoever from treatment with ICS.

Patients with moderate COPD in general should in my opinion not automatically be put on inhaled steroids, although this seems to be the current clinical practice in many countries. There seems to be little evidence that inhaled corticosteroids are helpful in managing patients with an FEV_1 above 1.5 L.

In my opinion, only patients with marked airflow limitation who experience frequent exacerbations and who also have a low health status definitely benefit from treatment. 'Marked airflow limitation' can be defined from ISOLDE as $FEV_1 < 1.25$ L, or $<40\%$ predicted. These patients by definition have severe COPD. There are, however, a few patients with moderate disease who fit the description of having frequent exacerbations and low health status, and these patients should probably be considered for treatment as well. It is not clear whether patients with severe disease but infrequent exacerbations will benefit from ICS, but it is most likely that they will not.

References

1 Jackevicius CA, Chapman KR. Prevalence of inhaled corticosteroid use among patients with chronic obstructive pulmonary disease: a survey. *Ann Pharmacother* 1997; **31**: 160–4.

2 Fletcher CM, Peto R, Tinker CM, Speizer FE. *The Natural History of Chronic Bronchitis and Emphysema*. Oxford: Oxford University Press, 1976.

3 Kanner RE, Anthonisen NR, Connett JE. Lower respiratory illnesses promote FEV_1 decline in current smokers but not ex-smokers with mild chronic obstructive pulmonary disease. *Am J Respir Crit Care Med* 2001; **164**: 358–64.

4 Seemungal T, Donaldson GC, Bhowmik A, Jeffries DJ, Wedzicha JA. Time course and recovery of exacerbations in patients with chronic obstructive pulmonary disease. *Am J Respir Crit Care Med* 2000; **161**: 1608–13.

5 Postma DS, Steenhuis EJ, van der Weele LT, Sluiter HJ. Severe chronic airflow obstruction: can corticosteroids slow down progression ? *Eur J Respir Dis* 1985; **67**: 56–64.

6 Postma DS, Peters I, Steenhuis EJ, Sluiter HJ. Moderately severe chronic airflow obstruction: can corticosteroids slow down progression? *Eur Respir J* 1988; **1**: 22–6.

7 Kerstjens HAM, Brand PLP, Hughes MD *et al*. A comparison of bronchodilator therapy with or without inhaled corticosteroid therapy for obstructive airways disease. *N Engl J Med* 1992; **327**: 1413–19.

8 Renkema TEJ, Schouten JP, Köeter GH, Postma DS. Effects of long-term treatment with corticosteroids in COPD. *Chest* 1996; **109**: 1156–62.

9 van Grunsven PM, van Schayck CP, Derenne JP *et al*. Long-term effects of inhaled corticosteroids in chronic obstructive pulmonary disease: a meta-analysis. *Thorax* 1999; **54**: 7–14.

10 Derenne JP. Effects of high-dose inhaled beclomethasone on the rate of decline in FEV_1 in patients with chronic obstructive pulmonary disease: results of a 2-year prospective multicentre study. *Am J Respir Crit Care Med* 1995; **151**: A463.

11 Bourbeau J, Rouleau MY, Boucher S. Randomised controlled trial of inhaled corticosteroids in patients with chronic obstructive pulmonary disease. *Thorax* 1998; **53**: 477–82.

12 Paggiaro PL, Dahle R, Bakran I *et al*. Multicentre randomised placebo-controlled trial of inhaled fluticasone propionate in patients with chronic obstructive pulmonary disease. *Lancet* 1998; **351**: 773–80.

13 Vestbo J, Sørensen T, Lange P *et al*. Long-term effect of inhaled budesonide in mild and moderate chronic obstructive pulmonary disease: a randomised,

controlled trial. *Lancet* 1999; **353**: 1819–23.

14 Pauwels RA, Löfdahl CG, Laitinen LA *et al*. Long-term treatment with inhaled budesonide in persons with mild chronic obstructive pulmonary disease who continue to smoke. *N Engl J Med* 1999; **340**: 1948–53.

15 Burge PS, Calverley PMA, Jones PW *et al*. Randomised, double-blind, placebo controlled study of fluticasone propionate in patients with moderate to severe chronic obstructive pulmonary disease; the ISOLDE trial. *BMJ* 2000; **320**: 1297–303.

16 Seemungal TAR, Donaldson G, Paul EA *et al*. Effect of exacerbation on quality of life in patients with chronic obstructive pulmonary disease. *Am J Respir Crit Care Med* 1998; **157**: 1418–22.

17 Jarad NA, Wedzicha JA, Burge PS, Calverley PMA, ISOLDE study group. An observational study of inhaled corticosteroid withdrawal in stable chronic obstructive pulmonary disease. *Respir Med* 1999; **93**: 161–6.

18 O'Brien A, Russo-Magno P, Karki A *et al*. Effects of withdrawal of inhaled steroids in men with severe irreversible airflow obstruction. *Am J Respir Crit Care Med* 2001; **164**: 365–71.

19 Lung Health Study Group. Effect of inhaled triamcinolone on the decline in pulmonary function in chronic obstructive pulmonary disease. *N Engl J Med* 2000; **343**: 1902–9.

20 Anthonisen NR, Connett JE, Kiley JP *et al*. Effects of smoking intervention and the use of an inhaled anticholinergic bronchodilator on the rate of decline of FEV_1. The Lung Health Study. *JAMA* 1994; **272**: 1497–505.

21 Lacoste JY, Bousquet J, Chanez P *et al*. Eosinophilic and neutrophilic inflammation in asthma, chronic bronchitis, and chronic obstructive pulmonary disease. *J Allergy Clin Immunol* 1993; **92**: 537–48.

22 Keatings VM, Barnes PJ. Granulocyte activation markers in induced sputum: comparison between chronic obstructive pulmonary disease, asthma, and normal subjects. *Am J Respir Crit Care Med* 1997; **155**: 449–53.

23 Sin DD, Tu JV. Inhaled corticosteroids and the risk of mortality and readmission in elderly patients with COPD. *Am J Respir Crit Care Med* 2001; **164**: 580–4.

24 Vestbo J. Another piece of the inhaled-corticosteroids-in-COPD puzzle. *Am J Respir Crit Care Med* 2001; **164**: 514–15.

25 Hansen EF, Phanareth K, Laursen LC, Kok-Jensen A, Dirksen A. Reversible and irreversible airflow obstruction as predictor of overall mortality in asthma and chronic obstructive pulmonary disease. *Am J Respir Crit Care Med* 1999; **159**: 1267–71.

26 Dirksen A, Christensen H, Evald T *et al*. Bronchodilator and corticosteroid reversibility in ambulatory patients with airways obstruction. *Dan Med Bull* 1991; **38**: 486–9.

27 Chanez P, Vignola AM, O'Shaugnessy T *et al*. Corticosteroid reversibility in COPD is related to features of asthma. *Am J Respir Crit Care Med* 1997; **155**: 1529–34.

28 Pedersen B, Dahl R, Karlström R, Peterson CG, Venge P. Eosinophil and neutrophil activity in asthma in a one-year trial with inhaled budesonide: the impact of smoking. *Am J Respir Crit Care Med* 1996; **153**: 1519–29.

29 Lenfant C, ed. *Global Strategy for Asthma Management and Prevention: NHBLI/WHO Workshop Report* Bethesda, MD: National Heart, Lung, and Blood Institute, 1995. (NIH Publication No. 95–3659.)

30 Wisniewski AF, Lewis SA, Green DJ *et al*. Cross-sectional investigation of the effect of inhaled corticosteroids on bone density and bone metabolism in patients with asthma. *Thorax* 1997; **52**: 853–60.

31 Cumming RG, Mitchell P, Leeder SR. Use of inhaled corticosteroids and the risk of cataracts. *N Engl J Med* 1997; **337**: 8–14.

32 Garbe E, Suissa S, LeLorier J. Association of inhaled corticosteroid use with cataract extraction in elderly patients. *JAMA* 1998; **280**: 539–43.

33 Price MJ, Hurrell C, Medley HV, Efthimiou J. Cost-effectiveness of fluticasone propionate in the management of symptomatic COPD patients. *Eur Respir J* 1999; **14** (Suppl. 30): 379s.

34 Price MJ, Hurrell C, Medley HV, Efthimiou J. Health care costs of treating exacerbations of chronic obstructive pulmonary disease (COPD). *Eur Respir J* 1999; **14** (Suppl. 30): 380s.

11: What are the future treatments for COPD?

Peter Barnes

Introduction

Anticholinergic and β_2-agonist bronchodilators are the mainstay of drug therapy in chronic obstructive pulmonary disease (COPD), but other treatments are also used and may have a place in particular patients. Inhaled corticosteroids are disappointing and have no effect on the accelerated decline in lung function seen in COPD, although they may have a small effect in reducing exacerbations. This chapter discusses some of the other treatments used for COPD and considers some of the novel approaches to treatment that may be used in the future.

Does theophylline have a role in COPD management?

Theophylline has been used for a long time in the management of COPD, but has not been formally studied in large randomized controlled trials [1]. Theophylline is used as a bronchodilator, with doses that give plasma concentrations of 10–20 mg/L. At these doses, theophylline results in reduced symptoms and a small improvement in lung function and exercise capacity [2,3]. In one study, theophylline improved dyspnoea by a reduction in hyperinflation, without significant changes in spirometry [4]. This may indicate an effect of the orally administered drug on small-airway function. Whether theophylline improves respiratory muscle function in patients with COPD is controversial, and there is little evidence that respiratory muscle weakness contributes to symptomatology in the chronic stable state.

There is increasing evidence that theophylline may have anti-inflammatory or immunomodulatory effects in asthma, and that these may be seen at lower doses than needed for bronchodilatation [5,6] (Fig. 11.1). The molecular basis for these effects is still uncertain, although some effects are mediated via a non-selective inhibition of phosphodiesterases (PDE) in inflammatory and immune cells. This has not yet been explored in COPD. In a recent study, theophylline (mean plasma level approximately 10 mg/L) was

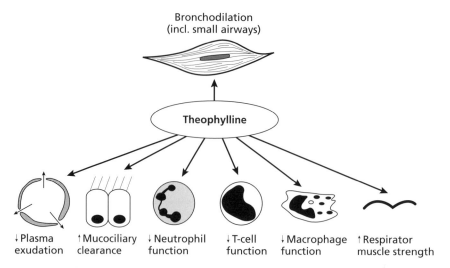

Bronchodilation
(incl. small airways)

Theophylline

| ↓Plasma exudation | ↑Mucociliary clearance | ↓Neutrophil function | ↓T-cell function | ↓Macrophage function | ↑Respirator muscle strength |

Fig. 11.1 Mechanisms of action of theophylline in chronic obstructive pulmonary disease (COPD).

shown to decrease the proportion of neutrophils and the concentration of myeloperoxidase, an index of neutrophil activation, in induced sputum of patients with COPD [7]. This effect may be mediated by an inhibitory effect of theophylline on PDE4, the predominant PDE in neutrophils. However, the antiinflammatory effect of theophylline may be mediated by some other molecular mechanism, since the inhibitory effect on PDE activity is very small at these concentrations of theophylline. Interestingly, recent studies have demonstrated that therapeutic concentrations of theophylline decrease neutrophil survival *in vitro*, whereas PDE4 inhibitors have the reverse effect [8]. An additional mechanism that might contribute to a beneficial effect of theophylline in COPD is an increase in interleukin-10 (IL-10) release, as has been demonstrated in asthmatic patients [9]. IL-10 is a potent anti-inflammatory cytokine that inhibits the release of inflammatory cytokines such as tumour necrosis factor-α (TNF-α) and IL-8, as well as increasing the expression of antiproteases. These studies suggest that theophylline might have an anti-inflammatory effect in COPD and that it may theoretically reduce the decline in lung function. However, it is unlikely that the necessary long-term randomized controlled trial will be conducted, as these drugs are cheap and pharmaceutical companies may be unwilling to invest in such expensive studies.

Side effects have been the main problem in the clinical use of theophylline in COPD patients. Side effects, particularly nausea, vomiting and headaches, occur increasingly as plasma concentrations rise from 10 to 20 mg/L and may be commoner in elderly patients. Benefit may be obtained at concentrations below 10 mg/L, so that aiming for a therapeutic concentration of 5–10 mg/L, as in patients with asthma, may be adequate.

Overall, theophylline is a useful additional treatment for patients with COPD, improving symptoms and lung function and may have the additional benefit of reducing the inflammatory response. More long-term studies and further investigation of its anti-inflammatory effect are now indicated.

What is the role of antileukotriene drugs in COPD?

There are no published studies on the effects of leukotriene receptor antagonists or 5′-lipoxygenase inhibitors in COPD. There is evidence for increased formation of leukotriene B_4 (LTB_4) in COPD patients [10], suggesting that inhibition of LTB_4 synthesis by a 5′-lipoxygenase inhibitor or blockage of LTB_4-receptors on neutrophils by a receptor antagonist may be of potential benefit. Although a 5′-lipoxygenase inhibitor, zileuton, is available for the treatment of asthma in some countries, its effects in COPD have not yet been reported. Several potent LTB_4-receptor antagonists have now been developed for clinical use and some are in clinical trial in COPD.

Cysteinyl-leukotrienes, as well as causing bronchoconstriction, also induce plasma extravasation and increase mucus secretion. However, the effects of cys-LT antagonists, such as montelukast ands zafirlukast, have not yet been studied in COPD. The major source of these mediators in asthmatic patients are likely to be mast cells and eosinophils, which are not likely to play an important role in the inflammatory process in COPD, so that there is less rationale for their use in COPD than in asthma.

Should mucolytics be used routinely?

Because mucus hypersecretion is a prominent feature of chronic bronchitis, various mucolytic therapies have been used to increase the ease of mucus expectoration, in the belief that this will improve lung function. Stopping smoking is the most effective way to reduce mucus hypersecretion. Anticholinergics may decrease mucus hypersecretion, although most studies have failed to show an effect of inhaled anticholinergics on mucociliary clearance. β_2-agonists and theophylline may improve mucus clearance. Steam inhalation (with or without aromatics) may provide symptomatic relief, but there is no evidence that it improves lung function or long-term symptom control.

Several drugs, such as N-acetylcysteine, carbocysteine, bromhexol and ambroxol, reduce mucus viscosity *in vitro*, but there is little evidence from controlled trials that they improve lung function in patients with COPD, and cannot be recommended as routine therapy. A systematic review of randomized controlled trials has recently shown that mucolytics have a modest bene-

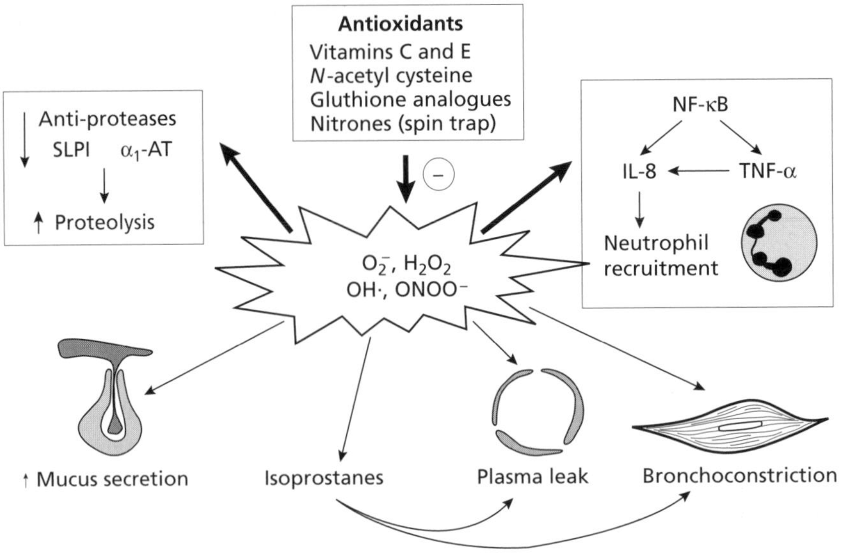

Fig. 11.2 Oxidative stress in chronic obstructive pulmonary disease (COPD).

fit on the frequency and duration of exacerbations in comparison with place-
bos, although there was a small but significant reduction in lung function [11].
The benefits could not entirely be explained by N-acetylcysteine, which is also
an antioxidant.

Expectorants, such as guanifeniesin and potassium iodide, similarly have
no proven beneficial effects. Recombinant human DNAase (alfadornase) has
beneficial effects in some patients with cystic fibrosis, but its role in COPD is
not yet clear. Until there is clear evidence of benefit in COPD, it should not be
used, in view of its high cost.

Do antioxidants have any activity in COPD?

Since oxidant damage may be critical in the pathophysiology of COPD,
antioxidant therapy is a logical approach [12]. Reactive oxygen species may
be inhaled in cigarette smoke or generated by activated inflammatory cells
within the lung, leading to reduced activity of antiproteases, increased production of inflammatory cytokines and direct inflammatory effects (Fig.
11.2). N-acetylcysteine was originally developed as a mucolytic, but has well
documented antioxidant effects. Controlled trials have demonstrated that it
reduces the frequency and severity of acute exacerbations of COPD [13], and
in an open study it significantly reduced the rate of decline in lung function
[14]. It may therefore be useful in long-term management of COPD, but is not

currently available on prescription in the UK. Further trials are indicated in patients with COPD who have more frequent exacerbations.

No studies with other antioxidants, such as vitamins C and E, have been reported in COPD. More effective antioxidants are now in development and should undergo clinical trials in COPD. It is likely that antioxidants may reduce the inflammation and proteolysis of COPD, resulting in reduced exacerbations, improved symptom control and a slowing of disease progression.

Which vaccines are effective in COPD?

Polyvalent pneumococcal vaccine is used in many countries to protect against the development of pneumococcal lung infections [15], but there is little evidence that it is specifically beneficial in patients with COPD, and it therefore cannot be routinely recommended.

Influenza vaccine is usually recommended, as patients with COPD are subject to severe exacerbations with this infection. Neuraminidase inhibitors, such as inhaled zanamivir or oral oseltamivir, are now becoming available for the treatment and prevention of influenza A and B infections [16]. However, it has not yet been shown that they specifically reduce the duration of exacerbations in patients with COPD, and they would only be of value during an influenza epidemic.

OM85-BV (Broncho-Vaxom) is a mixture of bacterial products that activate macrophage function (the advantage of which is obscure). There is some evidence that it may reduce the severity of acute exacerbations, but it cannot be recommended as a routine treatment [17].

Treatment of dyspnoea

Breathlessness is a problem in many patients, particularly 'pink puffers'. Several drugs, including nebulized opiates, dihydrocodeine and benzodiazepines, reduce the sensation of dyspnoea, but the reduction in ventilatory drive is potentially dangerous and these drugs should be avoided, particularly during exacerbations.

Respiratory stimulants

There is no role for respiratory stimulants, such as doxapram or almitrine, in the long-term management of COPD, since there is no evidence that central ventilatory drive is impaired. Ventilation is limited by mechanical rather than neurophysiological factors.

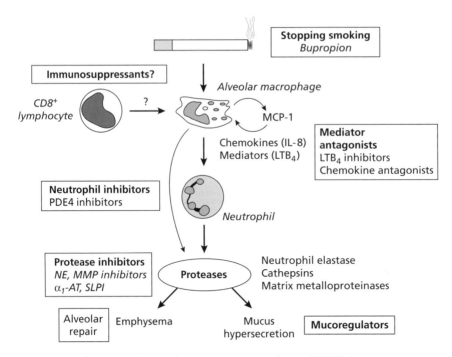

Fig. 11.3 Novel targets for chronic obstructive pulmonary disease (COPD) therapy.

Which new drugs are in development?

There have been relatively few advances in the therapeutic options for the treatment of COPD, but a better understanding of the molecular mechanisms involved in the pathogenesis of COPD will undoubtedly lead to improved therapies in the future [18,19]. COPD involves an active inflammatory process and progressive destruction of the lungs, so that it should be possible to develop drugs that are able to halt this process and prevent the accelerated decline in lung function that characterizes the disease. Better understanding of the cellular and molecular mechanisms involved in COPD has identified several novel therapeutic targets (Fig. 11.3).

New bronchodilators

Bronchodilators are the mainstay of current management of COPD, and the major recent advances have been in the development of long-acting bronchodilators. Tiotropium bromide is a very promising new anticholinergic drug that has a very long duration of action. It has a high affinity and dissociates very slowly from M_1 and M_3-muscarinic receptors in the human lung, and it produces long-term blockade of cholinergic neural bronchoconstriction in human airway smooth muscle. However, its effects on acetylcholine release are short-lived, confirming functional selectivity for M_3-receptors compared to M_2-receptors. In studies of patients with COPD, tiotropium bromide gives prolonged bronchodilatation, lasting over 24h [20,21]. This suggests that tiotropium bromide will be suitable for once-daily dosing, and it is now in advanced clinical trials as a once-daily dry powder inhalation.

Mediator antagonists

Several mediators are involved in the pathophysiology of COPD, and antagonists to individual mediators have now been developed or are in development. LTB_4 antagonists and 5'-lipoxygenase inhibitors are discussed above. Several cytokines are involved in the pathophysiology of COPD, including TNF-α and IL-8 [22]. There are now several inhibitors of TNF-α, including monoclonal antibodies and soluble receptors, that have been developed for the treatment of rheumatoid arthritis and inflammatory bowel disease, that might be beneficial in COPD. IL-8, which is chemotactic for neutrophils, may be blocked by receptor antagonists, such as the SB 225002, that may therefore reduce the neutrophilic inflammation in COPD airways.

New anti-inflammatory treatments

COPD is characterized by inflammation of the airways, with increased numbers of activated macrophages, neutrophils and CD8+ T lymphocytes. Corticosteroids are largely ineffective at suppressing this inflammatory process, prompting the search for new anti-inflammatory drugs. There are several approaches to inhibiting neutrophilic inflammation (Table 11.1).

PDEs break down cyclic nucleotides (cyclic adenosine monophosphate, cAMP and cyclic guanosine monophosphate, cGMP) which regulate cellular

Table 11.1 Inhibitors of neutrophilic inflammation.

- LTB_4 antagonists (LY 29311, SC-53228, CP-105,696, SB 201146)
- Interleukin-8 inhibitors (IL-8 synthesis inhibitors, CXC receptor antagonists)
- Antioxidants (N-acetylcysteine, glutathione analogues, vitamins C and E, nitrones)
- TNF inhibitors (monoclonal antibodies, soluble receptors, TNF convertase inhibitors)
- Phosphodiesterase-4 inhibitors (SB 207499, CP 80633, CDP-840)
- NF-κB inhibitors (IκB kinase inhibitors, IκB-α gene transfer)
- Adhesion molecule inhibitors (anti CD11/CD18, anti-ICAM-1, E-selectin inhibitors)
- Prostaglandin E analogues (misoprostol, butaprost)
- Interleukin-10
- Colchicine
- Macrolide antibiotics (erythromycin, clarithromycin, roxithromycin)

ICAM-1, intercellular adhesion molecule-1; LTB_4, leukotriene B_4; NF-κB, nuclear factor-κB; TNF, tumour necrosis factor.

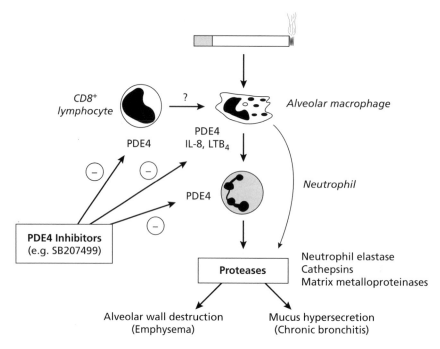

Fig. 11.4 Effects of phosphodiesterase 4 (PDE4) inhibitors in chronic obstructive pulmonary disease (COPD).

activity. Inhibition of these enzymes results in inhibition of inflammatory cells and relaxation of smooth muscle. Over 10 families of PDEs are now recognized, but the family most relevant to COPD inflammation is PDE4, since PDE4 inhibitors inhibit neutrophilic inflammation, but also inhibit macrophage and T-lymphocyte function [23] (Fig. 11.4). PDE4 inhibitors also have a bronchodilator action. A selective PDE4 inhibitor has recently been shown improve lung function and symptoms in patients with COPD [24]. The disadvantage of PDE4 inhibitors is that they cause nausea and vomiting, but more selective drugs have now been developed which are better tolerated.

The transcription factor nuclear factor-κB (NF-κB) is of critical importance for the persistence of chronic inflammation [25]. It regulates the synthesis of IL-8 and TNF-α, as well as adhesion molecules such as intercellular adhesion molecule-1 (ICAM-1), suggesting that NF-κB inhibitors might be beneficial in COPD. Several approaches to inhibition of NF-κB are now in development, but there are concerns that effective inhibition of NF-κB might impair host defence.

Neutrophil recruitment into the lungs and respiratory tract is dependent on adhesion molecules expressed on neutrophils and endothelial cells in the pulmonary and bronchial circulations. Neutrophil adhesion in response to chemotactic factors is characterized by expression of the β_2 integrins CD11a/CD18 (LFA-1) and CD11b/CD18 (Mac-1) on the surface of the neutrophil and their interaction with their counterreceptors, including intercellular adhesion molecule-1 (ICAM-1), on endothelial cells. E-selectin on endothelial cells also interacts with sialyl-Lewis[x] on neutrophils. Bronchial biopsies of patients with COPD have demonstrated increased expression of E-selectin on vessels and ICAM-1 on epithelial cells [26]. Drugs that interfere with these adhesion molecules should therefore inhibit neutrophil inflammation in COPD and well tolerated selectin inhibitors have now been developed for clinical studies. However, there are concerns about this therapeutic approach for a chronic disease, as an impaired neutrophilic response may increase the susceptibility to infections.

There is increasing recognition that mitogen-activated protein (MAP) kinases may play an important role in chronic inflammation. One MAP kinase, p38 MAP kinase is important in release of inflammatory mediators such as TNF-α, and small molecule inhibitors of this enzyme have now been developed that might be useful in COPD if these drugs are well tolerated [27].

Protease inhibitors

Emphysema may result from an imbalance between excessive protease activity and deficient endogenous antiproteases (Fig. 11.5, Table 11.2). A logical

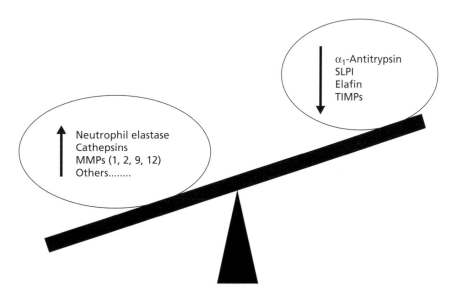

Fig. 11.5 Imbalance between proteases and antiproteases in chronic obstructive pulmonary disease (COPD).

Table 11.2 Protease inhibitors

- Neutrophil elastase inhibitors (ICI 200355, ONO-5046)
- Cathepsin inhibitors (suramin)
- Matrix metalloproteinase inhibitors (batimastat, marimastat, selective MMP inhibitors)
- α_1-Antitrypsin (purified, human recombinant, gene transfer)
- Elafin
- Secretory leukoprotease inhibitor (human recombinant)

MMP, matrix metalloproteinase.

approach to treatment is to inhibit endogenous proteases or to supplement endogenous antiproteases.

As neutrophil elastase is a major constituent of lung elastolytic activity and also potently stimulates mucus secretion, it is a potential target for inhibition. Several potent neutrophil elastase inhibitors have been developed, including peptide inhibitors, such as ICI 200355, and non-peptide inhibitors, such as ONO-5046. There are few clinical studies in COPD; the neutrophil elastase inhibitor MR889 administered for 4 weeks showed no overall effect on plasma elastin-derived peptides or urinary desmosine (markers of elastolytic activity) [28]. It may be difficult to inhibit enzyme activity, as neutrophils adhere to connective tissue, so that access of the enzyme inhibitor may be a problem. Intracellular inhibitors may be more effective.

Although neutrophil elastase is likely to be the major mechanism mediating elastolysis in patients with α_1-antitrypsin (α_1-AT) deficiency, it may well not be the major elastolytic enzyme in smoking-related COPD, and it is important to consider other enzymes, such as cathepsins and proteinase-3, as targets for inhibition.

Matrix metalloproteinases (MMPs) derived from macrophages, neutrophils and epithelial cells may also play a role in connective tissue destruction, suggesting that MMP inhibitors may be beneficial. Several MMPs are increased in COPD and have the capacity to destroy lung elastin fibres. Several MMP inhibitors are now in development, but non-selective inhibitors have been associated with musculoskeletal side effects, so that more selective drugs may be needed in the future.

The association of α_1-AT deficiency with early onset emphysema suggested that this endogenous inhibitor of neutrophil elastase may be of therapeutic benefit in COPD. Cigarette smoking may inactivate α_1-AT, resulting in unopposed activity of neutrophil elastase and cathepsins. Extraction of α_1-AT from human plasma is very expensive and extracted α_1-antitrypsin is only available in a few countries. This treatment has to be given intravenously and has a half-life of only 5 days. Human α_1-AT has now been available for over 10 years, but even in patients with severe α_1-AT deficiency and emphysema, there is only a marginal effect on the rate of decline in forced expiratory volume in 1 s (FEV$_1$) [29]. Inhaled α_1-AT formulations, although these are inefficient and expensive [30]. Recombinant α_1-AT with amino acid substitutions to increase stability may result in a more stable product. Gene therapy is another possibility using an adenovirus vector or liposomes, but there have been major problems in developing efficient delivery systems. There is a particular problem with gene transfer in α_1-AT deficiency, in that large amounts of protein (1–2 g) need to be synthesized each day. There is no evidence that α_1-AT treatment would halt the progression of COPD and emphysema in patients who have normal plasma concentrations.

Other serum protease inhibitors (serpins), such as elafin, may also be important in counteracting elastolytic activity in the lung. Elafin, an elastase-specific inhibitor is found in bronchoalveolar lavage and is synthesized by epithelial cells in response to inflammatory stimuli. Serpins may not be able to inhibit neutrophil elastase at the sites of elastin destruction, due to tight adherence of the inflammatory cell to connective tissue. Furthermore, these proteins may become inactivated by the inflammatory process and the action of oxidants, so that they may not be able to adequately counteract elastolytic activity in the lung unless used in conjunction with other therapies. Secretory leukoprotease inhibitor (SLPI) is a 12-kDa serpin that appears to be a major inhibitor of elastase activity in the airways and is secreted by epithelial cells. *In vitro*, recombinant human SLPI is more effective at inhibiting neutrophil mediated proteolysis than α_1-AT [31]. Recombinant human SLPI given by aerosolization increases antineutrophil elastase activity in epithelial lining fluid for over 12 h, indicating potential therapeutic use [32].

Drugs affecting remodelling

Since a major mechanism of airway obstruction in COPD is loss of elastic recoil due to proteolytic destruction of lung parenchyma, it seems unlikely that this could be reversible by drug therapy, although it might be possible to reduce the rate of progression by preventing the inflammatory and enzymatic disease process.

Retinoic acid increases the number of alveoli in rats and, remarkably, reverses the histological and physiological changes induced by elastase treatment [33]. It is not certain whether such alveolar proliferation is possible in adult human lungs, however. Retinoic acid activates intracellular retinoic acid receptors, which act as transcription factors to regulate the expression of many genes. The molecular mechanisms involved and whether this can be extrapolated to humans is not yet known. Several retinoic acid receptor subtype agonists have now been developed that may have a greater selectivity for this effect.

Hepatic growth factor (scatter factor) appears to be a major growth factor responsible for alveolar development, and alveolar cells respond to it during lung development [34]. If responsiveness could be restored, this might be a strategy for repairing damaged lung.

Monitoring the effects of therapy

Several drugs are now in development may be useful in COPD. These include LTB$_4$ antagonists and 5-lipoxygenase inhibitors, PDE4 inhibitors, new anti-oxidants and neutrophil elastase and MMP inhibitors. It will be difficult to demonstrate the efficacy of such treatments as determination of the effect of any drug on the rate of decline in lung function will require large studies over at least 2 years. There is an urgent need to develop surrogate markers, such as analysis of sputum parameters (cells, mediators, enzymes), that may predict the clinical usefulness of such drugs.

Drug delivery in COPD

By analogy with asthma, a disease that affects all airways, it has been presumed that the inhaled route of delivery is preferred for the treatment of patients with COPD. However, the disease process in COPD is predominantly in small airways and in the lung parenchyma, which may not be efficiently targeted by the inhalers designed to treat asthma. This may lead to the development of new inhaler devices with particles that have the optimal distribution for peripheral lung delivery. Furthermore, there is a strong argument in favour of oral drug delivery, in order to target lung parenchyma. A further approach is to develop cell-directed therapies. For example, alveolar macrophages appear to play a critical role in COPD and may be targeted by drugs that are designed to be engulfed by these cells, using specially designed liposomes or coated particles of drug. Much more research is needed to optimize drug delivery in COPD patients.

References

1 Kerstjens HA. Stable chronic obstructive pulmonary disease. *BMJ* 1999; 319: 495–500.
2 Taylor DR, Buick B, Kinney C, Lowry RC, McDevitt DG. The efficacy of orally administered theophylline, inhaled salbutamol, and a combination of the two as chronic therapy in the management of chronic bronchitis with reversible airflow obstruction. *Am Rev Respir Dis* 1985; 131: 747–51.

3 Murciano D, Avclair MH, Parievte R, Aubier M. A randomized controlled trial of theophylline in patients with severe chronic obstructive pulmonary disease. *N Engl J Med* 1989; 320: 1521–5.
4 Chrystyn H, Mulley BA, Peake MD. Dose–response relation to oral theophylline in severe chronic obstructive airway disease. *BMJ* 1988; 297: 1506–10.
5 Barnes PJ, Pauwels RA. Theophylline in

asthma: time for reappraisal? *Eur Respir J* 1994; **7**: 579–91.

6 Evans DJ, Taylor DA, Zetterstrom O *et al.* A comparison of low-dose inhaled budesonide plus theophylline and high-dose inhaled budesonide for moderate asthma. *N Engl J Med* 1997; **337**: 1412–18.

7 Culpitt SV, de Matos C, Russell RE *et al.* Effect of theophylline on induced sputum inflammatory indices and neutrophil chemotaxis in COPD. *Am J Respir Crit Care Med* 2002; **165**: 1371–6.

8 Yasui K, Hu B, Nakazawa T, Agematsu K, Komiyama A. Theophylline accelerates human granulocyte apoptosis not via phosphodiesterase inhibition. *J Clin Invest* 1997; **100**: 1677–84.

9 Mascali JJ, Cvietusa P, Negri J, Borish L. Anti-inflammatory effects of theophylline: modulation of cytokine production. *Ann Allergy Asthma Immunol* 1996; **77**: 34–8.

10 Hill AT, Bayley D, Stockley RA. The interrelationship of sputum inflammatory markers in patients with chronic bronchitis. *Am J Respir Crit Care Med* 1999; **160**: 893–8.

11 Poole PJ, Black PN. Oral mucolytic drugs for exacerbations of chronic obstructive pulmonary disease: systematic review. *BMJ* 2001; **322**: 1271–4.

12 Repine JE, Bast A, Lankhorst I. Oxidative stress in chronic obstructive pulmonary disease. *Am J Respir Crit Care Med* 1997; **156**: 341–57.

13 Grandjean EM, Berthet P, Ruffmann R, Leuenberger P. Efficacy of oral long-term *N*-acetylcysteine in chronic bronchopulmonary disease: a meta-analysis of published double-blind, placebo-controlled clinical trials. *Clin Ther* 2000; **22**: 209–21.

14 Lundback B, Lindstrom M, Jonsson E, Anderson S, van Herwaarden C. Effect of *N*-acetylcysteine on the decline in lung function in patients with COPD. *Eur Respir J* 1995; **5** (Suppl. 15): 895.

15 Fedson DS, Shapiro ED, LaForce FM *et al.* Pneumococcal vaccine after 15 years of use: another view. *Arch Intern Med* 1994; **154**: 2531–5.

16 Cox NJ, Hughes JM. New options for the prevention of influenza [editorial]. *N Engl J Medical* 1999; **341**: 1387–8.

17 Collet JP, Shapiro P, Ernst P *et al.* Effects of an immunostimulating agent on acute exacerbations and hospitalizations in patients with chronic obstructive pulmonary disease. The PARI-IS Study Steering Committee and Research Group. Prevention of Acute Respiratory Infection by an Immunostimulant. *Am J Respir Crit Care Med* 1997; **156**: 1719–24.

18 Barnes PJ. Future advances in COPD therapy. *Respiration* 2001; **68**: 441–8.

19 Barnes PJ. New treatments for COPD. *Nature Rev Drug Disc* 2002; **1**: 437–45.

20 Disse B, Speck GA, Rominger KL, Witek TJ, Hammer R. Tiotropium (Spiriva): mechanistical considerations and clinical profile in obstructive lung disease. *Life Sci* 1999; **64**: 457–64.

21 Barnes PJ. Tiotropium bromide. *Expert Opin Invest Drugs* 2001; **10**: 733–40.

22 Keatings VM, Collins PD, Scott DM, Barnes PJ. Differences in interleukin-8 and tumor necrosis factor-α in induced sputum from patients with chronic obstructive pulmonary disease or asthma. *Am J Respir Crit Care Med* 1996; **153**: 530–4.

23 Torphy TJ. Phosphodiesterase isoenzymes. *Am J Respir Crit Care Med* 1998; **157**: 351–70.

24 Compton CH, Gubb J, Nieman R *et al.* Cilomilast, a selective phosphodiesterase-4 inhibitor for treatment of patients with chronic obstructive pulmonary disease: a randomised, dose-ranging study. *Lancet* 2001; **358**: 265–70.

25 Barnes PJ, Karin M. Nuclear factor-κB: a pivotal transcription factor in chronic inflammatory diseases. *N Engl J Med* 1997; **336**: 1066–71.

26 Di Stefano A, Maestrelli P, Roggeri A *et al.* Upregulation of adhesion molecules in the bronchial mucosa of subjects with chronic obstructive bronchitis. *Am J Respir Crit Care Med* 1994; **149**: 803–10.

27 Underwood DC, Osborn RR, Bochnowicz S *et al.* SB 239063, a p38 MAPK inhibitor, reduces neutrophilia, inflammatory cytokines, MMP-9, and fibrosis in lung. *Am J Physiol Lung Cell Mol Physiol* 2000; **279**: L895–L902.

28 Luisetti M, Sturani C, Sella D *et al.* MR889, a neutrophil elastase inhibitor, in patients with chronic obstructive pulmonary disease: a double-blind, randomized, placebo-controlled clinical trial. *Eur Respir J* 1996; **9**: 1482–6.

29 Seersholm N, Wencker M, Banik N *et al.* Does α_1-antitrypsin augmentation therapy slow the annual decline in FEV$_1$ in patients with severe hereditary α_1-

antitrypsin deficiency. *Eur Respir J* 1997; **10**: 2260–3.

30 Hubbard RC, Crystal RG. Strategies for aerosol therapy of alpha 1-antitrypsin deficiency by the aerosol route. *Lung* 1990; **168** (Suppl.): 565–78.

31 Llewellyn-Jones CG, Stockley RA. Effect of fluticasone propionate on neutrophil chemotaxis, superoxide generation and extracellular proteolytic activity *in vitro*. *Thorax* 1994; **49**: 207–12.

32 McElvaney NG, Doujaiji B, Moan MJ *et al*. Pharmacokinetics of recombinant secretory leukoprotease inhibitor aerosolized to normals and individuals with cystic fibrosis. *Am Rev Respir Dis* 1993; **148**: 1056–60.

33 Massaro G, Massaro D. Retinoic acid treatment abrogates elastase-induced pulmonary emphysema in rats. *Nature Med* 1997; **3**: 675–7.

34 Ohmichi H, Koshimizu U, Matsumoto K, Nakamura T. Hepatocyte growth factor (HGF) acts as a mesenchyme-derived morphogenic factor during fetal lung development. *Development* 1998; **125**: 1315–24.

12: What is the role of rehabilitation in COPD?

Peter Wijkstra, Nick ten Hacken, Johan Wempe and Gerard Koeter

What are the basic elements in pulmonary rehabilitation?

Nowadays, the scientific foundations for pulmonary rehabilitation have been clearly established, and rehabilitation programmes have therefore become an essential part of the management of patients with chronic obstructive pulmonary disease (COPD). This has led to a new statement by the American Thoracic Society, in which they adopted the following definition: 'Pulmonary rehabilitation is a multidisciplinary programme of care for patients with chronic respiratory impairment that is individually tailored and designed to optimize physical and social performance and autonomy' [1]. In common practice, this means that pulmonary rehabilitation aims to reduce symptoms, increase functional capacity and increase quality of life, with an awareness and acceptance of the fact that the level of impairment may not be changed. The term 'impairment' is derived from the World Health Organization (WHO), which in 1980 structured the various aspects of chronic disease by introducing the international classification of impairments, disabilities, and handicaps [2]. This chapter explains how we can measure impairment, disability, and handicap in patients with COPD, and afterwards discusses several issues of pulmonary rehabilitation based on what is known in the literature.

According to the WHO, impairment is any loss or abnormality of psychological, physiological or anatomic structure or function [2]. In respiratory patients, we measure impairment mostly by lung function tests, including forced expiratory volume in 1 s (FEV_1) the ratio FEV_1/vital capacity (VC) and diffusion capacity. Inspiratory and peripheral muscle function are related to symptoms and may therefore also be important parameters for assessing the level of impairment. These measurements have become even more important, because in contrast to irreversible airflow obstruction, they can be improved by adequate training.

Disability is any restriction or lack (resulting from an impairment) of ability to perform an activity in the manner or within the range considered to be normal for a human being [2]. As mentioned above, impaired lung function may lead to disability; however, the relation between the two is not very strong [3,4]. Therefore, the level of disability has to be assessed directly by exercise tests. These tests can be divided into two types: maximal exercise tests, usually performed on a bicycle ergometer, and submaximal tests such as walking tests for a given time or shuttle walking tests. These exercise tests are objective measurements, while disability is also a term used to describe the patient's feeling of the impact of COPD during his or her daily activities. A number of measures of subjective feelings of disability are used in COPD, which mostly include dyspnoea, such as the Borg ratio of perceived exertion [5], Mahler's dyspnoea index [6], the Medical Research Council (MRC) dyspnoea scale [7], and the Oxygen Cost Diagram (OCD) [8]. Findings of low correlations between spirometry, on the one hand, and objective and subjective disability measurements on the other, may indicate a need to investigate disability directly both by exercise tests and subjective measurements.

Handicap is defined by the WHO as a disadvantage for a given individual resulting from an impairment or disability that limits or prevents the fulfilment of a role that is normal (depending on age, gender and social and cultural factors) for that individual [2]. It has been shown that impaired lung function may result in an impaired quality of life [9–11], which can represent the subjective experience of a handicap.

Interestingly, health-care use by COPD patients appears to be more related to an impaired quality of life than to the severity of the lung disease itself [12]. Therefore, it is important to assess quality of life as an important aspect of a chronic disease. Two general health measurements, the Quality of Well-Being Scale [13] and the Sickness Impact Profile [14] have been used in COPD patients. As these instruments are not sensitive enough to detect small changes [15] after therapy, Guyatt and co-workers developed the Chronic Respiratory Questionnaire (CRQ) [16], a disease-specific questionnaire, which was found to be sensitive in this respect. A disadvantage of the CRQ is that the questionnaire is not a standardized one, as the dimension 'dyspnoea' is strictly individualized—i.e. every patient has to quantify dyspnoea during activities that are important in their day-to-day life. This means that it is difficult to compare different studies by using the CRQ. For this reason, Jones and co-workers [15] developed a standardized disease specific questionnaire, the St George's Hospital Respiratory Questionnaire (SGRQ), which was found to be valid, repeatable, and sensitive. Neither the CRQ nor the SGRQ showed a strong relationship with lung function measurements or measurements of disability. The shared variance between the change in the CRQ with changes in walking distance was 27%, while the shared variance between CRQ and the MRC dyspnoea scale was only 10% [17]. The shared variance between the SGRQ, on the one hand, and forced vital capacity (FVC) and 6-min walking distance on the other, was 18% and 37%, respectively [15]. Therefore, it is not possible to predict the level of disability or quality of life for individual patients from their lung function [15,17,18]. This may not be entirely surprising, since patients may adapt to their disabilities and handicaps. Sometimes quality of life is surprisingly well maintained despite severe impairments and disabilities. As a consequence, one has to assess disability and quality of life directly.

By assessing all three aspects of a chronic disease—i.e. impairment, disability, and handicap—it is possible to focus on the specific problems of a patient and to determine which interventions in rehabilitation may be beneficial.

Which patients should be included in pulmonary rehabilitation?

Pulmonary rehabilitation is indicated for patients with a respiratory impairment who still are dyspnoeic despite optimal medical management, have reduced exercise tolerance, and have a handicap due to this pulmonary disorder. This means that all patients with complaints due to pulmonary diseases might be included in programmes. However, in this chapter we will focus on patients with COPD only. In the recent position paper of the American Thoracic Society (ATS), some indications were given for referral for pulmonary rehabilitation (Table 12.1) [1]. The problem with these indications is that they are general and therefore not easy to use in clinical practice. Only a few studies have focused on assessing which patients with COPD are ideal candidates for rehabilitation. Zu Wallack *et al.* included in their study patients with a mean FEV_1 of 1.0 L, and offered them a rehabilitation programme consisting of 12 3-h sessions given over 6 weeks [19]. The patients were supervised by a team consisting of nurse, respiratory therapist, dietitian, physical therapist, and occupational therapist. The most important part of the programme was exercise training (treadmill, bicycle training, upper extremity training, breathing exercises). After 6 weeks, the patients with the lowest 12-min walking distance (12-MWD) and the best FEV_1 at baseline showed the largest improvement in walking distance (Fig. 12.1). The authors conclude that patients with less airflow obstruction can exercise on a higher workload, and thereby derive more

Table 12.1 Common indications for referral for pulmonary rehabilitation [1].

Anxiety engaging in activities
Breathlessness with activities
Limitations with:
   Social activities
   Leisure activities
   Indoor and/or outdoor chores
   Basic or instrumental activities of daily living
Loss of independence

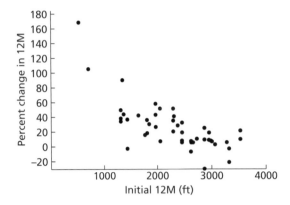

Fig. 12.1 Percentage improvement in 12-min walking distance in relation to the initial 12-minute walking distance ($r = -0.71$; $P < 0.0001$) [19].

aerobic benefit from rehabilitation. This suggests that lung function might be an important predictor of the outcome of rehabilitation. However, a study by Maltais *et al.* showed contradictory results [20]. In this study, 42 patients with a moderately severe airflow obstruction (mean FEV_1 38% of predicted) received a 12-week endurance programme. The effects of training were compared in patients with a FEV_1 <40% of predicted and FEV_1 >40% of predicted. Percent changes in VO_{2max}, W_{max}, and V_E were significant and of similar magnitude in both groups. They concluded that a physiological training effect could be achieved even in patients with severe COPD.

Another way to identify ideal candidates is to look at whether some of the underlying basic problems can be improved by rehabilitation. There is growing evidence that COPD patients have muscle weakness and that this is related to exercise tolerance [21,22]. Pure strength training was found to be beneficial in improving quality of life [23] and exercise tolerance [24] in these patients. Therefore, it might be concluded that patients with impaired muscle function are good candidates for rehabilitation, because it is possible to improve their functional status by training their muscles. Finally, there is now also clear evidence that rehabilitation improves quality of life and dyspnoea, suggesting that patients with a poor quality of life and severe dyspnoea complaints are good candidates too [25,26].

Unfortunately, only a few studies have been carried out to investigate patient profiles in order to characterize patients who are suitable for a rehabilitation programme. Based on what we know at present, it seems that patients with an impaired muscle function, decreased exercise tolerance, severe complaints of dyspnoea, and poor quality of life might be good candidates for inclusion. However, all results are derived from groups of patients, and we do not know how to interpret them in an individual patient. Moreover, although we have the impression that motivation is a very important factor in this

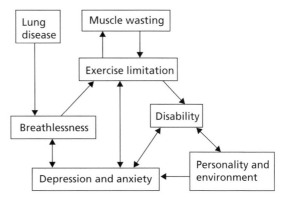

Fig. 12.2 Model of the pathways involved in the development of impaired health or quality of life in patients with chronic obstructive pulmonary disease [27].

respect, no data are available. Further prospective studies are therefore need-ed to identify individuals who are good candidates.

In what setting can we organize rehabilitation?

Impaired health in patients with COPD is determined by several factors (Fig. 12.2) [27]. Figure 12.2 illustrates some of the elements linking lung disease to impaired quality of life and shows that the pathways between them may be complex. The task of a rehabilitation team is to unravel these links and to structure the specific problems in an individual patient with COPD. A possible strategy is to assess the three aspects of COPD—i.e. impairment, disability, and handicap. This makes it possible to focus on the specific problems of the patient, leading to the most effective type of intervention. This determines the staffing and consequently the kind of setting for rehabilitation. A European Respiratory Society (ERS) task force has recently published selection criteria for three types of programme: in-patient; outpatient; and home rehabilitation [28].

   Several criteria for in-patient rehabilitation have been formulated:
1   Need for 24-h supervised monitoring management plan, including training.
2   Behavioural intervention to correct psychosocial problems.
3   Need for specific interventions, such as nutrition.
4   Pre- and postoperative rehabilitation programmes.
5   Identification of a need for long-term oxygen or long-term home mechanical ventilation.
6   Logistic reasons for outpatient rehabilitation not being possible, such as distance.
These criteria mean that a patient who is largely disabled and who has a severe handicap needs different types of intervention. On the other hand, a patient

who has undergone lung volume reduction surgery needs a very intensive physical programme, which can only take place in an in-patient setting.

Specific criteria for outpatient rehabilitation include:

1 The patients are in a stable state.
2 They are capable of maintaining an independent lifestyle.
3 They have no major psychological problems.
4 They have no extrapulmonary disease.

The main goals here are to alleviate dyspnoea, increase exercise tolerance and improve the quality of life. All targets can be achieved by exercise training, although other types of intervention are available in this setting when needed.

Inclusion criteria for home rehabilitation are, for example:

1 Newly diagnosed patients and those hospitalized for the first time .
2 Patients with recurrent exacerbations.
3 Patients who have previously received formal in-patient or outpatient rehabilitation.

When severe extrapulmonary disease and severe desaturation during exercise have been excluded, patients who meet the criteria for outpatient rehabilitation can also be included for home rehabilitation. Several studies have been published recently showing that rehabilitation in the home setting may improve exercise tolerance, dyspnoea and quality of life [29–32]. Some studies compared rehabilitation in the home setting with outpatient rehabilitation in different settings. Strijbos [32] *et al.* showed that after 12 weeks of rehabilitation in the home setting, long-term benefits can be achieved for walking distance and maximal exercise capacity. In contrast, patients who carried out the same programme in an outpatient setting could not maintain the positive initial effects. Puente-Maestu *et al.* compared a high-intensity training programme with frequent supervision in the outpatient setting with a low-intensity training programme (self-administered) in the home setting [33]. Patients who received supervised training in the outpatient setting showed a significantly higher VO_{2max} in the incremental test and an increased endurance time in comparison with the self-administered group. However, no significant differences in the effect on the quality of life were observed between the two groups. This suggests that high-intensity training is necessary to increase VO_{2max} and endurance capacity, while a low-intensity, self-administered programme is necessary to enhance the quality of life.

In summary, the complexity of the medical, psychological and social problems faced by a patient with COPD determines the staff needed for a rehabilitation programme and thus determines the appropriate setting. When the situation is less complex and less equipment/intervention is needed, patients can be trained both in an outpatient setting and at home.

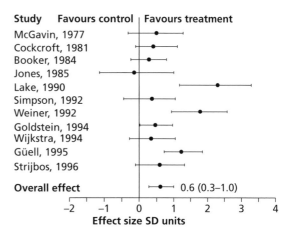

Study   Favours control Favours treatment
McGavin, 1977
Cockcroft, 1981
Booker, 1984
Jones, 1985
Lake, 1990
Simpson, 1992
Weiner, 1992
Goldstein, 1994
Wijkstra, 1994
Güell, 1995
Strijbos, 1996

Overall effect   0.6 (0.3–1.0)

        −2   −1   0   1   2   3   4
              Effect size SD units

Fig. 12.3 Effects of pulmonary rehabilitation in different studies on functional exercise tolerance (6-min walking distance) in chronic obstructive pulmonary disease patients. The effect size is shown with standard deviation [34].

What are the short-term effects of pulmonary rehabilitation?

A number of randomized controlled trials have shown that rehabilitation leads to short-term effects in patients with COPD [29,30,32,34]. In this chapter, we consider studies with a duration of a maximum of 6 months to be short-term. Important in this respect is to interpret these results in the light of the minimal clinically important difference (MCID). Looking at the MCID, it has been shown that rehabilitation relieves dyspnoea and improves control over COPD [35]. Although most rehabilitation studies do also report increased exercise tolerance, the value of this improvement is less clear (Fig. 12.3). In contrast, Celli concluded on basis of a number of controlled randomized trials that rehabilitation does improve exercise tolerance, dyspnoea and quality of life [36].

Positive results have been shown in different settings. Goldstein *et al.* set up a randomized controlled trial in which they assigned 89 patients (FEV_1 35% of predicted) to either an in-patient rehabilitation programme for 8 weeks, followed by an outpatient programme of 16 weeks, or to a conventional care programme consisting of medication alone [34]. Patients in the rehabilitation group showed an improved endurance capacity compared to the control group. In addition, they found a decrease in dyspnoea, fewer complaints with regard to emotional function and better control over the disease. Wijkstra *et al.* showed that patients after 12 weeks of home rehabilitation (FEV_1 44% of predicted; $n=30$) had significantly better exercise tolerance, a better quality of life, and fewer dyspnoea complaints during exercise compared to the controls [29]. It seems, therefore, that rehabilitation is equally successful in different settings. One Dutch study is important in this respect. Strijbos *et al.* compared home rehabilitation ($n=15$), outpatient rehabilitation ($n=15$)

and a control group ($n=15$) in COPD (FEV_1 41% of predicted) [32]. Patients received a 12-week programme consisting of visiting the physiotherapist twice weekly either at the outpatient clinic (outpatient group) or in their home town (home group). In addition, a nurse and a physician supervised the patients once a month. After 12 weeks, improved exercise tolerance and decreased dyspnoea were observed in both rehabilitation groups compared to the control group. In addition, both Dutch studies found a clinically relevant improvement in health status after 12 weeks of training. In contrast to the studies by Wijkstra and Strijbos, Wedzicha *et al.* showed that health status did not improve after home-based rehabilitation in patients with a FEV_1 of 0.9 L, which is lower than in the above-mentioned studies [37]. In this study, the patients were stratified according to their disability assessed by the MRC dyspnoea scale. The patients were randomized to receive outpatient rehabilitation if their dyspnoea was graded 3–4. They received home rehabilitation if their dyspnoea was graded as 5, meaning that they were too breathless to leave the house. Sixty patients were randomly assigned to the outpatient group, 30 received rehabilitation and 30 patients were included in the control group. Another 60 were included for home-based rehabilitation—i.e. 30 patients received exercise training by a local physiotherapist, while 30 patients were randomized to the control group. Patients receiving outpatient rehabilitation significantly improved their exercise tolerance and health status, assessed using the SGRQ, compared to the control group after 8 weeks of training. Although it is debatable whether the training intensity in the home rehabilitation group was high enough to achieve benefits, no significant improvements were shown in this group. This is the only study that has stratified patients according the severity of disability on the MRC dyspnoea scale, which makes this study unique. The study shows that the level of disability may influence the effects of rehabilitation, although it may be arguable whether these patients with complex problems (MRC dyspnoea scale 5) are the best candidates for home-based rehabilitation. Such patients might be better candidates for inpatient rehabilitation, as a multidisciplinary approach is needed. Still, the study by Wedzicha raises an important point, which may be particularly helpful in developing strategies to find good candidates for adequate rehabilitation in an appropriate setting.

What are the long-term effects?

Only a few studies are available investigating the long-term effects of pulmonary rehabilitation. Recently, an uncontrolled Italian study investigated the effects of an outpatient rehabilitation programme after 12 months [38]. The study included both asthmatics (FEV_1 64% of predicted) and COPD patients (FEV_1 43% of predicted). Patients received three 3-h sessions per week

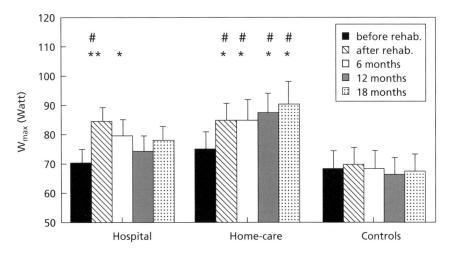

Fig. 12.4 Mean values (SEM) for maximal workload (W_{max}) reached during incremental symptom-limited cycle testing at visits 1–5. *, $P <0.05$; **, $P <0.005$ compared with baseline; #, $P <0.05$ compared with the control group [32].

for 8–10 weeks, including exercise training, upper and lower limb exercises, education and a nutritional programme. After 10 weeks, exercise tolerance and quality of life improved significantly in the COPD patients. However, only the improvements in quality of life were still present after 1 year. In contrast, Strijbos *et al.* did show more positive effects after home-based rehabilitation after 18 months [32]. This controlled trial compared home-based rehabilitation and outpatient rehabilitation with a control group. Patients received a programme of 12 weeks consisting of visiting the physiotherapist twice weekly either at the outpatient clinic (outpatient group) or in their own environment (home group). In addition, a nurse and a physician supervised the patients once a month. After this period of 12 weeks, no supervision was given. After 18 months, the home-based rehabilitation group showed a significantly improved maximal workload compared to the control group (Fig. 12.4), and a significantly improved walking distance compared to baseline. Both groups showed a significant improvement in well-being after 18 months. Another Dutch study that investigated the long-term effects of rehabilitation at home showed that health status improved, but exercise tolerance remained the same (Fig. 12.5) [39,40]. In contrast, exercise tolerance in the control group decreased significantly, whereas the health status remained unchanged.

Recently, a very interesting study was published by Griffiths *et al.* Two hundred patients with COPD, with a mean FEV_1 of 0.9 ± 0.4 L, were randomly assigned to a 6-week multidisciplinary outpatient rehabilitation programme (18 visits) or standard medical management [41]. After 1 year, there

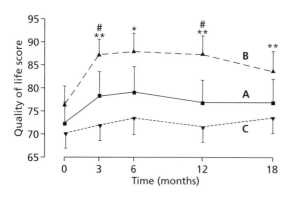

Fig. 12.5 Quality of life. Group A (rehabilitation group follow-up once a week); Group B (rehabilitation group follow-up once a month); Group C (control group, no rehabilitation at all). *, $P<0.05$; **, $P<0.01$ compared with baseline; #, $P<0.05$ compared with the control group [39].

was no difference between the rehabilitation group ($n=99$) and the control group ($n=101$) in the number of hospitalizations, but a significant difference was found in the number of days spent in hospital (mean 10.4±9.7 vs. 20.7± 20.7; $P=0.022$). Compared with the control group, the rehabilitation group also showed greater improvements in walking distance and in both general and specific health status.

Another randomized controlled trial was conducted in patients with moderate to severe COPD (FEV_1 35% of predicted) [42]. Thirty patients randomized to rehabilitation received 3 months of outpatient breathing retraining and chest physiotherapy, 3 months of daily supervised exercise and 6 months of weekly supervised breathing exercises. Significant differences were found between the groups in perception of dyspnoea, 6-minute walking distance, and day-to-day dyspnoea, fatigue and emotional function measured by the Chronic Respiratory Questionnaire. The improvements were maintained for a total period of 2 years. In addition, the rehabilitation group experienced a significant reduction in exacerbations.

At present only two studies have been published investigating the effects of pulmonary rehabilitation after 5 years. In the study by Ries *et al.*, 119 patients with COPD (FEV_1 1.2 L) were randomly assigned to either an 8-week comprehensive outpatient rehabilitation programme or an 8-week education programme [43]. Rehabilitation consisted of 12 4-h sessions including education, physical and respiratory care instruction, psychosocial support and supervised exercise training. Monthly supervision was given during the first year. The education group received four 2-h sessions about education. After 2 months, maximal exercise tolerance, endurance capacity, perceived breathlessness, and muscle fatigue all improved significantly compared to the education group. However, although these effects were still present after 1 year, they tended to diminish afterwards. A recently published abstract reported positive effects 5 years after home rehabilitation [44]. In this study, Strijbos *et al.* presented follow-up data from an earlier study [32] comparing home-based rehabilitation, outpatient rehabilitation, and a control group. After 5 years, the walking distance in the home rehabilitation group was still increased compared to the control group.

In summary, there is now enough evidence that rehabilitation leads to short-term benefits in quality of life, exercise tolerance and dyspnoea in patients with COPD. However, the long-term benefits are less clear. Home-based rehabilitation may be an attractive approach for maintaining long-term benefits, as the patients can incorporate what they learn into their daily lives more easily [1]. On the other hand, some patients with severe disability and handicap need a more multidisciplinary approach. These patients may be better candidates for rehabilitation in a centre (in-patient or outpatient).

What are the essential components of pulmonary rehabilitation?

A comprehensive rehabilitation programme consists of different components. The literature reports usually include the following elements: exercise training, specific limb training, respiratory muscle training, education, nutritional therapy, and psychosocial intervention. While everybody has the feeling that a multidisciplinary treatment is needed in some patients, there is no evidence yet that all components of rehabilitation are equally effective in reducing the level of disability or handicap.

Exercise training

Exercise training has been shown to be an effective element in several studies. An important study in this respect was by Ries *et al.*, comparing a comprehensive rehabilitation programme, including exercise training, with an educational programme [43]. After 2 months, the rehabilitation group showed improved exercise tolerance, exercise endurance, perceived breathlessness, and perceived muscle fatigue in comparison with the education group. Earlier, Toshima and colleagues came to similar conclusions [45]. This is very important, as it appears that exercise training can improve not only exercise tolerance but also dyspnoea, which is a important complaint in COPD.

Another issue is how patients with COPD should be trained. For a long time, it was commonly thought that no real physiological training response was possible in patients with COPD. A study by Casaburi *et al.* was very important in this respect. Exercise training at a high level of intensity (70% maximal workload) improved the maximal and submaximal exercise capacity more than exercise training at a lower level (30% maximal workload) [46]. The study also showed that a reduction in ventilation was significantly related to a decrease in lactate. The drawback of this study was that the patients only had moderate COPD (FEV_1 54% of predicted). The study by Maltais *et al.* is thus even more relevant, as it included patients with a FEV_1 of 1.0 L [47]. The authors showed that a 12-week leg cycling test resulted in a significant decrease in ventilation and lactate at the same workload. In addition, they showed that after training, the oxidative enzymes of the quadriceps muscle were increased, suggesting a true physiological training benefit. From these studies, it is known that patients with COPD can be trained in a physiological way and that the effects are greater when the training intensity is higher. The question is whether training continuously at a high level is of most benefit to a patient with severe COPD, when in view of the fact that interval training resembles the daily activity pattern best. A recent study by Coppoolse *et al.*, comparing continuous training with interval training, is interesting in this respect. Different physiological response patterns were shown, reflecting specific types of training in either oxidative or glycolytic pathways [48]. It is of interest to determine which type of exercise programme is beneficial to the individual patient.

On the basis of the literature reports, the ATS adopted the following training strategy [1]: a rehabilitation programme should contain exercise training for at least 4 weeks, and patients should receive endurance training for 20–30 min three to five times a week at a level of 60% of the maximal workload. However, not all patients can train at this high level. In these patients, interval training consisting of 2–3 min at high intensity (60–80% of the maximal workload), with equal periods of rest, might be an alternative approach.

Limb training

The endurance training discussed above is mostly carried out using walking, treadmill, and cycling exercises. Strength training of the lower limbs is an attractive approach, because peripheral muscle weakness contributes to exercise limitation in patients with COPD [21,22]. Two studies have investigated this issue. Simpson *et al.* showed that specific strength training improved muscle function by 16–40%, depending on the specific muscle that was trained [23]. They also found an increased endurance capacity and an improved quality of life. Clark *et al.* showed that a programme of low-intensity leg and arm exercises leads to an improved walking distance and demonstrated a physiological training response by showing a reduced ventilatory equivalent for oxygen and carbon dioxide [24].

Upper limb training is now generally recommended as part of the rehabilitation programme [1]. The beneficial effects of this training are reflected in reduced metabolic and ventilatory requirements, leading to an increase in endurance capacity in arm exercises [49,50]. However, there is no conclusive evidence that upper limb training is beneficial in addition to exercise training in improving functional status.

Inspiratory muscle training

Inspiratory muscle function may be impaired in patients with COPD, which may lead to dyspnoea [51], impaired exercise tolerance [23] and hypercapnia [52]. Several studies have therefore investigated the effects of inspiratory muscle training (IMT) on these parameters. IMT is generally started at a specific percentage of the maximal inspiratory pressure (PI_{max}). The minimum load for achieving a real training effect is 30% of the PI_{max}, which can be increased to 60–80%. Although most studies showed improved function of the inspiratory muscles after IMT [53–57], only a minority found a decrease in dyspnoea [55] or an improvement in exercise tolerance [54]. The reasons for these disappointing results might be an inadequate training protocol or not including appropriate patients in the study [58]. Gosselink and Decramer suggested that patients with ventilatory limitation might be ideal candidates [59]. In contrast to this, both Larson *et al.* [60] and Sanchez Riera *et al.* [61] recently showed positive results of IMT on both dyspnoea and exercise performance in patients with COPD in whom a ventilatory limitation was not established.

In summary, there is at present no strong evidence that IMT is beneficial in all patients with COPD. It might be beneficial in a specific group of patients with a ventilatory limitation. To further clarify the role of IMT in a rehabilitation programme, more needs to be known about the optimal candidates and how these patients should be trained.

Education

All rehabilitation programmes include education as an important component. Important topics normally addressed in educational programmes are: the anatomy and physiology of the lung, breathing strategies, medication, self-management skills, psychological factors (coping, anxiety, panic control), and smoking cessation [1]. Education may improve patients' active participation in a programme, improve understanding of the disease, and help patients and their family members to cope with the disabilities and handicaps due to the pulmonary disease [1]. However, no clear evidence has so far been found for the effects of education alone. Two studies, mentioned above, did not show any change in exercise tolerance or symptoms with education alone [43,45]. However, in these studies the education groups served mostly as control group in a trial of more comprehensive rehabilitation. At present, there has only been one randomized and controlled study comparing education sessions with written material only [62]. The authors found that the education sessions significantly improved the domains of social disability and knowledge of COPD. However, neither exercise parameters nor health-related quality of life were measured in this study.

Thus, although it is widely assumed that education is beneficial in rehabilitation, the influence of education as a sole component has not clearly been demonstrated. A possible explanation for these disappointing results is that sensitive tools are not available for measuring the effects of pure education adequately. It might be interesting to investigate whether education is effective as an adjunct to exercise training when such tools have been developed.

Nutrition

Weight loss is an important issue in patients with COPD. About 20–30% of COPD patients are underweight [63]. In addition, although some patients have normal weight, they may have a low fat-free mass (FFM) [64]. FFM and body weight are very important, as it has been shown that these are related to survival and exercise capacity [64,65]. Nutritional support was found to be beneficial in patients with COPD in improving respiratory and peripheral muscle strength, as well as improving exercise tolerance. In a large trial, Schols *et al.* investigated the physiological effects of daily nutritional supplements, alone or in combination with anabolic steroids, as an integrated part of a rehabilitation programme [66]. Treatment with exercise and nutrition resulted in increased weight, fat-free mass and PI_{max}. Another finding in this study was that not all patients responded to therapy—i.e. some did not gain weight or improve their respiratory muscle strength. It appeared that weight gain and increase in PI_{max} were related to improved survival. Cox regression analysis showed that weight gain and body mass index were significant predictors of survival (Fig. 12.6) [67]. In the recent ATS statement, it was therefore concluded that nutritional supplementation should be considered for patients with COPD suffering from involuntary weight loss and for all depleted patients. It is recommended to give oral or enteral protein and caloric support to achieve a positive energy balance, in combination with exercise as an anabolic stimulus to enhance FFM. The reason for the failure to respond to nutrition is not clear, but some hypermetabolic patients showed elevated levels of acute-phase proteins, suggesting that systemic inflammation is responsible for tissue depletion [68]. If this hypothesis is correct, it means that caloric support alone is not sufficient to increase weight and FFM.

Psychosocial intervention

Psychosocial intervention is mostly needed in a rehabilitation programme when there are problems such as anxiety, depression and difficulties in coping

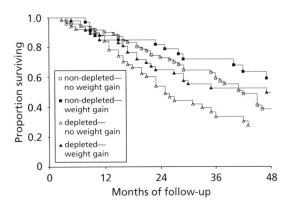

Fig. 12.6 Weight gain (>2 kg/8 weeks) after intervention predicts improved survival in patients with chronic obstructive pulmonary disease [62].

with the chronic disease. Intervention can be given in the form of a regular education session, on an individual basis or in a group. The effectiveness of this type of intervention is not clearly established. Ries *et al.* found no significant changes in depression after outpatient rehabilitation, although the self-assessed efficacy for walking distance improved [43]. In contrast, Dekhuijzen *et al.* showed a beneficial effect on anxiety and depression [69]. These studies, however, used different outcome measures, so that it is difficult to draw conclusions. At present, although it is assumed that psychological interventions are needed in some patients, there is no convincing evidence in the literature that this is beneficial.

What are the effects of pulmonary rehabilitation on health-care costs and survival?

The costs of caring for patients with COPD are extremely high in comparison with those with asthma, mostly due to the high costs of hospitalization and chronic oxygen therapy in patients with COPD. It is therefore important to look very carefully at all treatments that might reduce the number and duration of hospitalizations. Several uncontrolled trials suggest that pulmonary rehabilitation is effective in decreasing the number of hospital days and number of hospitalizations [70–72]. Hudson *et al.* followed up 64 patients for 4 years [70]. They showed that for the 44 patients who were alive after 4 years, the total number of days of hospitalization decreased from 529 in the year prior to the study to 207 in the last year of the study. Recently, an Italian uncontrolled study also showed a significant reduction in the number of hospitalizations compared to the period before rehabilitation started [38]. However, these positive effects have not yet been confirmed in controlled studies. The most important study in this respect is by Ries *et al.* [43]. Patients received either an 8-week comprehensive outpatient rehabilitation programme or an 8-week

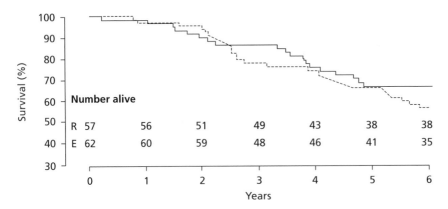

Fig. 12.7 Survival in patients with chronic obstructive pulmonary disease following a rehabilitation programme (R, solid line) and control COPD patients following an education programme (E, dashed line). No significant differences were found between the two groups [40].

education programme. During the first year, the patients were supervised once a month. The study showed that the rehabilitation group tended to have fewer hospitalization days after rehabilitation compared to the education group, but the difference did not reach significance ($P=0.2$). Also, there was no difference in the survival between the two groups (Fig. 12.7).

Recently, Griffiths *et al.* investigated the difference in mean costs and in quality-adjusted life years (QALYs) of 12 months of care after either a 6-week outpatient multidisciplinary programme or standard medical treatment [73]. They showed that the programme resulted in an increase in the mean number of QALYs of 0.03 per patient ($P=0.03$). Their conclusion was that the programme was cost-effective and even more effective in comparison with the programme used by Goldstein *et al.* [74], which incorporated a substantial period of in-patient care.

There have also been a few studies carrying out cost–benefit analyses of home-based rehabilitation. Campbell-Haggerty *et al.* [72] included 20 patients with a mean FEV_1 of 700 mL in a so-called 'respi-care' programme, which was coordinated by a hospital-based pulmonary nurse specialist, advised by a pulmonologist. The 'respi-care' service included nursing visits every week and respiratory therapy and social service every 2 weeks. The mean time that the patients participated in the study was 19 months (range 6–37 months). Each subject was matched for an equal length of time before entering the programme. The 'respi-care' programme resulted in a significant decrease in hospital days and emergency room visits and a reduction in costs of $328 per patient per month. These results were supported by the study by Roselle *et al.* [75], who included 418 patients with COPD in a programme consisting of home visits by a professional nurse at a minimum of once every 30 days. The patients were also visited by a respiratory therapist, as determined by the patient's needs. Compared to the period before the patients entered the programme, there was a significant decrease in the length of hospital stay (from 18.3 days to 6.1 days), resulting in cost savings of $2625 per patient for 1 year. In our own study [39], we retrospectively examined the costs of a home programme and compared them with the costs of an outpatient programme. The costs of a home programme, with a local physiotherapist visiting once a week for 18 months, were 50% lower compared to a once-weekly visit to the outpatient clinic ($2300 versus $4250 per patient for 18 months). The difference was mainly due to the costs for the patients of travelling to the hospital for the outpatient programme.

What are the conclusive effects of rehabilitation and what questions remain?

Although there is no ideal candidate for rehabilitation, it seems that patients with impaired muscle function, decreased exercise tolerance, severe complaints of dyspnoea, and a poor quality of life may be good candidates for inclusion. Based on the level of disability and handicap, the patients must receive an individually tailored programme, supervised by the staff they need. The complexity of medical and psychosocial factors determines the appropriate setting for rehabilitation—in-patient, outpatient, or home-based.

There is now conclusive evidence that rehabilitation is effective in improving dyspnoea, exercise tolerance, and quality of life. However, these positive effects are generally not maintained for a long period. More attention therefore needs to be given to long-term adherence to rehabilitation measures. Although some deterioration is certainly due to the progress of the disease, the question is whether this process can be stopped with maintenance exercise programmes.

Exercise training is the cornerstone of any type of rehabilitation programme. Although it can be assumed that other components such as education and nutrition are probably beneficial, scientific evidence for this is lacking. Further investigations should focus on the additional aspects of education, breathing retraining, psychosocial interventions, nutrition and specific muscle training.

COPD patients with severe respiratory insufficiency can sometimes not be trained adequately. These patients might benefit from giving the muscles some rest during the night with non-invasive positive-pressure ventilation (NIPPV). The results so far have not been encouraging, but in a selected group of patients—i.e. those with increasing hypercapnia during the night—beneficial effects have been found.

Some studies have suggested that rehabilitation is cost-effective and that outpatient rehabilitation may be cheaper than in-patient programmes, but it is still too early for firm conclusions to be drawn.

Finally, the primary goal of pulmonary rehabilitation is to optimize the patient's social performance and autonomy, as stated in the definition at the beginning of this chapter. This means that we must focus in further research on developing sensitive instruments that can measure changes in activities of daily living (ADL) after rehabilitation. Rehabilitation is beneficial for individual patients with severe COPD if their ADL can be increased, thereby improving their level of independence.

References

1 American Thoracic Society. Pulmonary rehabilitation: 1999. *Am J Respir Crit Care Med* 1999; **159**: 1666–82.

2 World Health Organization. *The International Classification of Impairments, Disabilities and Handicaps.* Geneva: WHO, 1980.

3 Wijkstra PJ, Tenvergert EM, van der Mark TW *et al*. Relation of lung function, maximal inspiratory pressure, dyspnoea, and quality of life with exercise capacity in patients with chronic obstructive pulmonary disease. *Thorax* 1994; **49**: 468–72.

4 Swinburn CR, Wakefield JM, Jones PW. Performance, ventilation and oxygen consumption in three different types of exercise tests in patients with chronic lung disease. *Thorax* 1985; **40**: 581–6.

5 Borg G. Psychophysical bases of perceived exertion. *Med Sci Sports Exerc* 1982; **5**: 377–81.

6 Mahler DA, Weinberg DH, Wells CK, Feinstein AR. The measurement of dyspnea: contents, interobserver correlates of two new clinical indices. *Chest* 1985; **85**: 751–8.

7 O'Reilly JF, Shaylor JM, Fromings KM, Harrison BDW. The use of the 12 minute walking test in assessing the effect of oral steroid therapy in patients with chronic airways obstruction. *Br J Dis Chest* 1982; **76**: 374–82.

8 McGavin CR, Artvinli M, Naoe H, McHardy GJR. Dyspnea, disability and distance walked: comparison of estimates of exercise performance in respiratory disease. *BMJ* 1978; **2**: 241–3.

9 McSweeny AJ, Grant I, Heaton RK, Adams KM, Timms RM. Life quality of patients with chronic obstructive pulmonary disease. *Arch Intern Med* 1982; **142**: 473–8.

10 Prigatano GP, Wright EC, Levin D. Quality of life and its predictors in patients with mild hypoxemia and chronic obstructive pulmonary disease. *Arch Intern Med* 1984; **144**: 1613–19.

11 Schrier AC, Dekker FW, Kaptein AA, Dijkman JH. Quality of life in elderly patients with chronic non-specific lung disease in family practice. *Chest* 1990; **98**: 894–9.

12 Traver GA. Measures of symptoms and quality of life to predict emergent use of institutional health care resources in chronic obstructive pulmonary disease. *Heart Lung* 1988; **17**: 689–97.

13 Kaplan RM, Atkins CJ, Timms R. Validity of a well-being scale as an outcome measure in chronic obstructive pulmonary disease. *J Chron Dis* 1984; **37**: 85–95.

14 Bergner M, Bobbitt RA, Carter WB, Gilson BS. The Sickness Impact Profile: development and final revision of a health status measure. *Med Care* 1981; **19**: 787–805.

15 Jones PW, Quirk FH, Baveystock CM, Littlejohns P. A self-complete measure of health status for chronic airflow limitation. *Am Rev Respir Dis* 1992; **145**: 1321–7.

16 Guyatt GH, Berman LB, Townsend M, Pugsley SO, Chambers LW. A measure of quality of life for clinical trials in chronic lung disease. *Thorax* 1987; **42**: 773–8.

17 Guyatt GH, Townsend M, Pugsley SO *et al*. Measuring functional status in chronic lung disease: conclusions from a

randomized control trial. *Respir Med* 1989; **83**: 293–7.

18 Morgan AD, Peck DF, Buchanan DR, McHardy GJR. Psychological factors contributing to disproportionate disability in chronic bronchitis. 1983; **27**: 259–63.

19 Zu Wallack RL, Patel K, Reardon Z *et al*. Predictors of improvement in the 12-MWD following a six-week outpatient pulmonary rehabilitation programme. *Chest* 1991; **99**: 805–8.

20 Maltais F, Leblanc P, Jobin J *et al*. Intensity of training and physiologic adaptation in patients with COPD. *Am J Crit Care Med* 1997; **155**: 555–61.

21 Hamilton N, Killian KJ, Summers E, Jones NL. Muscle strength, symptom intensity, and exercise capacity in patients with cardiorespiratory disorders. *Am J Respir Crit Care Med* 1995; **152**: 2021–31.

22 Gosselink R, Troosters T, Decramer M. Peripheral muscle weakness contributes to exercise limitation in COPD. *Am J Respir Crit Care Med* 1996; **153**: 976–80.

23 Simpson K, Killian KJ, McCartney N *et al*. Randomised controlled trial of weightlifting exercise patients with chronic airflow limitation. *Thorax* 1992; **47**: 70–5.

24 Clark CJ, Cochrane JE, Mackay E. Low intensity peripheral muscle conditioning improves exercise tolerance and breathlessness in COPD. *Eur Respir J* 1996; **9**: 2590–6.

25 Celli BR. Pulmonary rehabilitation in patients with COPD. *Am J Respir Crit Care Med* 1995; **152**: 861–4.

26 American College of Chest Physicians, American Association of Cardiovascular and Pulmonary Rehabilitation. Pulmonary rehabilitation: joint ACCP/AACVPR evidence-based guidelines. ACCP/AACVPR Pulmonary Rehabilitation Guidelines Panel. *Chest* 1997; **112**: 1363–96.

27 Wijkstra PJ, Jones PW. Quality of life in patients with COPD. *Eur Respir Mon* 1998; **7**: 235–46.

28 Donner CF, Muir JF. Selection criteria and programmes for pulmonary rehabilitation with in COPD patients. Rehabilitation and Chronic Care Scientific Group. *Eur Respir J* 1997; **10**: 744–57.

29 Wijkstra PJ, van Altena R, Kraan J *et al*. Quality of life in patients with chronic obstructive pulmonary disease improves after rehabilitation at home. *Eur Respir J* 1994; **7**: 269–73.

30 Wijkstra PJ, Van de Mark THW, Kran J. Effects of home rehabilitation on physical performance in patients with COPD. *Eur Respir J* 1996; **9**: 104–10.

31 Cambach W, Chadwick-Straver RVM, Wagenaar RC, Keimpema van ARJ, Kemper HCG. The effects of a community-based pulmonary rehabilitation programme on exercise tolerance and quality of life: a randomized controlled trial. *Eur Respir J* 1997; **10**: 104–13.

32 Strijbos JH, Postma DS, Altena van R, Gimeno F, Koëter GH. A comparison between an outpatient hospital-based pulmonary rehabilitation programme and home-care pulmonary rehabilitation programme in patients with COPD. *Chest* 1996; **109**: 366–72.

33 Puente-Maestu L, Sanz ML, Sanz P *et al*. Comparison of effects of supervised versus self-monitored training programmes in patients with chronic obstructive pulmonary disease. *Eur Respir J* 2000; **15**: 517–25.

34 Goldstein RS, Gort EH, Stubbing H *et al*. Randomised controlled trial of respiratory rehabilitation. *Lancet* 1994; **344**: 1394–7.

35 Lacasse Y, Wong E, Guyatt GH *et al*. Meta-analysis of respiratory rehabilitation in COPD. *Lancet* 1996; **348**: 1115–19.

36 Celli BR. Is pulmonary rehabilitation an effective treatment for COPD? [editorial]. *Am J Respir Crit Care Med* 1997; **155**: 781–3.

37 Wedzicha JA, Bestall JC, Garrod R *et al*. Randomized controlled trial of pulmonary rehabilitation in severe chronic obstructive pulmonary disease patients stratified with the MRC dyspnoea scale. *Eur Respir J* 1998; **12**: 363–9.

38 Foglio K, Bianchi L, Bruletti G *et al*. Long term effectiveness of pulmonary rehabilitation in patients with chronic airway obstruction. *Eur Respir J* 1999; **13**: 125–32.

39 Wijkstra PJ, van der Mark THW *et al*. Long-term effects of home rehabilitation on physical performance in chronic obstructive pulmonary disease. *Am J Respir Crit Care Med* 1996; **153**: 1234–41.

40 Wijkstra PJ, TenVergert EM, van Altena R et al. Long-term effects of rehabilitation at home on quality of life and exercise tolerance in patients with chronic obstructive pulmonary disease. *Thorax* 1995; **50**: 824–8.

41 Griffiths TL, Burr ML, Campbell IA et al. Results at 1 year of outpatient multidisciplinary pulmonary rehabilitation: a randomised controlled trial. *Lancet* 2000; **355**: 362–8.

42 Guell R, Casan P, Belda J et al. Long-term effects of outpatient rehabilitation of COPD: a randomized trial. *Chest* 2000; **117**: 976–83.

43 Ries AL, Kaplan RM, Limberg TM, Prewitt LM. Effects of pulmonary rehabilitation on physiologic and psychosocial outcomes in patients with chronic pulmonary disease. *Ann Intern Med* 1995; **122**: 823–32.

44 Strijbos JH, Wijkstra PJ, Postma DS, Koeter GH. Five year effects of rehabilitation at different settings in patients with COPD [abstract]. *ERS Madrid* 1999; **209**: 15s.

45 Toshima MT, Kaplan RM, Ries AL. Experimental evaluation of rehabilitation in chronic obstructive pulmonary disease: the short term effects on exercise tolerance and health status. *Health Psychol* 1990; **9**: 237–52.

46 Casaburi R, Patessio A, Ioli F et al. Reductions in exercise lactic acidosis and ventilation as a result of exercise training in patients with obstructive lung disease. *Am Rev Respir Dis* 1991; **143**: 9–18.

47 Maltais F, Leblanc P, Simard J et al. Skeletal muscle adaptation to endurance training in patients with COPD. *Am J Respir Crit Care Med* 1996; **154**: 442–7.

48 Coppoolse R, Schols AMWJ, Baarends EM et al. Interval versus continuous training in patients with severe COPD: a randomised clinical trial. *Eur Respir J* 1999; **14**: 258–63.

49 Celli B, Criner G, Rassulo J. Ventilatory muscle recruitment during unsupported arm exercise in normal subjects. *J Appl Physiol* 1988; **64**: 1936–41.

50 Martinez FJ, Couser JI, Celli BR. Respiratory response to arm elevation in patients with chronic airflow limitation. *Am Rev Respir Dis* 1991; **143**: 476–80.

51 Killian KJ, Jones NL. Respiratory muscles and dyspnoea. *Clin Chest Med* 1988; **9**: 237–48.

52 Begin P, Grassino A. Inspiratory muscle dysfunction and chronic hypercapnia in COPD. *Am Rev Respir Dis* 1991; **143**: 905–12.

53 Belman MJ, Shadmehr R. Targeted resistive ventilatory muscle training in chronic pulmonary disease. *J Appl Phys* 1988; **65**: 2726–35.

54 Dekhuijzen PN, Folgering HTM, van Herwaarden CL. Target-flow inspiratory muscle training during pulmonary rehabilitation in patients with COPD. *Chest* 1991; **99**: 128–33.

55 Harver A, Mahler DA, Daubenspeck JA. Targeted inspiratory muscle training improves respiratory muscle function and reduces dyspnoea in patients with COPD. *Ann Intern Med* 1989; **111**: 117–24.

56 Preusser B, Winningham ML, Clanton TL. High versus low-intensity inspiratory muscle interval training in patients with COPD. *Chest* 1994; **105**: 106–17.

57 Weiner P, Azgad Y, Ganam R, Weiner M. Inspiratory muscle training in patients with bronchial asthma. *Chest* 1992; **102**: 1357–61.

58 Smith K, Cook D, Guyatt GH et al. Respiratory muscle training in chronic airflow obstruction. *Am Rev Respir Dis* 1992; **145**: 533–9.

59 Gosselink R, Decramer M. Inspiratory muscle training: where are we? *Eur Respir J* 1994; **7**: 2103–5.

60 Larson JL, Covey MK, Wirtz SE et al. Cycle ergometer and inspiratory muscle training in chronic obstructive pulmonary disease. *Am J Respir Crit Care Med* 1999; **160**: 500–7.

61 Sanchez Riera H, Montemayor Rubio T, Ortega Ruiz F et al. Inspiratory muscle training in patients with COPD: effect on dyspnea, exercise performance, and quality of life. *Chest* 2001; **120**: 748–56.

62 Ashikaga T, Vacek PM, Lewis SO. Evaluation of a community based education programme for individuals with COPD. *J Rehabil* 1980; **46**: 23–7.

63 Engelen MKPJ, Schols AMWJ, Baken WC et al. Nutritional depletion in relation to respiratory and peripheral muscle function in outpatients with COPD. *Eur Respir J* 1993; **7**: 1793–7.

64 Schols AMWJ, Soeters PB, Dingemans AMC. Prevalence and characteristics of

nutritional depletion in patients with stable COPD eligible for pulmonary rehabilitation. *Am Rev Respir Dis* 1993; **147**: 1151–6.

65 Schols AMWJ, Mostert R, Soeters PB. Body composition and exercise performance in patients with COPD. *Thorax* 1991; **46**: 695–9.

66 Schols AMWJ, Soeters PB, Mostert R *et al*. Physiologic effect of nutritional support and anabolic steroids in patients with COPD: a placebo controlled randomised trial. *Am J Respir Crit Care Med* 1995; **152**: 1268–74.

67 Schols AMWJ, Slangen J, Volovics A, Wouters EFM. Weight loss is a reversible factor of COPD. *Am J Respir Crit Care Med* 1998; **157**: 1791–7.

68 Schols AM, Buurman WA, Staal van den Brekel AJ, Dentener MA, Wouters EF. Evidence for a relation between metabolic derangements and increased levels of inflammatory mediators in a subgroup of patients with chronic obstructive pulmonary disease. *Thorax* 1996; **51**: 819–24.

69 Dekhuijzen PNR, Beek MML, Folgering HTHM, Herwaarden van CLA. Psychological changes during pulmonary rehabilitation and target-flow inspiratory muscle training in COPD patients with a ventilatory limitation during exercise. *Int J Rehab Res* 1990; **13**: 109–17.

70 Hudson LD, Tyler ML, Petty TL. Hospitalization needs during outpatient rehabilitation for severe chronic airway obstruction. *Chest* 1976; **70**: 606–10.

71 Petty T, Nett LM, Finigan MM *et al*. A comprehensive program for chronic airway obstruction: methods and preliminary evaluation of symptomatic and functional improvement. *Ann Intern Med* 1969; **70**: 1109–20.

72 Campbell-Haggerty M, Stockdale-Woolley R, Nair S. Respi-care: an innovative home care program for the patient with chronic obstructive pulmonary disease. *Chest* 1991; **100**: 607–12.

73 Griffiths TL, Phillips CJ, Davies S, Burr ML, Campbell IA. Cost-effectiveness of an outpatient multidisciplinary pulmonary rehabilitation programme. *Thorax* 2001; **56**: 779–84.

74 Goldstein RS, Gort EH, Guyatt GH *et al*. Economic analysis of respiratory rehabilitation. *Chest* 1997; **112**: 370–9.

75 Roselle S, D'Amico FJ. The effect of respiratory therapy on hospital readmission rates of patients with chronic obstructive pulmonary disease. *Respir Care* 1982; **27**: 1194–9.

13: Oxygen therapy — is it possible to prescribe rationally and objectively?

Louise Restrick

Background

Oxygen therapy, when prescribed rationally, is an extremely important and effective intervention in chronic obstructive pulmonary disease (COPD). It is the only treatment, apart from stopping smoking, that reduces mortality. It is imperative that patients with COPD who would benefit from oxygen therapy are identified and treated. There are four principal situations in which oxygen therapy is used in patients with COPD and hypoxaemia. These are:
- Acutely, during exacerbations
- Long-term oxygen therapy (LTOT)
- Short-burst therapy
- Ambulatory oxygen

The rationales for treatment, and hence the objectives of therapy, are different in each of these situations. Each therefore needs to be considered separately.

Acute oxygen therapy in COPD

In the acute situation, the aim of oxygen prescription is to correct severe or life-threatening hypoxaemia, without causing unacceptable hypercapnia. The use of controlled oxygen therapy in acute severe exacerbations of COPD, or pneumonia in COPD, is well established. For patients with hypercapnoeic respiratory failure, it may be used with non-invasive ventilation and/or respiratory stimulants to prevent dangerous hypercapnoea when the respiratory drive is lost as hypoxaemia is corrected. As the focus of this chapter is on oxygen therapy in the community, either as long-term regular treatment or as intermittent therapy, acute oxygen therapy in hospital will not be considered further. However, patients' and, sometimes, health-care professionals' experiences of acute oxygen therapy in hospital often determine expectations for oxygen therapy in chronic stable situations where the objectives of treatment are different and do not involve the correction of severe, life-threatening hypoxaemia.

Long-term oxygen therapy

The rationale of long-term oxygen therapy (LTOT) for patients with COPD is based on a theoretical desirability of correcting chronic hypoxaemia over the long term, rather than on concern about acute hypoxaemia. Patients with severe COPD develop chronic hypoxaemia, which leads to pulmonary hypertension, cor pulmonale, secondary polycythaemia and reduced survival. The rationale for LTOT is to prevent or slow these complications of chronic hypoxaemia and improve survival. Two large randomized trials demonstrated that LTOT does indeed improve survival in hypoxaemic patients with COPD [1,2]. The aim of LTOT is to improve survival by the regular use of oxygen for sufficient hours to prevent the complications of chronic hypoxaemia in COPD. The aim of LTOT is commonly misunderstood; it is not to improve breathlessness, nor for the majority of patients is it needed to correct life-threatening hypoxaemia. A domiciliary oxygen concentrator is the most commonly used method for providing LTOT.

Short-burst therapy

Many patients with COPD also have oxygen cylinders, which they use for short-burst therapy. The rationale for this treatment is symptomatic improvement of episodes of breathlessness. Oxygen is used for short periods during episodes of increased breathlessness, or before or after exercise.

Ambulatory oxygen therapy

This is oxygen carried by the patient, either as a lightweight cylinder of gaseous oxygen, or a liquid oxygen cylinder, and used on exercise. The aim of ambulatory oxygen therapy is to increase exercise tolerance and reduce breathlessness on exercise. Its main purpose is not to increase the hours of use of LTOT, nor to correct life-threatening hypoxaemia, although these may be reasons for use in some patients.

Assessment and rational prescribing of LTOT, short-burst therapy, or ambulatory oxygen all need to be based on the different objectives for use in each of these situations, where there is evidence to support the practice. The UK Department of Health commissioned the Royal College of Physicians of London to produce clinical guidelines and advice for prescribers in the UK on domiciliary oxygen therapy services in COPD and other diseases, which were published in 1999 [3]. These comprehensive guidelines cover LTOT, short-burst therapy and ambulatory therapy. The guidelines for LTOT, which are largely evidence-based, have hardly changed since the original guidelines for the prescription of domiciliary oxygen concentrators were introduced in 1985. In contrast, many of the recommendations—particularly relating to short-burst therapy and ambulatory oxygen—are largely based on consensus expert opinion, as is acknowledged in the report.

Are the UK guidelines for prescription of LTOT correct?

The British Medical Research Council (MRC) study [1] and the American Nocturnal Oxygen Therapy Trial (NOTT or NOT Trial) [2], published in the early 1980s, demonstrated that oxygen for more than 15 h per day improved survival in hypoxaemic patients with severe COPD. This led to the original definition of LTOT as 'the provision of oxygen for 15 h or more a day for a prolonged period'. Most patients using LTOT do not need to be on continuous oxygen with the associated implications of restricted mobility, although survival with LTOT improves as the hours of daily use are increased from 15 h to 20 h [1,2]. However, there is a small group of patients with COPD who have very severe chronic hypoxaemia, and in these patients oxygen, provided by a concentrator (and cylinders), is used continuously in an attempt to correct life-threatening hypoxaemia as well as to prevent the complications of chronic hypoxaemia.

The recommended [3] indications for LTOT in COPD are that:

1   PaO_2 is less than 7.3 kPa (55 mmHg); or
2   PaO_2 is between 7.3 kPa and 8 kPa (55 mmHg and 60 mmHg), with:
  (a)   Secondary polycythaemia
  (b)   Peripheral oedema
  (c)   Pulmonary hypertension
  (d)   Nocturnal hypoxaemia.

The patient should be assessed when breathing air and clinically stable for the previous 4 weeks. These recommendations are mainly derived from the MRC study of 87 patients and the NOT Trial involving 203 patients [1,2]. These landmark studies used different designs, but in neither was the patient blinded to the treatment. This would have required a comparison with 'sham' oxygen, i.e. air, delivered to the patient, in comparison with oxygen. In the MRC study [1], oxygen prescribed for at least 15 h per day was compared with a control group who did not have oxygen. Mortality over 5 years was reduced from 67% in the control group to 45% in the group treated with oxygen. While the treated group was prescribed at least 15 h of oxygen, actual use was not measured. In the NOT Trial [2], nocturnal oxygen therapy was compared with continuous oxygen therapy. Mortality was halved at 2 years, from 44% in the group receiving oxygen overnight to 22% in the group receiving continuous oxygen therapy. Mean oxygen use in the NOT Trial was 12 h in the nocturnal oxygen therapy group and 18 h in the continuous oxygen use group over an average period of 19 months.

Arterial oxygen tension (PaO_2) less than 7.3 kPa (55 mmHg)

A PaO_2 of up to 8 kPa (60 mmHg) was the entry criterion for PaO_2 for the MRC study [1]. The main entry criterion for PaO_2 for the NOT Trial was a PaO_2 below 7.3 kPa (55 mmHg), although patients with a PaO_2 of up to 8 kPa (60 mmHg) were included if they also had oedema, secondary polycythaemia, or significant pulmonary hypertension [2]. The mean PaO_2 of patients entering both studies was 6.8 kPa (51 mmHg). The widely used cut-off PaO_2 of 7.3 kPa (55 mmHg) for the prescription of LTOT in guidelines therefore describes the majority of patients entering these two studies in which LTOT improved survival.

PaO_2 between 7.3 kPa and 8 kPa (55 mmHg and 60 mmHg)

The range of PaO_2 between 7.3 and 8 kPa (55 mmHg and 60 mmHg) remains a grey area. From the MRC and NOT Trial, it is not clear whether LTOT has a beneficial effect on prognosis for these patients. This question was addressed by a randomized controlled trial in 135 Polish patients with COPD [4]. These patients had a PaO_2 between 7.4 kPa (55.5 mmHg) and 8.7 kPa (65.3 mmHg), with mean PaO_2 8 kPa (60 mmHg). LTOT, over at least 3 years, was not associated with a survival benefit, and there was no difference in survival between the patients with a PaO_2 above or below 8 kPa (60 mmHg). However, the mean daily use of oxygen was only 13.5 h.

Patients with a PaO_2 between 7.3 kPa and 8 kPa (55 mmHg and 60 mmHg) and secondary polycythaemia, peripheral oedema, evidence of pulmonary hypertension or nocturnal hypoxaemia (defined as oxygen saturation (SaO_2) below 90% for at least 30% of the night [5]), are specifically recommended for LTOT [3].

Secondary polycythaemia and peripheral oedema are relatively easy to detect clinically and were features of the patients in the MRC study and the NOT Trial [1,2]. This is not the case for either pulmonary hypertension or nocturnal hypoxaemia. Patients with pulmonary hypertension were included in the NOT Trial, but not in the MRC study. Pulmonary hypertension was defined electrocardiographically by a 3-mm P pulmonale in leads II, III and aVF [2]. The diagnosis of pulmonary hypertension clinically is imprecise and is left at the discretion of the clinician in the 1999 UK guidelines [3]. The majority of patients with severe COPD and a PaO_2 of less than 8 kPa (60 mmHg) will have some pointers of pulmonary hypertension—for example, prominent pulmonary arteries on their chest radiograph. Those clinicians wanting to prescribe LTOT for patients with a PaO_2 up to 8 kPa (60 mmHg) can therefore do so within the guidelines, by choosing a lower threshold for making a clinical diagnosis of pulmonary hypertension. However, there is no direct evidence for

LTOT being of benefit in this group of patients with a clinical diagnosis of pulmonary hypertension.

The specific criterion of nocturnal hypoxaemia with a PaO_2 between 7.3 kPa and 8 kPa (55 mmHg and 60 mmHg) for the provision of LTOT is more controversial. Nocturnal hypoxaemia due to nocturnal hypoventilation is well recognized in COPD and can lead to pulmonary hypertension [6,7]. There are two randomized controlled trials of nocturnal oxygen in patients with COPD and nocturnal hypoxaemia [8,9]. However, in both studies, the mean PaO_2 at entry was above 8 kPa (60 mmHg). In the Fletcher et al. study of seven patients treated with nocturnal oxygen and nine patients given sham oxygen, with a mean PaO_2 at entry of about 10 kPa (75 mmHg), there was no effect of oxygen on mortality over 3 years [8]. There were no significant differences in pulmonary artery pressure between the nocturnal oxygen and control groups, either at the start or end of the study. However, at 3 years there was a small increase in pulmonary artery pressure in the untreated group and a small reduction in pulmonary artery pressure in the group treated with nocturnal oxygen; the change in pulmonary artery pressure was significantly different between the groups.

In the second larger study of 76 patients with nocturnal desaturation, with a mean PaO_2 at entry of 8.4 kPa (63 mmHg), there was also no difference in mortality at 2 years between patients receiving nocturnal oxygen and those who did not [9]. Nocturnal oxygen did not allow delay in the prescription of LTOT and had no effect on pulmonary haemodynamics in this study. There are no controlled trials of patients with nocturnal hypoxaemia and a daytime PaO_2 between 7.3 kPa and 8 kPa (55 mmHg and 60 mmHg). While LTOT may prevent, delay, or reverse the progression of pulmonary hypertension [10], this may not be of large enough benefit to translate into improved survival. The main determinant of survival in COPD is the severity of airway obstruction, and the only measure that has an effect on progression of airway obstruction is smoking cessation.

The recommendation to prescribe LTOT for patients with moderate hypoxaemia—PaO_2 between 7.3 kPa and 8 kPa (55 mmHg and 60 mmHg)—and clinically determined pulmonary hypertension or nocturnal hypoxaemia is therefore based on extrapolation of physiological data, rather than data showing improved survival. This recommendation has service and cost implications that need to be taken into account.

The implication of including nocturnal hypoxaemia as a criterion for prescribing LTOT in COPD is that patients with a daytime PaO_2 between 7.3 kPa and 8 kPa (55 mmHg and 60 mmHg) will have to be screened for nocturnal hypoxaemia with overnight oximetry. The prevalence of nocturnal hypoxaemia in this group is high, and its severity is directly related to the severity of the daytime hypoxaemia [7]. Nocturnal hypoxaemia was present in 43% of patients with a daytime PaO_2 between 8 kPa and 9.3 kPa (60 mmHg and 69.8 mmHg) [5]. The prevalence is likely to be even higher in those with a daytime PaO_2 between 7.3 kPa and 8 kPa (55 mmHg and 60 mmHg). This will therefore require significant resources to implement.

A more cost-effective use of resources to improve prognosis in COPD is likely to be screening for severe hypoxaemia in patients with severe COPD in the community, so that all patients with a PaO_2 less than 7.3 kPa (55 mmHg) receive LTOT. It has been estimated that there may be 60 000 individuals with COPD in England and Wales who would meet the criteria for the prescription of LTOT [11]. However, the numbers of patients on LTOT are much less than the estimates [12]. Currently, there are approximately 20 000 patients in the UK with oxygen concentrators. Screening by oximetry in the community has been shown to be effective in practice [13], and the benefit of LTOT for this group of patients is proven. The Cochrane review [14] of LTOT for patients with COPD and a PaO_2 below 7.3 kPa (55 mmHg) calculated a number needed to treat (NNT) of 4.5 from the MRC study [1], i.e. treating five patients with LTOT would save one life over 5 years. Identifying and treating those patients with COPD who are not on LTOT and should be is a serious problem that can and needs to be addressed as a high priority.

Patients with COPD and additional reasons for nocturnal hypoxaemia — e.g. previous thoracoplasty, obstructive sleep apnoea — need to have formal sleep studies performed, as oximetry is not sufficient to evaluate these patients [15]. Nocturnal oxygen therapy may be prescribed with non-invasive ventilation (NIV) or continuous positive airway pressure (CPAP) for some of these patients.

Other criteria for prescription of LTOT

It is important that patients are assessed when they are clinically stable. The gradual improvement in PaO_2 after an acute exacerbation is well recognized [1]. Nonetheless, in the UK significant numbers of prescriptions are still inappropriately initiated when the patient is unstable, often at the time of hospital discharge. Of 176 patients on LTOT in London, 25% did not meet the criteria for hypoxaemia [16]. Out of more than 500 Scottish patients on LTOT, 61% were assessed when unstable and 33% were assessed as in-patients following an exacerbation [17]. The pressure to start patients with COPD on LTOT at the time of hospital discharge, when they are not yet stable, needs to be countered by raising awareness of the natural history of COPD and the rationale for LTOT.

Both the original and 1999 UK guidelines recommend arterial blood gas tensions should be measured on two occasions not less than three weeks apart when the patient is stable. This guideline has not been followed for 15 years and needs examining critically. In one study only 6% of patients had arterial blood gases repeated [17]. A bigger problem is that 15–25% of patients are prescribed LTOT without arterial blood gases at all, let alone while stable [16,17]. The appropriate focus should be on ensuring all patients are formally assessed for LTOT, and that this is done with one set of arterial blood gas tensions measured when the patient meets the clinical definition of stability. Clinical stability is defined as the absence of an exacerbation of COPD and of peripheral oedema for the previous 4 weeks [3]. It is unrealistic and unnecessary to insist on two sets of arterial blood gases, provided the patient is assessed when clinically stable.

Guidelines also recommend that arterial blood gas tensions are repeated after breathing oxygen for 30 min to confirm that the PaO_2 increases above 8 kPa (60 mmHg). This is also poorly done in practice. It was only measured in 59% of patients in one study [17], and in another study follow-up oximetry on oxygen showed undercorrection in 17% of patients [16]. As the aim of LTOT is to improve survival, it is rational that there should be formal arrangements for follow-up of these patients to ensure adequate correction of hypoxaemia, optimize compliance, detect deterioration, and identify continuing requirement for LTOT. The majority of patients, 92–97%, are already under follow-up [16,17], although more than 40% do not have arterial blood gases repeated [17]. There are no randomized studies to indicate whether active follow-up improves prognosis or reduces inappropriate use of LTOT. Currently, follow-up is patchy, with no systematic arrangements in the UK, although this is improving as respiratory nurse specialists take on this role in many centres.

A further problem has been poor communication about patients on LTOT between clinicians in the community and hospital [16]. The use of a register for patients on LTOT with standardized forms providing a two-way flow of information is one suggested way for improving this situation [3].

The benefits of LTOT are evidenced-based. Therefore it should be possible for the prescription of LTOT to be rational and objective. We need to make sure that patients with COPD are not missing out on the only treatment (apart from stopping smoking) that reduces mortality.

All patients with severe COPD should be screened with oximetry. Those with a resting SaO_2 of 92% or below need to have arterial blood gases performed on one occasion when stable. If the PaO_2 is below 7.3 kPa (55 mmHg), LTOT should be prescribed for as much time as possible in 24 h, but at least 15 h. Patients with a PaO_2 between 7.3 and 8 kPa (55 mmHg and 60 mmHg), and with secondary polycythaemia or peripheral oedema, should also be prescribed LTOT. The evidence for treating patients with moderate hypoxaemia and pulmonary hypertension, or nocturnal hypoxaemia detected by overnight screening oximetry, is not compelling, although such treatment is recommended in the latest UK guidelines [3]. Patients on LTOT should have annual follow-up as a minimum and correction of hypoxaemia should be confirmed.

When is short-burst oxygen justified—if at all?

Short-burst oxygen therapy has been traditionally used for symptomatic relief of breathlessness at rest, to preoxygenate before exercise and to alleviate breathlessness after exercise. Although this pattern of use is widespread, the evidence for its efficacy is limited. Assessing symptomatic improvement in breathlessness is difficult and this pattern of use is often driven by patients' requests for an oxygen cylinder. In 1989, nearly 1 million oxygen cylinders were supplied to patients' homes in England and Wales [12]. These 1360-L cylinders last about 10 h at 2 L/min, but individual daily use has been shown to be low [18].

A small randomized controlled trial showed that short-burst oxygen used for 10 min reduced breathlessness in patients with COPD and chronic hypoxaemia at rest [19]. However, there are no good data in patients who are breathless at rest but not hypoxaemic. Oxygen given for 5 or 15 min before exercise was found to be beneficial in one double-blind cross-over study in 10 patients with severe COPD [20]. These patients walked significantly further, on both 6-min walking tests and treadmill walks, with a 10% increase in distance walked (20–30 m improvement). Patients predosed with oxygen were also less breathless on treadmill walking. The patients were all 'pink puffers', with a mean PaO_2 at rest of 9.7 kPa (73 mmHg), but saturation during exercise was not measured. There is also one study of 18 patients with severe COPD, known to have exercise-induced desaturation, demonstrating a beneficial effect of oxygen for 5 min either before or after climbing stairs in reducing the severity of breathlessness and desaturation [21]. However, when the patients were asked their views, there was no significant preference for oxygen over air. A further difficulty is that the effects of oxygen may not be reproducible with time [22].

The recommendations in the 1999 UK guidelines acknowledge that the evidence for short-burst therapy is inadequate [3]. Oxygen is recommended for episodic breathlessness not relieved by other treatments, with demonstration of improvements in breathlessness and/or exercise tolerance. A trial of 5 min of oxygen therapy either before or after exercise for patients with COPD known to have exercise-induced desaturation, with continued short-burst therapy if there is symptomatic benefit, is indicated on current evidence. However, education about oxygen therapy needs to include information on the situations, such as short-burst therapy, where benefit is small or has not been demonstrated, so that prescribing of short-burst oxygen therapy is kept to a minimum and for clearly defined reasons.

Is ambulatory oxygen a viable option and if so how should the oxygen be made available?

Ambulatory oxygen is the provision of oxygen therapy during exercise. The main aims of ambulatory oxygen are to reduce effort-induced breathlessness and increase exercise tolerance. With the increasing use of pulmonary rehabilitation, which has been shown to achieve both these aims for patients with COPD, the role of ambulatory oxygen in training programmes also needs to be defined.

The terms ambulatory oxygen and portable oxygen are often confused. Ambulatory oxygen is carried by the patient, while portable oxygen is transported with the patient, but is not 'on their person'. Portable oxygen includes the smaller cylinders that can be carried on a wheelchair or transported by car for severely hypoxaemic patients, who require continuous oxygen to correct dangerous hypoxaemia, rather than to reduce breathlessness and improve walking distances. As ambulatory oxygen needs to be used by mobile patients outside the home, the practicalities of equipment are important.

Randomized controlled trials are essential to evaluate the effects of ambulatory oxygen because of the large placebo effect, the effect of training, and variable individual responses. However, there are relatively few such studies. One study in 26 patients with severe COPD demonstrated that oxygen improved endurance but not maximal work rate on a treadmill [23]. Ambulatory oxygen resulted in a 13% increase in the distance walked during a 6-min walking test and reduced breathlessness on exercise in a randomized controlled study in 10 patients with severe COPD [20]. A further study of 50 patients confirmed that the increase in distance walked with ambulatory oxygen is around 10% when compared to an air cylinder [24]. However, the placebo effect alone of an ambulatory cylinder can be a 6–9% improvement in the distance walked [24,25]. The mechanism for the beneficial effect of oxygen on exercise endurance is, at least in part, by reduction in minute ventilation [26].

Predicting who will walk further with ambulatory oxygen is difficult, as there is no direct relationship between reduction in breathlessness and improved walking distance [20,24,25]. In part, this is explained by the observation that ambulatory oxygen reduces the severity of breathlessness for a given level of exercise [26].

Patients with COPD who desaturate on exercise as a group tend to improve their distance walked with ambulatory oxygen [24,27]. The 1999 UK guidelines recommend that only patients who show arterial oxygen desaturation on exercise of at least 4% below 90% during a baseline walking test breathing air should be assessed for ambulatory oxygen [3]. In one study of 20 patients with COPD who desaturated on exercise, the 6-min distance walked improved by 22% and breathlessness decreased by 36% with ambulatory oxygen, compared to patients who did not desaturate, in whom breathlessness was also reduced (by 47%) but there was no effect on the distance walked [27]. However, the situation is more complex, in that only a proportion of patients who desaturate on exercise will show reduced breathlessness and/or extended walking distances on ambulatory oxygen, and some patients who do not desaturate on exercise will improve with ambulatory oxygen [24,27]. Hence, oxygen desaturation during exercise is not a reliable criterion for selection for ambulatory oxygen.

Ambulatory oxygen should only be provided for patients who show an improvement of at least 10% in walking distance and/or visual analogue score for breathlessness when walking with an oxygen cylinder compared with an air cylinder. The proportion of patients who will fulfil the criteria for ambulatory oxygen using this protocol will vary, but was 58% in the original study using these criteria [24].

The role of ambulatory oxygen during training, i.e. pulmonary rehabilitation, remains unclear. The argument for using oxygen is that it improves outcomes by allowing training at greater intensity; against is that training under hypoxic conditions allows adaptation. One randomized, placebo-controlled study of 25 patients with COPD (mean PaO_2 8.5 kPa/63.8 mmHg) showed that while ambulatory oxygen during pulmonary rehabilitation reduced breathlessness at the end of rehabilitation, it had no effect on exercise tolerance or health status [28]. Furthermore, the group without oxygen increased their exercise tolerance during pulmonary rehabilitation, with no ill effects from significant desaturation during exercise (minimum SaO_2 of 85%). This small study suggests that the extra inconvenience of training with oxygen is not justified [28].

Ambulatory oxygen is provided in the UK at present by small oxygen cylinders that can be carried (capacity 230 L, weight 2.3 kg). These only deliver 80 min of oxygen at 2 L/min in practice [24] and are not currently prescribable.

An alternative method of providing ambulatory oxygen is liquid oxygen, allowing up to 8 h oxygen from a lightweight cylinder. When full, this may weigh 3.4 kg, but the patient only needs to fill it for the required hours of use, making it lighter than this in practice. A large tank of liquid oxygen is kept at the patient's home for refilling the cylinder and is replaced regularly (about every 3 weeks). In theory, liquid oxygen is a more practical way of delivering ambulatory oxygen, although it is more expensive. One randomized study in the UK comparing ambulatory oxygen provided by gaseous cylinders with liquid oxygen cylinders found that the majority of patients preferred liquid oxygen and used it more [29]. However, this study did not show a marked increase in the time patients spent away from home.

Availability of the systems for provision of ambulatory oxygen partly determines patterns of use in different countries. In the United States, liquid oxygen is available and much more widely used, based on the criteria of exercise desaturation alone. It is also used to increase the hours of use of LTOT in mobile patients. A few patients with COPD, like many of those with pulmonary fibrosis, require a higher flow rate on exercise to correct desaturation and in these patients liquid oxygen may be the only practical solution, as ambulatory gaseous cylinders only last about half an hour at 4 L/min.

The equipment used to deliver oxygen from an ambulatory source is also important. Most patients use nasal cannulae. However, other systems may be more efficient, including transtracheal oxygen catheters and oxygen-conserving devices [30]. Transtracheal catheters reduce the dead space of the upper airway, and once in place are a much less obtrusive method of oxygen delivery. They are used in the United States, but have not become standard practice in the UK, partly because of the reluctance to use an invasive procedure to deliver oxygen and partly because of complications associated with their use. Oxygen-conserving devices, including reservoirs and pulsed-flow oxygen delivery systems, can be twice to seven times as economical on oxygen use [30]. Studies comparing these different methods of delivering oxygen are lacking.

The issues of efficacy, practicality and cost are closely intertwined when evaluating the rational use of ambulatory oxygen. The case for liquid oxygen is strongest for patients with pulmonary fibrosis who require high flow rates to correct exercise-induced oxygen desaturation. The theoretical advantages of liquid oxygen for patients with COPD still need to be established in large randomized controlled trials. The best method of delivery for ambulatory oxygen during pulmonary rehabilitation needs to be defined, if found to be appropriate.

Evidence that ambulatory oxygen improves exercise tolerance in some patients with COPD is well established [20,24–27]. There is an urgent need for ambulatory oxygen therapy in some form to be prescribable in the UK to appropriate patients with COPD. Even being able to prescribe gaseous cylinders, which are the cheaper alternative at present, would have a big impact on quality of life for many patients with COPD. It is not rational that large cylinders, used for short-burst oxygen therapy, for which there is much less evidence of benefit, are prescribable but that ambulatory oxygen, even when it has been shown to benefit individual patients following assessment, is not.

Should oxygen therapy be prescribed to smokers?

Prescribing oxygen to patients who smoke is controversial. The two issues are whether oxygen therapy is effective and whether it is safe. In the MRC study, more than a quarter of the control subjects and more than half of the treated subjects were smokers [1], providing evidence that LTOT reduces mortality in patients who smoke. From the safety point of view, an oxygen concentrator is a low flow system with a lower risk of fire than a pressurized oxygen cylinder. The UK guidelines suggest that LTOT should not be prescribed to patients who continue to smoke. However, the evidence does not support this recommendation. In practice, smoking is prevalent among patients on LTOT; 14–19% admitted to smoking in recent studies [16,17]. While every attempt should be made at smoking cessation, patients who continue to smoke should not be discriminated against. LTOT via a concentrator should be prescribed for any patient with a PaO_2 below 7.3 kPa (55 mmHg). In contrast, ambulatory oxygen and short-burst therapy, are usually provided by high-pressure cylinders and there is a significant fire hazard associated with smoking; hence they should not be prescribed for smokers.

Conclusions

We still have a long way to go towards the aim of rational and objective prescription of oxygen. We need further well-conducted randomized trials to extend the 20-year-old results of the MRC and NOT Trials. A benefit of LTOT in moderate hypoxaemia has not been shown. The role of ambulatory oxygen therapy is starting to be defined, but large studies are needed, including studies on its role in pulmonary rehabilitation. There is limited evidence for the use of short-burst oxygen therapy. If used, it should be recommended for 5 min before or after exercise in patients who desaturate on exercise and describe symptomatic benefit with its use.

While we await evidence in these areas, there is much that can be done. The evidence for survival benefit of LTOT is clear and guidelines are established, yet prescription is woefully inadequate. We need to increase awareness of the benefits of appropriate oxygen therapy and ensure evidence-based prescribing by all clinicians who care for patients with severe COPD. The practicalities of oxygen provision urgently need to be sorted out. Which equipment can be prescribed needs to be put on a rational basis; in particular, ambulatory oxygen, either as gaseous cylinders or liquid oxygen, should be prescribable for patients who have been formally assessed and found to benefit [3]. Oxygen services need to be defined, organized and funded, including arrangements for detecting hypoxaemic patients in the community, so that LTOT is provided for those patients with severe COPD who could benefit from it.

References

1 Long term domiciliary oxygen therapy in chronic hypoxic cor pulmonale complicating chronic bronchitis and emphysema: report of the Medical Research Council Working Party. *Lancet* 1981; i: 681–6.

2 Nocturnal Oxygen Therapy Trial Group. Continuous or nocturnal oxygen therapy in hypoxemic chronic obstructive lung disease: a clinical trial. *Ann Intern Med* 1980; **93**: 391–8.

3 Domiciliary Oxygen Therapy Services. *Clinical Guidelines and Advice for Prescribers*. London: Royal College of Physicians, 1999.

4 Gorecka D, Gorzelak K, Sliwinski P, Tobiasz M, Zielinski J. Effect of long-term oxygen therapy on survival in patients with chronic obstructive pulmonary disease with moderate hypoxaemia. *Thorax* 1997; **52**: 674–9.

5 Levi-Valensi P, Aubry P, Rida Z. Nocturnal hypoxemia and long-term oxygen therapy in COPD patients with daytime PaO_2 60–70 mmHg. *Lung* 1990; **168** (Suppl.): 770–5.

6 Douglas NJ, Calverley PM, Leggett RJ *et al.* Transient hypoxaemia during sleep in chronic bronchitis and emphysema. *Lancet* 1979; i: 1–4.

7 Catterall JR, Douglas NJ, Calverley PM *et al.* Transient hypoxemia during sleep in chronic obstructive pulmonary disease is not a sleep apnea syndrome. *Am Rev Respir Dis* 1983; **128**: 24–9.

8 Fletcher EC, Luckett RA, Goodnight WS *et al.* A double-blind trial of nocturnal supplemental oxygen for sleep desaturation in patients with chronic obstructive pulmonary disease and a daytime PaO_2 above 60 mm Hg. *Am Rev Respir Dis* 1992; **145**: 1070–6.

9 Chauoat A, Weitzenblum E, Kessler R *et al.* A randomised trial of nocturnal oxygen therapy in chronic obstructive pulmonary disease patients. *Eur Respir J* 1999; **14**: 997–9.

10 Weitzenblum E, Sautegeau A, Ehrhart M, Mammosser M, Pelletier A. Long-term oxygen therapy can reverse the progression of pulmonary hypertension in patients with chronic obstructive pulmonary disease. *Am Rev Respir Dis* 1985; **131**: 493–8.

11 Williams BT, Nicholl JP. Prevalence of hypoxaemic chronic obstructive lung disease with reference to long-term oxygen therapy. *Lancet* 1985; ii: 369–72.

12 Williams B, Nicholl J. Recent trends in the use of domiciliary oxygen in England and Wales. *Health Trends* 1991; **23**: 166–7.

13 Roberts CM, Franklin J, O'Neill A *et al.* Screening patients in general practice with COPD for long-term domiciliary oxygen requirement using pulse oximetry. *Respir Med* 1998; **92**: 1265–8.

14 Crockett AJ, Cranston JM, Moss JR, Alpers JH. Domiciliary oxygen for chronic obstructive pulmonary disease (Cochrane Review). *Cochrane Library* 2002: 1. Oxford: Update Software.

15 Douglas NJ, Flenley DC. Breathing during sleep in patients with obstructive lung disease. *Am Rev Respir Dis* 1990; **141**: 1055–70.

16 Restrick LJ, Paul EA, Braid GM *et al.* Assessment and follow up of patients prescribed long term oxygen treatment. *Thorax* 1993; **48**: 708–13.

17 Morrison D, Skwarski K, MacNee W. Review of the prescription of domiciliary long term oxygen therapy in Scotland [published erratum appears in *Thorax* 1995; **50**: 1327]. *Thorax* 1995; **50**: 1103–5.

18 Okubadejo AA, Paul EA, Wedzicha JA. Domiciliary oxygen cylinders. indications, prescription and usage. *Respir Med* 1994; **88**: 777–85.

19 Swinburn CR, Mould H, Stone TN, Corris PA, Gibson GJ. Symptomatic benefit of supplemental oxygen in hypoxemic patients with chronic lung disease. *Am Rev Respir Dis* 1991; **143**: 913–15.

20 Woodcock AA, Gross ER, Geddes DM. Oxygen relieves breathlessness in 'pink puffers'. *Lancet* 1981; i: 907–9.

21 Killen JWW, Corris PA. A pragmatic assessment of the placement of oxygen when given for exercise induced dyspnoea. *Thorax* 2000; **55**: 544–6.

22 Evans TW, Waterhouse JC, Carter A, Nicholl JF, Howard P. Short burst oxygen treatment for breathlessness in chronic obstructive airways disease. *Thorax* 1986; **41**: 611–15.

23 Bradley BL, Garner AE, Billiu D, Mestas JM, Forman J. Oxygen-assisted exercise in chronic obstructive lung disease. *Am Rev Respir Dis* 1978; **118**: 239–43.

24 Lock SH, Paul EA, Rudd RM, Wedzicha JA. Portable oxygen therapy. assessment and usage. *Respir Med* 1991; **85**: 407–12.

25 Waterhouse JC, Howard P. Breathlessness and portable oxygen in chronic obstructive airways disease. *Thorax* 1983; **38**: 302–6.

26 O'Donnell DE, D'Arsigny C, Webb KA. Effects of hyperoxia on ventilatory limitation during exercise in advanced chronic obstructive pulmonary disease. *Am J Respir Crit Care Med* 2001; **163**: 892–8.

27 Jolly EC, Di Boscio V, Aguirre L *et al.* Effects of supplemental oxygen during activity in patients with advanced COPD without severe resting hypoxemia. *Chest* 2001; **120**: 437–43.

28 Garrod R, Paul EA, Wedzicha JA. Supplemental oxygen during pulmonary rehabilitation in patients with COPD with exercise hypoxaemia. *Thorax* 2000; **55**: 539–44.

29 Lock SH, Blower G, Prynne M, Wedzicha JA. Comparison of liquid and gaseous oxygen for domiciliary portable use. *Thorax* 1992; **47**: 98–100.

30 Tiep B. Portable oxygen therapy with oxygen conserving devices and methodologies. *Monaldi Arch Chest Dis* 1995; **50**: 51–7.

14: Chronic obstructive lung disease: what is the role of surgery?

Thomas Waddell and Roger Goldstein

Introduction

Surgeons encounter patients with chronic obstructive pulmonary disease (COPD) in a variety of contexts. For example, some patients develop mass lesions that require surgery to advance their diagnosis or management. In others, a spontaneous pneumothorax demands prompt surgical assistance. These are standard surgical roles with which every thoracic surgeon and pulmonary specialist is familiar. In contrast, surgical contributions to the management of end-stage emphysema have a long and fascinating history [1]. A number of once exciting procedures fell into disfavour for lack of evidence of their efficacy among an extremely high-risk group of patients. Such procedures include costochondrectomy, phrenic nerve crush, pneumoperitoneum and resection of the carotid body. Other procedures, based on sounder physiological principles, have enjoyed more success. In this chapter, we will comment on the role of surgery in the management of COPD, with particular emphasis on approaches that remove or replace emphysematous tissue. These include bullectomy, lung volume reduction and lung transplantation.

Why bullectomy?

Bullectomy for resection of compressive giant bullae is clearly beneficial, provided patients are selected carefully. Criteria for consideration of surgery include the presence of a localized giant bulla, defined as occupying more than one-third of the hemithorax, in the presence of compression of the surrounding, relatively 'normal' lung. Whereas there has never been a randomized controlled trial of bullectomy, early surgical case series reported favourable experience with minimal mortality and functional improvement [2]. Laros *et al.* reported long-term results in 27 patients followed for 10 years after surgical resection [3]. They noted improvements in forced expiratory volume in 1 s (FEV_1) when the bulla communicated with the bronchial tree. Resection of a closed bulla resulted in a larger increase in forced vital capacity (FVC). Older patients with more advanced lung disease had significant palliation, with a mean survival time of 7 years. There were no recurrent bullae. The techniques and indications for surgery for this relatively rare opportunity do not require extensive discussion. Bullectomy is usually performed through a thoraco-tomy, for a unilateral procedure, although recently video-assisted thoracic surgery (VATS) has been used. The operation is often simplified if several bullae are on one pedicle. Selection criteria vary from one-third to two-thirds of the hemithoracic volume, provided that there is significant dyspnoea and compression of the remaining lung. The boundary between a giant bulla and heterogeneous diffuse emphysema can occasionally be difficult, but is increas-ingly becoming only a semantic discrimination. Chronic bronchitis and hypercapnia remain important risk factors [4].

What are the options for patients with generalized emphysema?

Several overviews regarding the surgical management of COPD have recently been published [5,6]. For patients with more generalized emphysema, resec-tion of lung parenchyma improves elastic recoil and chest wall mechanics. Advances in preoperative diagnostic imaging, thoracic anaesthesia, surgical technique and critical care have led to great interest in this area. As with resec-tion of large bullae, lung volume reduction has specific indications and is not appropriate for most patients with COPD. Transplantation of one or both lungs provides the best restoration of pulmonary function. Unlike bullectomy or volume reduction, transplantation is independent of the anatomic subtypes of emphysema. However, transplantation has its own indications, limitations and exclusion criteria that must be taken into account to identify those most likely to benefit from this procedure.

What is the role of lung volume reduction surgery?

The role of lung volume reduction (LVR) in the management of end-stage em-physema remains controversial. In carefully selected patients, surgery has been associated with statistically significant improvements in lung volumes, expiratory flow rates, exercise capacity and work of breathing [7–11]. It has also been shown to improve subjective measures of dyspnoea and health-related quality of life (HRQL) beyond that which could be achieved by pul-monary rehabilitation alone [12]. In a randomized controlled trial of LVR sur-gery among subjects with stable, severe COPD, surgery did not influence survival compared with the control group. It is therefore considered primarily for its potential benefit on quality of life. The duration of these improvements

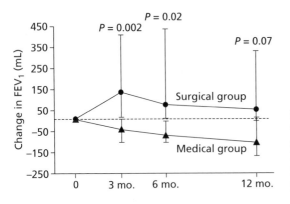

Fig. 14.1 Median changes in forced expiratory volume in 1 s in the groups receiving surgical and medical treatment. *P* values are for the comparison between groups at each time point. Bars show the 95% confidence intervals. From [13], with permission.

is unclear. Clinical trials will answer important issues such as duration, selection criteria, precise outcomes and best technique.

Several clinical trials have recently been published. In two of them, patients participated in a program of rehabilitation prior to being randomized to receive surgery or continued medical treatment [13,14]. In a third, patients received either rehabilitation or surgery [15]. In these three trials, only surgical treatment significantly improved the FEV_1. Improved exercise capacity occurred after rehabilitation, with further improvements after LVR. Pompeo *et al.* noted a reduction in dyspnoea following surgery [15] and Geddes *et al.* (Fig. 14.1) reported improvements in a generic measure of quality of life [13], sustained for 12 months. In the Geddes trial, high mortality in the surgical arm was modified after the entry criteria were changed during the trial [13]. In the Criner *et al.* trial, significance was only reached after the control group crossed over to receive surgical management [14]. Other randomized trials currently in progress will enable the effects of surgery on functional exercise capacity and health-related quality of life to be compared with rehabilitation alone. The largest ongoing trial is the US National Emphysema Treatment Trial, which has so far only reported on high-risk patients. Last year, the group conducting the trial cautioned that patients with an FEV_1 below 20% predicted and either a carbon monoxide diffusing capacity below 20% predicted or a homogeneous distribution of emphysema were at high risk for death after surgery. Those who did survive had only small changes in pulmonary function and exercise capacity, with no improvements in their quality of well-being, compared with medically treated patients [16].

Although LVR surgery was never intended as a life-sustaining or life-extending procedure, it will be of importance to know whether it might improve survival. Meyers *et al.* reported on a group of patients who were considered suitable for the procedure, but who did not undergo it as funding had been withheld by Medicare pending the results of controlled trials [17]. Compared to a similar group of patients who were funded for surgery, the survival in the non-funded group was decreased. Brenner *et al.* [18] reported that in patients who experienced an increase in $FEV_1 > 0.56\,L$, survival exceeded 95%, whereas survival was <80% for those with a lesser FEV_1 response. These inconclusive observations are interesting and suggest hypotheses for further research.

How does LVR work?

Resection of highly compliant lung increases the elastic recoil of the remaining lung. Airflow is increased, work of breathing is decreased and dyspnoea is improved [19]. These changes occur promptly following surgery [20]. The correlation between improved lung mechanics, reduced dyspnoea and improved health-related quality of life is weak. Brenner *et al.* [7] noted that although 28% of the patients in their study had minimal improvements in FEV_1, many improved in their dyspnoea scores. Leyenson *et al.* also reported on the poor correlations between quality of life, spirometry and dyspnoea [10]. For some patients, improved ventilation–perfusion relationships after surgery have resulted in improved oxygenation, to the extent that the patient no longer required long-term oxygen therapy [12]. It has become clear that the improvements in HRQL and functional exercise capacity following LVR must be distinguished from the improvements that occur after rehabilitation [12].

How should LVR be done?

The conceptual simplicity of the operation belies the reality. The operation is best performed in specialized centres, as success is dependent on excellent anaesthesia, perioperative analgesia, experienced nursing care and physical therapy, given that the patients are very impaired. Although the operation was first reported as a bilateral procedure via a median sternotomy [21], surgeons quickly progressed to using a thoracoscopic approach, initially unilateral, or staged bilateral procedures, but more recently as bilateral procedures. Direct comparisons have suggested greater benefits following bilateral procedures than following unilateral operations [11,22,23]. Our approach is to offer bilateral volume reduction via a thoracoscopic approach. Patients with upper-lobe predominance are placed in the supine position. Patients requiring lower-lobe resection are placed in the lateral position, which requires turning and redraping between sides. In the absence of a randomized trial comparing median sternotomy with thoracoscopic volume reduction, clinical experience is that VATS is associated with reduced morbidity, less pain, earlier mobilization, a shorter hospital stay and a more rapid return to an exercise program [24–26].

Preoperative rehabilitation is important. We therefore enroll all prospec-

Table 14.1 Criteria for lung volume reduction surgery.

Inclusion criteria	Exclusion criteria
'Physiological' age < 75	'Physiological' age > 75
Class III or IV dyspnoea	$PaCO_2 > 55$
Significant impairment of ADL	Previous thoracic surgery on operable side
FEV_1 15%-40%	Steroid use 10 mg/day or more
TLC > 120%	RVSP > 50 mmHg
RV > 180%	Significant CAD or left ventricular dysfunction
Destruction and distention on CXR and CT	Exacerbation episodes requiring antibiotics
Correlation between CT and V/Q scan	more than three times in the last 6 months
re heterogeneous target zones	Homogeneous disease

ADL, activities of daily living; CAD, coronary artery disease; CT, computed tomography; CXR, chest X-ray; FEV_1, forced expiratory volume in 1 s; TLC, total lung capacity; RV, right ventricle; RVSP, right ventricular systolic pressure.

tive surgical candidates for at least 6 weeks of supervised rehabilitation. Post-operatively, we offer supervised rehabilitation for the more marginal patients, but encourage a maintenance program for all patients. This ensures compliance with good health-care habits.

Who should have lung volume reduction surgery?

Criteria for LVR surgery include stable patients with severe emphysema and minimal bronchitis, hyperinflation with gas trapping at total lung capacity and dyspnoea during activities of daily living. More specific criteria are summarized in Table 14.1. We confirm emphysema by high-resolution computed tomography (CT)—with blinded grading on a five-point scale by an experienced radiologist—and identify heterogeneity both by CT and by ventilation–perfusion scan. Ventilation curves are displayed separately for each zone (upper middle and lower) on both sides. Perfusion (%) and the slope of the xenon washout curve (visual) are helpful in identifying target zones.

Although patients with homogeneous disease will respond to LVR surgery [27], patients in whom the distribution of emphysema is heterogeneous tend to experience greater improvements in postoperative FEV_1 than those with homogeneous disease. We therefore include heterogeneity among our selection criteria. Upper-lobe predominance appears to result in greater improvements than lower-lobe predominance [28], although patients with lower-lobe disease (especially α_1-antitrypsin-deficient patients) have derived benefit from the procedure. Patients with the most preoperative hyperinflation appear to enjoy the greatest improvements in dyspnoea [7]. High inspiratory flow resistance has been associated with a limited benefit from LVR surgery [29].

Who should not have lung volume reduction?

Previous lung surgery, extensive pleural adhesions, pulmonary hypertension, hypercapnia and very severe impairments (FEV_1 <0.4 L) or disability (6-min walk <250 m) are the main exclusion criteria (Table 14.1). We also exclude individuals in whom the presence of associated medical conditions such as cardiovascular disease, connective-tissue disease or severe osteoporosis might compromise their mobility or quality of life. As with any experimental procedure, clear guidelines are balanced by a careful patient assessment at a combined end-stage emphysema clinic in which each patient is seen by a thoracic surgeon and a respiratory specialist.

What is the role of lung transplantation?

Lung transplantation offers substantial palliation of dyspnoea and improved quality of life, although it may not extend survival [30]. It is usually reserved for patients with end-stage disease and severe dyspnoea despite maximal medical management. Most candidates are seriously considered when their FEV_1 falls below 20% of predicted. Single-lung transplantation (SLT) is the more frequently performed procedure, although bilateral sequential transplantation offers superior functional results and may improve long-term survival [31]. LVR may be offered prior to transplantation, or may be combined with SLT.

Should lung transplantation be unilateral or bilateral?

The operative mortality for bilateral lung transplantation varies widely. One transplant centre reported 30-day mortality rates of 10% for single-lung transplantation and 22% for bilateral lung transplantation [32]. Additional early mortality led to a very poor 1-year survival of only 35% after bilateral lung transplantation, although in this report one-third of the bilateral lung transplants were performed with the older *en-bloc* technique, which employs a single tracheal anastomosis. In contrast, another transplant centre reported excellent results following bilateral lung transplantation. The 60-day mortality was only 3.5%, as compared with 21.3% for single-lung transplants [33]. Divergent clinical experiences and multidisciplinary learning curves inevitably influence the selection of the procedure.

Actuarial 1-year survival rates of 93% for single-lung transplantation and 71% for bilateral lung transplantation have been reported [31]. Bilateral transplantation resulted in greater improvements in FEV_1 and FVC, although the FEV_1/FVC ratio, arterial blood gases and 6-min walk did not differ significantly between bilateral lung transplantation (BLT) and SLT. Functional equivalence between BLT and SLT has also been reported for exercise capacity, including measurements of dyspnoea at rest and during peak exercise [34]. Although SLT may provide sufficient pulmonary reserve to maintain normal blood gases, should the graft deteriorate, single-lung recipients become impaired more rapidly than double-lung recipients. Therefore, the long-term mortality appears to favour the bilateral procedure. Bilateral transplants can be performed with marginal lungs that are not always suitable for SLT [35]. Our centre currently uses bilateral procedures for 80% of transplantations for emphysema.

Who should have lung transplantation?

Candidates are required to be ambulatory and to have rehabilitation potential, as judged by their preoperative participation and progress in rehabilitation. Adequate nutritional status (preoperative weight within 80–120% of ideal body weight) is a prerequisite, as is a suitable psychosocial profile and support system. The goal of the selection process is to identify patients in the most appropriate risk category for whom current impairment, disability and handicap or dismal life expectancy justify the risk of operation. Put another way, patients must be severely compromised and deteriorating despite optimal medical management. Generally accepted objective guidelines for patients with emphysema include: New York Heart Association functional class III, $FEV_1 < 20\%$ of predicted, rapid decline in FEV_1, hypoxia, and hypercapnia [36]. Factors such as weight loss, frequent respiratory infections and repeated hospitalization are also considered.

Who should not have lung transplantation?

Contraindications to lung transplantation are not specific to emphysema. Absolute contraindications include current or recent malignancy, significant disease affecting other organ systems, extrapulmonary infection, substance abuse and significant psychiatric illness. Relative contraindications are becoming less prohibitive with additional surgical experience. For example, previous thoracic surgery complicates but does not prohibit transplantation. Moderate steroid usage is now considered acceptable. Combined coronary bypass and lung transplantation is possible for highly selected recipients. Ventilator dependence remains a contraindication, although a patient previously listed for transplantation who develops respiratory failure requiring ventilation will still be considered if a suitable organ becomes available soon after mechanical ventilation is initiated.

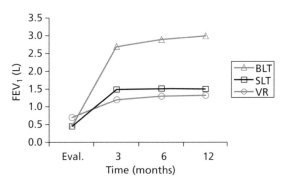

Fig. 14.2 Forced expiratory volume in 1 s before and after volume reduction (VR), single-lung transplantation (SLT) and bilateral lung transplantation (BLT). Modified from [37], with permission.

Do criteria for volume reduction and transplantation overlap?

Patients with COPD who met the criteria for lung transplantation have received LVR surgery [37]. *Post-hoc* analysis suggested that improvements following volume reduction were equivalent to improvements seen among LVR surgery patients who were not eligible for transplants (Fig. 14.2). At 6 months, FEV_1 increased by 59% in the 'transplant-eligible' group, compared to a 79% increase in the overall LVR surgery group. The 6-min walk test increased by 33% in 'transplant-eligible' subjects. This figure was intermediate between 28% for the overall group of LVR surgery patients and 47% for those who had received single-lung transplantations. The actual walking distance was 449 m for 'transplant-eligible' LVR surgery patients and 461 m post-SLT. Thus, although the LVR patients had a smaller improvement in their FEV_1 (0.55–0.87 L after LVR vs. 0.48–1.59 L after SLT), the improvements in functional exercise capacity were similar with the two procedures, without the risks or complications of SLT such as rejection and immunosuppression.

What are the future directions?

The value of surgery for giant bullae is well established and without question. Short-term randomized trials have demonstrated that LVR surgery is effective in improving pulmonary mechanics, decreasing dyspnoea, increasing exercise tolerance and improving quality of life. Longer-term studies will quantify the duration of benefit, appropriate selection criteria and best techniques. Animal models of emphysema [38] enable us to evaluate several potential endobronchial techniques that might improve pulmonary mechanics and health-related quality of life for patients with emphysema. This is likely to become an area of very active research. Transplantation will continue to be an option for a minority of patients with end-stage emphysema. More widespread use of transplantation will depend on significant improvements in immunosuppression as well as an expansion of the donor pool. Until that time, the balance for clinicians and patients remains the risk of early death or major complications, against the improvements in functional exercise capacity and health-related quality of life.

References

1 Cooper JD. The history of surgical procedures for emphysema. *Ann Thorac Surg* 1997; **63**: 312–19.
2 Potgieter PD, Benatar SR, Hewitson RP, Ferguson AD. Surgical treatment of bullous lung disease. *Thorax* 1981; **36**: 885–90.
3 Laros CD, Gelissen HJ, Bergstein PG et al. Bullectomy for giant bullae in emphysema. *J Thorac Cardiovasc Surg* 1986; **91**: 63–70.
4 Petro W, Hubner C, Greschuchna D, Maasen W, Konietzko N. Bullectomy. *Thorac Cardiovasc Surg* 1983; **31**: 342–5.
5 Maurer JR. Surgical approaches to end-stage disease: lung transplantation and volume reduction. *Clin Chest Med* 1997; **18**: 173–414.
6 Shrager JB, Kaiser LR, Edelman JD. Lung volume reduction surgery. *Curr Prob Surg* 2000; **37**: 253–317.
7 Brenner M, McKenna RJ, Gelb AF et al. Dyspnea response following bilateral thoracoscopic staple lung volume reduction surgery. *Chest* 1997; **112**: 916–23.
8 Cooper JD, Patterson GA, Sundaresan RS et al. Results of 150 consecutive lung volume reduction procedures in patients with severe emphysema. *J Thorac Cardiovasc Surg* 1996; **112**: 1319–30.
9 Keenan RJ, Landreneau RJ, Sciurba FC et al. Unilateral thoracoscopic surgical approach for diffuse emphysema. *J Thorac Cardiovasc Surg* 1996; **111**: 308–16.
10 Leyenson V, Furukawa S, Kuzma AM et al. Correlation of changes in quality of life after lung volume reduction surgery with changes in lung function, exercise, and gas exchange. *Chest* 2000; **118**: 728–35.
11 Lowdermilk GA, Keenan RJ, Landreneau RJ et al. Comparison of clinical results for unilateral and bilateral thoracoscopic lung volume reduction. *Ann Thorac Surg* 2000; **69**: 1670–4.
12 Moy ML, Ingenito EP, Mentzer SJ, Evans RB, Reilly J Jr. Health-related quality of

life improves following pulmonary rehabilitation and lung volume reduction surgery. *Chest* 1999; **115**: 383–9.
13 Geddes D, Davies M, Koyama H et al. Effect of lung volume reduction surgery in patients with severe emphysema. *N Engl J Med* 2000; **343**: 239–45.
14 Criner GJ, Cordova FC, Furukawa S et al. Prospective randomized trial comparing bilateral lung volume reduction surgery to pulmonary rehabilitation in severe chronic obstructive pulmonary disease. *Am J Respir Crit Care Med* 1999; **160**: 2018–27.
15 Pompeo E, Marino M, Nofroni I, Matteucci G, Mineo TC. Reduction pneumoplasty versus respiratory rehabilitation in severe emphysema: a randomized study. *Ann Thorac Surg* 2000; **70**: 948–54.
16 National Emphysema Treatment Trial Research Group. Patients at high risk of death after lung volume reduction surgery. *N Engl J Med* 2001; **345**: 1075–83.
17 Meyers BF, Yusen RD, Lefrak SS et al. Outcome of Medicare patients with emphysema selected for, but denied, a lung volume reduction operation. *Ann Thorac Surg* 1998; **66**: 331–6.
18 Brenner M, McKenna RJ, Chen JC et al. Survival following bilateral staple lung volume reduction surgery for emphysema. *Chest* 1999; **115**: 390–6.
19 Gelb AF, McKenna RJ, Brenner M et al. Contribution of lung and chest wall mechanics following emphysema resection. *Chest* 1996; **110**: 11–17.
20 Tschernko EM, Wisser W, Hofer S et al. The influence of lung volume reduction surgery on ventilatory mechanics in patients suffering from severe chronic obstructive pulmonary disease. *Anesth Analg* 1996; **83**: 996–1001.
21 Cooper JD, Trulock EP, Triantafillou AN et al. Bilateral pneumectomy (volume reduction) for chronic obstructive pulmonary disease. *J Thorac Cardiovasc Surg* 1995; **109**: 106–19.

22 McKenna RJ, Brenner M, Fischel RJ, Gelb AF. Should lung volume reduction for emphysema be unilateral or bilateral? *J Thorac Cardiovasc Surg* 1996; **112**: 1331–9.

23 Kotloff RM, Tino G, Palevsky HI *et al*. Comparison of short-term functional outcomes following unilateral and bilateral lung volume reduction surgery. *Chest* 1998; **113**: 890–5.

24 Wisser W , Tschernko E, Klepetko W *et al*. Functional improvement after volume reduction: sternotomy versus videoendoscopic approach. *Ann Thorac Surg* 1997; **63**: 822–8.

25 Kotloff RM, Tino G, Bavaria JE *et al*. Bilateral lung volume reduction surgery for advanced emphysema. *Chest* 1996; **110**: 1399–406.

26 Roberts JR, Bavaria JE, Wahl P *et al*. Comparison of open and thoracoscopic bilateral volume reduction surgery: complications analysis. *Ann Thorac Surg* 1998; **66**: 1759–65.

27 Thurnheer R, Engel H, Weder W *et al*. Role of lung perfusion scintigraphy in relation to chest computed tomography and pulmonary function in the evaluation of candidates for lung volume reduction surgery. *Am J Respir Crit Care Med* 1999; **159**: 301–10.

28 McKenna RJ, Brenner M, Fischel RJ *et al*. Patient selection criteria for lung volume reduction surgery. *J Thorac Cardiovasc Surg* 1997; **114**: 957–67.

29 Ingenito EP, Evans RB, Loring SH *et al*. Relation between preoperative inspiratory lung resistance and the outcome of lung-volume reduction surgery for emphysema. *N Engl J Med* 1998; **338**: 1181–5.

30 Hosenpud JD, Bennett LE, Keck BM, Edwards EB, Novick RJ. Effect of diagnosis on survival benefit of lung transplantation for end-stage lung disease. *Lancet* 1998; **351**: 24–7.

31 Sundaresan RS, Shiraishi Y, Trulock EP *et al*. Single or bilateral transplantation for emphysema. *J Thorac Cardiovasc Surg* 1996; **112**: 1485–95.

32 Bando K, Paradis IL, Keenan RJ *et al*. Comparison of outcomes after single and bilateral lung transplantation for obstructive lung disease. *J Heart Lung Transplant* 1995; **14**: 692–8.

33 Bavaria JE, Kotloff R, Palevsky H *et al*. Bilateral versus single lung transplantation for chronic obstructive pulmonary disease. *J Thorac Cardiovasc Surg* 1997; **113**: 520–8.

34 Orens JB, Becker FS, Lynch JP *et al*. Cardiopulmonary exercise testing following allogeneic lung transplantation for different underlying disease states. *Chest* 1995; **107**: 144–9.

35 Sundaresan S, Semenkovich J, Ochoa L *et al*. Successful outcome of lung transplantation is not compromised by the use of marginal donor lungs. *J Thorac Cardiovasc Surg* 1995; **109**: 1075–80.

36 Smith CM. Patient selection, evaluation, and preoperative management for lung transplant candidates. *Clin Chest Med* 1997; **18**: 183–98.

37 Gaissert HA, Trulock EP, Cooper JD, Sundaresan RS, Patterson GA. Comparison of early functional results after volume reduction or lung transplantation for chronic obstructive pulmonary disease. *J Thorac Cardiovasc Surg* 1996; **111**: 296–307.

38 Shrager JB, Kim DK, Hashmi YJ *et al*. Lung volume reduction surgery restores the normal diaphragmatic length–tension relationship in emphysematous rats. *J Thorac Cardiovasc Surg* 2001; **121**: 217–24.

15: What is an acute exacerbation of COPD?

Wisia Wedzicha

Exacerbations of chronic obstructive pulmonary disease (COPD) are an important cause of the considerable morbidity and mortality found in COPD and an important cause of hospital admission [1]. Some patients are prone to frequent exacerbations that have considerable impact on quality of life and activities of daily living [2]. COPD exacerbations are also associated with increased airway inflammatory changes [3] that are caused by a variety of factors such as viruses, bacteria and possibly common pollutants (Fig. 15.1). COPD exacerbations are commoner in the winter months and thus are an important cause of hospital admission and pressures on hospital beds occurring at that time [4].

How is a COPD exacerbation defined?

Definitions of exacerbations are important especially for standardization in intervention studies. Although there is no standardized definition of a COPD exacerbation, an exacerbation is often described as an acute worsening of respiratory symptoms. However, some symptoms are more important in the description of an exacerbation than others and Anthonisen and colleagues pointed out that the most important symptoms of exacerbations were increased dyspnoea, sputum volume and purulence [5]. Definitions based on symptoms have been used in other studies [2–4]. Other definitions of exacerbations have been based on health care utilization, e.g. unscheduled physician visits, changes or increases in medication, use of oral steroids at exacerbation and hospital admission, or using the combination of worsening of symptoms and health care utilization [6]. However, health care utilization in COPD varies widely and thus there may be considerable difficulty in standardizing such a definition.

How often do patients report COPD exacerbations?

A cohort of moderate to severe COPD patients was followed in East London,

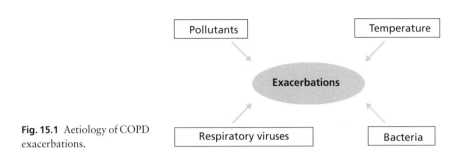

Fig. 15.1 Aetiology of COPD exacerbations.

UK (East London COPD Study) with daily diary cards and peak flow readings [2]. The patients were asked to report exacerbations as soon as possible after symptomatic onset [2]. The diagnosis of COPD exacerbation was based on criteria modified from those described by Anthonisen and colleagues [5], which require two symptoms for diagnosis, one of which must be a major symptom of increased dyspnoea, sputum volume or sputum purulence. Minor exacerbation symptoms included cough, wheeze, sore throat, nasal discharge or fever. The study found that about 50% of exacerbations were unreported to the research team, despite considerable encouragement being provided and were only diagnosed from diary cards, though there were no differences in major symptoms or physiological parameters between reported and unreported exacerbations [2]. Patients with COPD are accustomed to frequent symptom changes and thus may tend to under-report exacerbations to physicians. These patients have high levels of anxiety and depression and may accept their situation [7,8]. The tendency of patients to under-report exacerbations may explain the higher total rate of exacerbations at 2.7 per patient per year, which is higher than previously reported by Anthonisen and coworkers at 1.1 per patient per year [5]. However, in the latter study, exacerbations were unreported and diagnosed from patients' recall of symptoms.

What is the relation between exacerbation frequency and quality of life?

There is a close relationship between exacerbation frequency and quality of life measures. Using the median number of exacerbations as a cut-off point, COPD patients in the East London Study were classified as frequent and infrequent exacerbators. Quality-of-life scores measured using a validated disease specific scale—the St George's Respiratory Questionnaire (SGRQ), were significantly worse in all of its three component scores (symptoms, activities and impacts) in the frequent, compared to the infrequent, exacerbators. This suggests that exacerbation frequency is an important determinant of health status in COPD and is thus one of the important outcome measures in COPD. Factors predictive of frequent exacerbations included daily cough and sputum and frequent exacerbations in the previous year. An earlier study of acute infective exacerbations of chronic bronchitis found that one of the factors predicting exacerbation was also the number in the previous year [9].

What is the time course of a COPD exacerbation and do all exacerbations recover to baseline symptoms and physiological parameters?

In a study of 504 exacerbations, with daily monitoring being performed, there was some deterioration in symptoms, though no significant peak flow changes [10]. Falls in peak flow and FEV_1 at exacerbation were generally small and not useful in predicting exacerbations, but larger falls in peak flow were associated with symptoms of dyspnoea, presence of colds and related to a longer recovery time from exacerbations. The median time to recovery of peak flow was 6 days and 7 days for symptoms, but at 35 days peak flow had returned to normal in only 75% of exacerbations, while at 91 days, 7.1% of exacerbations had not returned to baseline lung function. Exacerbations took longer to recover in the presence of increased dyspnoea or symptoms of a common cold at exacerbation, suggesting that respiratory viruses lead to longer and thus more severe exacerbations. Another interesting finding is that the changes observed in lung function at exacerbation were smaller than those observed at asthmatic exacerbations, though the average length of an asthmatic exacerbation was longer at 9.6 days, compared to 6 or 7 days in COPD [11,12].

Are there airway inflammatory changes at COPD exacerbation?

Airway inflammatory changes are an important feature of COPD and it has been assumed that exacerbations are associated with increased airway inflammation. However, there has been little information available on the nature of any inflammatory changes, especially when studied close to an exacerbation, as performing bronchial biopsies at exacerbation is difficult in patients with moderate to severe COPD. The relation of any airway inflammatory changes to symptoms and physiological changes at exacerbations of COPD is also an important factor to consider.

In an Italian study, where biopsies were performed at exacerbation in patients with chronic bronchitis, increased airway eosinophilia was found, though patients described had only mild COPD [13]. With exacerbation, there were more modest increases observed in neutrophils, T lymphocytes (CD3) and TNF-α-positive cells, while there were no changes in CD4 or CD8 T cells, macrophages or mast cells. Sputum induction allows study of these patients at exacerbation and it has been shown that it is a safe and well tolerated

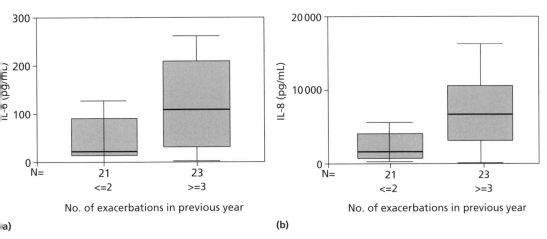

Fig. 15.2 Induced sputum levels of interleukin-6 (IL-6) (a) and IL-8 (b) in patients who are categorized as frequent exacerbators (≥3 exacerbations in the previous year) and those who are infrequent exacerbators (≤2 exacerbations in previous year). Data is expressed as medians (IQR). (Reproduced from Bhwomik *et al.* [3])

technique in COPD patients [14]. Levels of inflammatory cytokines had been previously shown to be elevated in induced sputum in COPD patients when stable [15]. In a cohort of COPD patients from the East London COPD study, the inflammatory markers in induced sputum were related to symptoms and physiological parameters both at baseline and at exacerbation [3]. There was a relation between exacerbation frequency and sputum cytokines, in that there was increased sputum interleukin-6 (IL-6) and IL-8 found in patients at baseline when stable with frequent exacerbations compared to those with infrequent exacerbations (Fig. 15.2), although there was no relation between cytokines and baseline lung function. As discussed below, exacerbations are triggered by viral infections, especially by rhinovirus, which is the cause of the common cold. Rhinovirus has been shown to increase cytokine production in an epithelial cell line [16] and thus repeated viral infection as occurs in patients with a history of frequent exacerbation may lead to up-regulation of cytokine airway expression.

There were increases at exacerbation in induced sputum IL-6 levels and the levels of IL-6 were higher when exacerbations were associated with symptoms of the common cold (Fig. 15.3). Studies where experimental rhinovirus infection has been induced in patients have found increases in sputum IL-6 in normal subjects and asthmatics [17–19]. However, rises in cell counts and IL-8 were more variable with exacerbation and not reaching statistical significance, suggesting marked heterogeneity in the degree of the inflammatory response at exacerbation. The exacerbation IL-8 levels were related to sputum neutrophil and total cell counts, indicating that neutrophil recruitment is

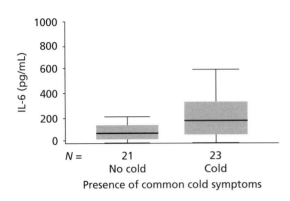

Fig. 15.3 Sputum interleukin-6 (IL-6) levels in COPD patients with the presence of a cold with the exacerbation and those without a cold. Sputum IL-6 levels are higher in the presence of a cold. Data is expressed as medians (IQR). From [3].

Table 15.1 Causes of COPD exacerbations.

Viruses
Rhinovirus (common cold)
Influenza
Parainfluenza
Coronavirus
Adenovirus
RSV

Bacteria
Haemophilus influenzae
Streptococcus pneumoniae
Branhamella cattarhalis
Staphylococcus aureus
Pseudomonas aeruginosa
Chlamydia pneumoniae

Common pollutants
Nitrogen dioxide
Particulates
Sulphur dioxide
Ozone

the major source of airway IL-8 at exacerbation. In comparison with asthma, COPD exacerbations are associated with generally less pronounced airway inflammatory responses [20], and this may explain the relatively reduced response compared to steroids seen at exacerbation in COPD patients [21–27].

What are the causes of COPD exacerbations?

The triggers of COPD exacerbations are shown in Table 15.1. Respiratory viral infections are the most important cause of exacerbations. COPD exacerbations are frequently triggered by upper respiratory tract infections and these are commoner in the winter months, when there are more respiratory viral in-

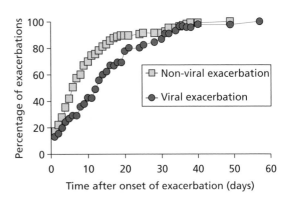

Fig. 15.4 Graph showing the cumulative percentage of viral and non-viral exacerbations recovering with respect to time after onset during 150 COPD exacerbations. $P = 0.006$, Mann–Whitney U-test. Data adapted from Seemungal *et al.* [36]).

fections in the community. COPD patients have been found to have increased hospital admissions, suggesting increased exacerbations when increasing environmental pollution occurs. During the December 1991 pollution episode in the UK, COPD mortality was increased together with an increase in hospital admissions of elderly COPD patients [28]. However, common pollutants especially oxides of nitrogen and particulates may interact with viral infections to precipitate an exacerbation rather than acting alone [29].

Viral infections

Studies in childhood asthma have shown that viruses, especially rhinovirus, can be detected by polymerase chain reaction from a large number of these exacerbations [30]. Rhinovirus has not hitherto been considered to be of much significance during exacerbations of COPD. In a study of 44 chronic bronchitics, Stott and colleagues found rhinovirus in 13 (14.9%) of 87 exacerbations of chronic bronchitis [31]. In 25 chronic bronchitics with 116 exacerbations over 4 years, Gump *et al.* found that only 3.4% of exacerbations could be attributed to rhinoviruses [32]. In a more recent study of 35 episodes of COPD exacerbation using serological methods and nasal samples for viral culture, little evidence was found for a rhinovirus aetiology of COPD exacerbation [33].

A number of studies have now shown that at least 50% of COPD exacerbations were associated with viral infections, and that the majority of these were due to rhinovirus [34–36]. Viral exacerbations were associated with symptomatic colds and prolonged recovery (Fig. 15.4) [10,36]. Seemungal and colleagues showed that that rhinovirus can be recovered from induced sputum more frequently than from nasal aspirates at exacerbation, suggesting that natural rhinovirus can infect the lower airway and be a cause of inflammatory changes at exacerbation [34]. Exacerbations associated with the presence of rhinovirus in induced sputum had larger increases in airway IL-6 levels [35], suggesting that viruses increase the severity of airway inflammation at exacerbation. This finding is in agreement with the data that respiratory viruses produce longer and more severe exacerbations and have a major impact on health care utilization [10,34]. Other viruses that may be important in triggering exacerbations are shown in Table 15.1.

Bacterial infection

Lower airway bacterial colonization has been shown to be common in COPD and has been found overall in approximately 30% of COPD patients. Colonization has been shown to be related to the degree of airflow obstruction and current cigarette smoking status [37]. Bacteria that have been usually associated with exacerbation are *Haemophilus influenzae* and *Streptococcus pneumoniae*. Some studies have shown increasing bacterial counts during exacerbation, while others have not confirmed these findings [38,39]. Soler and colleagues showed that the presence of potentially pathogenic organisms in bronchoalveolar lavage from COPD patients at bronchoscopy was associated with a greater degree of inflammation [40]. In a larger study, Hill and colleagues showed that the airway bacterial load was related to inflammatory markers [41]. They also found that the bacterial species was related to the degree of inflammation, with *Pseudomonas aeruginosa* colonization showing greater myeloperoxidase activity (an indirect measure of neutrophil activation).

Thus bacterial colonization in COPD is an important determinant of airway inflammation and further long-term studies are required to investigate whether bacterial colonization predisposes to the decline in lung function characteristic of COPD. Patel and colleagues have recently shown that patients with frequent exacerbations have increased sputum bacterial colonization, compared to patients with less frequent exacerbations [42] and this may explain the higher cytokine levels observed in the frequent exacerbator patient group [3].

How are bronchodilator therapies used at exacerbation?

Bronchodilators, especially inhaled β_2-agonists and anticholinergic agents, are frequently used in the treatment of acute exacerbations of COPD. In patients with stable COPD, symptomatic benefit can be obtained with bronchodilator therapy in COPD, even without significant changes in spirometry. This is probably due to a reduction in dynamic hyperinflation that is characteristic of COPD and hence leads to a decrease in the sensation of dyspnoea especially during exertion [43]. In stable COPD greater bronchodilatation has been demonstrated with anticholinergic agents than with beta-agonists. However, studies investigating bronchodilator responses in acute exacerbations of COPD have shown no differences between agents used and no significant additive effect of the combination therapy, even though combination of an anticholinergic and bronchodilator has benefits when patients are stable [44,45]. This difference in effect between the acute and stable states may be due to the fact that the larger doses of drug delivered in the acute setting produce maximal bronchodilatation, whereas the smaller doses administered in the stable condition may be having a submaximal effect.

Methylxanthines, e.g. theophylline, are sometimes used in the management of acute exacerbations of COPD. Although there is some evidence that theophyllines are useful in COPD, the main limiting factor is the frequency of toxic side-effects. The therapeutic action of theophylline is thought to be due to its inhibition of phosphodiesterase which breaks down cyclic AMP, an intracellular messenger, thus facilitating bronchodilatation. However, studies of intravenous aminophylline therapy in acute exacerbations of COPD have shown no significant beneficial effect over and above conventional therapy [46]. It is possible that some of the new phosphodiesterase inhibitors in development may have advantages, be more specific and possess a more favourable side-effect profile.

What is the role of steroids at acute exacerbation?

In patients with stable COPD, only about 10–15% of patients show a positive response to oral corticosteroids using spirometry [47] and, unlike the situation in asthma, steroids have little effect on airway inflammatory markers in patients with COPD [48,49]. Corticosteroids have traditionally been used in the management of acute exacerbations of COPD, although there has only recently been evidence of their beneficial role in the acute situation [21–27].

A number of early studies have investigated the effects of corticosteroid therapy, though these studies were generally small. Thompson and colleagues gave a 9-day course of prednisolone or placebo in a randomized manner to out-patients presenting with acute exacerbations of COPD [25]. Unlike the previous studies, these patients were either recruited from out-patients or from a group that were pre-enrolled and self reported the exacerbation to the study team. In this study patients with exacerbations associated with acidosis or pneumonia were excluded, so exacerbations of moderate severity were generally included. Patients in the steroid-treated group showed a more rapid improvement in PaO_2, alveolar–arterial oxygen gradient, FEV_1, peak expiratory flow rate and a trend towards a more rapid improvement in dyspnoea in the steroid-treated group.

Seemungal and colleagues followed a cohort of COPD patients in the East London study and described the effect of therapy with prednisolone on COPD exacerbations diagnosed and treated in the community [10]. Exacerbations treated with steroids were more severe and associated with larger falls in peak flow rate. The treated exacerbations also had a longer recovery time to baseline for symptoms and peak flow rate. However, the rate of peak flow rate recovery was faster in the prednisolone-treated group, though not the rate of symptom score recovery. An interesting finding in this study was that steroids significantly prolonged the median time from the day of onset of the initial exacerbation to the next exacerbation from 60 days in the group not treated with prednisolone to 84 days in the patients treated with prednisolone. If short course oral steroid therapy at exacerbation does prolong the time to the next exacerbation, then this could be an important way to reduce exacerbation frequency in COPD patients.

In another recent study, Davies and colleagues randomized patients admitted to hospital with COPD exacerbations to treatment with prednisolone or placebo [26]. In the prednisolone-treated group, the FEV_1 rose faster until day 5, when a plateau was observed in the steroid-treated group. Changes in the prebronchodilator and postbronchodilator FEV_1 were similar suggesting that this is not just an effect on bronchomotor tone, but involves faster resolution of airway inflammatory changes or airway wall oedema with exacerbation. Length of hospital stay analysis showed that patients treated with prednisolone had a significantly shorter length of stay. Six weeks later, there were no differences in spirometry between the patient groups and health status was similar to that measured at 5 days after admission. Thus the benefits of steroid therapy at exacerbation are most obvious in the early course of the exacerbation.

Niewoehner and colleagues performed a randomized controlled trial of either a 2-week or 8-week prednisolone course at exacerbation compared to placebo, in addition to other exacerbation therapy [27]. The primary end point was a first treatment failure, including death, need for intubation, readmission or intensification of therapy. There was no difference in the results using the 2- or 8-week treatment protocol. The rates of treatment failure were higher in the placebo group at 30 days, compared to the combined 2- and 8-week prednisolone groups. As in the study by Davies and colleagues, the FEV_1 improved faster in the prednisolone-treated group, though there were no differences by 2 weeks. In contrast, Niewoehner and colleagues performed a detailed evaluation of steroid complications and found considerable evidence of hyperglycaemia in the steroid-treated patients. Thus steroids should be used at COPD exacerbation in short courses of no more than 2 weeks duration to avoid risk of complications.

Do antibiotics have benefit for COPD exacerbations?

As COPD exacerbations frequently present with increased sputum purulence and volume, antibiotics have traditionally been used as first-line therapy. However, viral infections may be the triggers in a significant proportion of acute infective exacerbations in COPD and antibiotics used for the consequences of secondary infection. A study investigating the benefit of antibiotics in over 300 acute exacerbations demonstrated a greater treatment success rate in patients treated with antibiotics, especially if their initial presentation was with the symptoms of increased dyspnoea, sputum volume and purulence [5]. A randomized placebo-controlled study investigating the value of antibiotics in patients with mild obstructive lung disease in the community concluded that antibiotic therapy did not accelerate recovery or reduce the number of relapses [50]. A meta-analysis of trials of antibiotic therapy in COPD identified only nine studies of significant duration and concluded that antibiotic therapy offered a small but significant benefit in outcome in acute exacerbations [51].

What are the various models of supported discharge at exacerbation of COPD patients?

COPD exacerbations are one of the most important causes of hospital admissions, especially during the winter months when they are most frequent. Thus there is a particular need to devise strategies to reduce the hospital admissions associated with exacerbations. There has arisen a need to develop different models of supported discharge, where patients are discharged back early to the community with increased support and care packages and a number of these have been evaluated [54–57].

In a randomized study, Cotton and colleagues allocated patients to discharge on the next day or usual management and observed no differences in mortality or readmission rates between the two groups [55]. There was a reduction in hospital stay from a mean of 6.1 days to 3.2 days. In another larger study by Skwarska and colleagues, patients were randomized to discharge on the day of assessment or conventional management [56]. Again there were no differences in readmission rates, although these were high at around 30% of the study populations at 3 months. There were no differences in visits to primary care physicians and health status measured 8 weeks after discharge was similar in the two groups. The authors also demonstrated that there were significant cost savings of around 50% for the home support group, compared to the admitted group. Davies and colleagues found no differences in mortality or readmission rate between the home and hospital treated group [57]. However, only about 25% of patients presenting for hospital admission with a COPD exacerbation are suitable for home therapy and thus selection is required [56,57]. Other considerations need to be taken into account in organizing an assisted discharge service, in that resources have to be released for the nurses to follow the patients and the benefits may be seasonal, as COPD admissions are a particular problem in the winter months.

Can COPD exacerbations be prevented?

As upper respiratory tract infections are common factors in causing exacerbation, influenza and pneumococcal vaccinations are recommended for all patients with significant COPD. A study that reviewed the outcome of influenza vaccination in a cohort of elderly patients with chronic lung disease found that influenza vaccination is associated with significant health benefits with fewer outpatient visits, fewer hospitalizations and a reduced mortality [58]. Early studies on long-term antibiotics in exacerbation prevention have not shown a benefit on exacerbation frequency. However, recent data suggests that lower airway bacterial colonization in COPD increases the exacerbation frequency [42]. The same study shows that patients with bacterial colonization were also more likely to have more severe exacerbations, as shown by a longer recovery time [42]. Thus with the introduction of new and more effective antibiotics, new and well designed studies are required to assess the effects of long-term antibiotics on exacerbation frequency in COPD.

Mucolytic agents have also been prescribed in COPD though their use worldwide is very variable with little use in the UK and more prescriptions in mainland Europe. A recent meta-analysis was published that assessed the effects of oral mucolytics in COPD [59]. A total of 23 randomized controlled trials were identified and the main outcome was that there was a 29% reduction in exacerbations with mucolytic therapy. The number of patients who had no exacerbations was greater in the mucolytic group and days of illness was also reduced, though mucolytics had no effect on lung function. The drug that contributed most to the beneficial results in the review was N-acetylcysteine, though the mechanism of action of N-acetylcysteine is not entirely clear and may be a combination of mucolytic and antioxidative effects. These early studies are mostly small and further large studies on the effects of mucolytics are in progress and the results will be available in the next few years.

In the ISOLDE study of long-term inhaled fluticasone in patients with moderate to severe COPD, a reduction in exacerbation frequency was shown. However, the overall exacerbation frequency was relatively low in that study and this was probably due to a retrospective assessment of exacerbations [60]. The effect of inhaled steroids was greater in patients with more impaired lung function, suggesting that this is the group to target with long-term inhaled steroid therapy. Another earlier study suggested that the severity of exacerbations may be reduced with inhaled steroid therapy [61]. An observational study showed that exacerbations were increased following withdrawal of inhaled steroids though this study was not placebo controlled [62]. Two recent studies have also shown that small reductions in exacerbations can be achieved with bronchodilator therapy, though both studies involved relatively short periods of therapy at 12 weeks [63,64]. Recently the new long-acting anticholinergic drug tiotropium has been shown to reduce exacerbations by 24% when studied over a 1-year period [65].

Do exacerbations contribute to disease progression in COPD?

Early epidemiological studies suggested that exacerbations do not contribute to decline in lung function and thus disease progression in COPD [1]. However, as discussed earlier not all exacerbations recover to baseline levels and this incomplete recovery from an exacerbation may lead to decline in lung function. Recent data from the Lung Health Study shows that in patients who continue to smoke cigarettes, decline in lung function is greater if they have had exacerbations [66]. In another recent study patients who had a history of frequent exacerbations had a faster decline in lung function than patients who had infrequent exacerbations, though the difference between FEV_1 decline in frequent and infrequent exacerbators was relatively small [67]. Overall probably only about 25% of the fall in lung function can be attributed to the effects of exacerbation. However, these data suggest that COPD exacerbation is an important target for therapy. Reduction of COPD exacerbation frequency may not only improve quality of life and reduce hospital admission, but it may have a more important role in reducing the progression of COPD.

References

1 Fletcher CM, Peto R, Tinker CM, Speizer FE. *Natural History of Chronic Bronchitis and Emphysema*. Oxford University Press, Oxford 1976.

2 Seemungal TAR, Donaldson GC, Paul EA, Bestall JC, Jeffries DJ, Wedzicha JA. Effect of exacerbation on quality of life in patients with chronic obstructive pulmonary disease. *Am J Respir Crit Care Med* 1998; 151: 1418–22.

3 Bhowmik A, Seemungal TAR, Sapsford RJ, Wedzicha JA. Relation of sputum inflammatory markers to symptoms and physiological changes at COPD exacerbations. *Thorax* 2000; 55: 114–200.

4 Donaldson GC, Seemungal T, Jeffries DJ, Wedzicha JA. Effect of environmental temperature on symptoms, lung function and mortality in COPD patients. *Eur Resp J* 1999; 13: 844–9.

5 Anthonisen NR, Manfreda J, Warren CPW, Hershfield ES, Harding GKM, Nelson NA. Antibiotic therapy in exacerbations of chronic obstructive pulmonary disease. *Ann Intern Med* 1987; 106: 196–20.

6 Rodriguez-Roisin R. Towards a consensus definition for COPD exacerbations. *Chest* 2000; 117: 398S–401S.

7 Okubadejo AA, Jones PW, Wedzicha JA. Quality of life in patients with COPD and

severe hypoxaemia. *Thorax* 1996; 51: 44–7.

8 Okubadejo AA, O'Shea L, Jones PW, Wedzicha JA. Home assessment of activities of daily living in patients with severe chronic obstructive pulmonary disease on long term oxygen therapy. *Eur Resp J* 1997; 10: 1572–55.

9 Ball P, Harris JM, Lowson D, Tillotson G, Wilson R. Acute infective exacerbations of chronic bronchitis. *Q J Med* 1995; 88: 61–8.

10 Seemungal TAR, Donaldson GC, Bhowmik A, Jeffries DJ, Wedzicha JA. Time course and recovery of exacerbations in patients with chronic obstructive pulmonary disease. *Am J Respir Crit Care Med* 2000; 161: 1608–13.

11 Reddel HS, Ware S, Marks G, Salome C, Jenkins C, Woolcock A. Differences between asthma exacerbations and poor asthma control. *Lancet* 1999; 353: 364–9.

12 Tattersfield AE, Postma DS, Barnes PJ *et al*. Exacerbations of asthma: a descriptive study of 425 severe exacerbations. *Am J Respir Crit Care Med* 1999; 160: 594–9.

13 Saetta M, Di Stefano A, Maestrelli P *et al*. Airway eosinophilia in chronic bronchitis during exacerbations. *Am J Respir Crit Care Med* 1994; 150: 1646–52.

14 Bhowmik A, Seemungal TAR, Sapsford RJ, Devalia JL, Wedzicha JA. Comparison of spontaneous and induced sputum for investigation of airway inflammation in chronic obstructive pulmonary disease. *Thorax* 1998; 53: 953–6.

15 Keatings VM, Collins PD, Scott DM *et al*. Differences in Interleukin-8 and umour Necrosis Factor in induced sputum from patients with chronic obstructive pulmonary disease and asthma. *Am J Respir Crit Care Med* 1996; 153: 530–4.

16 Subauste MC, Jacoby DB, Richards SM, Proud D. Infection of a human respiratory epithelial cell line with rhinoovirus. *J Clin Invest* 1995; 96: 549–57.

17 Fraenkel DJ, Bardin PG, Sanderson G, Dorward M, Lau C, Johnston SL, Holgate ST. Lower airways inflammation during rhinovirus colds in normal and in asthmatic subjects. *Am J Respir Crit Care Med* 1995; 151: 879–86.

18 Grunberg K, Smits HH, Timmers MC *et al*. Experimental rhinovirus 16 infection: effects on cell differentials and soluble markers in sputum of asthmatic subjects. *Am J Respir Crit Care Med* 1997; 156: 609–16.

19 Fleming HE, Little EF, Schnurr D *et al*. Rhinovirus-16 colds in healthy and asthmatic subjects. *Am J Respir Crit Care Med* 1999; 160: 100–8.

20 Pizzichini MM, Pizzichini E, Clelland L *et al*. Sputum in severe exacerbations of asthma: kinetics of inflammatory indices after prednisone treatment *Am J Respir Crit Care Medical* 1997; 155: 1501–8.

21 Albert RK, Martin TR, Lewis SW. Controlled clinical trial of methylprednisolone in patients with chronic bronchitis and acute respiratory insufficiency. *Ann Intern Med* 1980; 92: 753–8.

22 Emerman CL, Connors AF, Lukens TW, May ME, Effron D. A randomised controlled trial of methylprednisolone in the emergency treatment of acute exacerbations of chronic obstructive pulmonary disease. *Chest* 1989; 95: 563–7.

23 Bullard MJ, Liaw SJ, Tsai YH, Min HP. Early corticosteroid use in acute exacerbations of chronic airflow limitation. *Am J Emerg Med* 1996; 14: 139–43.

24 Murata GH, Gorby MS, Chick TW, Halperin AK. Intravenous and oral corticosteroids for the prevention of relapse after treatment of decompensated COPD. *Chest* 1990; 98: 845–9.

25 Thompson WH, Nielson CP, Carvalho P *et al*. Controlled trial of oral prednisolone in outpatients with acute COPD exacerbation. *Am J Respir Crit Care Med* 1996; 154: 407–12.

26 Davies L, Angus RM, Calverley PMA. Oral corticosteroids in patients admitted to hospital with exacerbations of chronnic obstructive pulmonary disease: a prospective randomised controlled trial. *Lancet* 1999; 354: 456–60.

27 Niewoehner DE, Erbland ML, Deupree RH *et al*. Effect of systemic glucocorticoids on exacerbations of chronic obstuctive pulmonary disease. *N Engl J Med* 1999; 340: 1941–7.

28 Anderson HR, Limb ES, Bland JM *et al*.

Health effects of an air pollution episode in London. *Thorax 1995* December 1991; 50: 1188–93.

29 Linaker CH, Coggon D, Holgate ST *et al*. Personal exposure to nitrogen dioxide and risk of airflow obstruction in asthmatic children with upper respiratory infection. *Thorax* 2000; 55: 930–3.

30 Johnston SL, Pattemore PK, Sanderson G *et al*. Community study of the role of viral infections in exacerbations of asthma in 9–11 year old children. *Br Med J* 1995; 310: 1225–9.

31 Stott EJ, Grist NR, Eadie MB. Rhinovirus infections in chronic bronchitis. isolation of eight possible new rhinovirus serotypes. *J Med Microbiol* 1968; 109: 117.

32 Gump DW, Phillips CA, Forsyth BR. Role of infection in chronic bronchitis. *Am Rev Respir Dis* 1976; 113: 465–73.

33 Philit FJ, Etienne A. Calvet *et al*. Infectious agents associated with exacerbations of chronic obstructive pulmonary disease and attacks of asthma. *Rev Mal Respir* 1992; 9: 191–6.

34 Greenberg SB, Allen M, Wilson J, Atmar RL. Respiratory viral infections in adults with and without chronic obstructive pulmonary disease Am J Respir Crit Care Medical 2000; 162: 167–73.

35 Seemungal TAR, Harper-Owen R, Bhowmik A, Jeffries DJ, Wedzicha JA. Detection of rhinovirus in induced sputum at exacerbation of chronic obstructive pulmonary disease. *Eur Resp J* 2000; 16: 677–83.

36 Seemungal TAR, Harper-Owen R, Bhowmik A *et al*. Respiratory viruses, symptoms and inflammatory markers in acute exacerbations and stable chronic obstructive pulmonary disease. *Am J Respir Crit Care Med* 2001; 164: 1618–23.

37 Zalacain R, Sobradillo V, Amilibia J *et al*. Predisposing factors to bacterial colonization in chronic obstructive pulmonary disease. *Eur Resp J* 1999; 13: 343–8.

38 Monso E, Rosell A, Bonet G *et al*. Risk factors for lower airway bacterial colonization in chronic bronchitis. *Eur Resp J* 1999; 13: 338–42.

39 Wilson R. Bacterial infection and chronic obstructive pulmonary disease. *Eur Respir J* 1999; 13: 233–5.

40 Soler N, Ewig S, Torres A, Filella X, Gonzalez J, Zaubet A. Airway inflammation and bronchial microbial patterns in patients with stable chronic obstructive pulmonary disease. *Eur Resp J* 1999; 14: 1015–22.

41 Hill AT, Campbell EJ, Hill SL, Bayley DL, Stockley RA. Association between airway bacterial load and markers of airway inflammation in patients with chronic bronchitis. *Am J Med* 2000; 109: 288–95.

42 Patel IS, Seemungal TAR, Wilks M, Lloyd Owen S, Donaldson GC, Wedzicha JA. Relationship between bacterial colonisation and the frequency, character and severity of COPD exacerbations Thorax 2002; 57: 759–64.

43 Belman MJ, Botnick WC, Shin JW. Inhaled bronchodilators reduce dynamic hyperinflation during exercise in patients with chronic obstructive pulmonary disease. *Am J Respir Crit Care Med* 1996; 153: 967–75.

44 Combivent Inhalation Aerosol Study Group. In chronic obstructive pulmonary disease, a combination of ipratropium and albuterol is more effective than either agent alone. *Chest* 1994; 105: 1411–9.

45 Rebuck AS, Chapman KR, Abboud R, Pare PD, Kreisman H, Wolkove N, Vickerson F. Nebulized anticholinergic and sympathomimetic treatment of asthma and chronic obstructive airways disease in the emergency room. *Am J Med* 1987; 82: 59–64.

46 Rice KL, Leatherman JW, Duane PG, Snyder LS, Harmon KR, Abel J, Niewoehner DE. Aminophylline for acute exacerbations of chronic obstructive pulmonary disease. A controlled trial. *Ann Intern Med* 1987; 107: 305–9.

47 Callahan CM, Cittus RS, Katz BP. Oral corticosteroid therapy for patients with stable chronic obstructive pulmonary disease: a meta-analysis. *Ann Intern Med* 1991; 114: 216–23.

48 Keatings VM, Jatakanon A, Worsdell Y, Barnes PJ. Effects of inhaled and oral glucocorticoids on inflammatory indices in asthma and COPD. *Am J Respir Crit Care Med* 1997; 155: 542–8.

49 Culpitt SV, Maziak W, Loukidis S *et al*. Effects of high dose inhaled steroids on cells, cytokines and proteases in induced

sputum in chronic obstructive pulmonary disease. *Am J Respir Crit Care Med* 1999; 160: 1635–9.

50 Sachs APE, Koeter GH, Groenier KH, Van der Waaij D, Schiphuis J, Meyboom-de Jong B. Changes in symptoms, peak expiratory flow and sputum flora during treatment with antibiotics of exacerbations in patients with chronic obstructive pulmonary disease in general practice. *Thorax* 1995; 50: 758–63.

51 Saint S, Bent S, Vittinghoff E, Grady D. Antibiotics in chronic obstructive pulmonary disease exacerbations. *A Meta-Anal JAMA* 1995; 273: 957–60.

52 Moser KM, Luchsinger PC, Adamson JS, McMahon SM, Schlueter DP, Spivack M, Weg JG. Respiratory stimulation with intravenous doxapram in respiratory failure. *N Engl J Med* 1973; 288: 427–31.

53 Angus RM, Ahmed AA, Fenwick LJ, Peacock AJ. Comparison of the acute effects on gas exchange of nasal ventilation and doxapram in exacerbations of chronic obstructive pulmonary disease. *Thorax* 1996; 51: 1048–50.

54 Gravil JH, Al-Rawas OA, Cotton MM *et al*. Home treatment of exacerbations of COPD by an acute respiratory assessment service. *Lancet* 1998; 351: 1853–5.

55 Cotton MM, Bucknall CE, Dagg KD *et al*. Early discharge for patients with exacerbations of COPD. a randomised controlled trial. *Thorax* 2000; 55: 902–6.

56 Skwarska E, Cohen G, Skwarski KM *et al*. A randomised controlled trial of supported discharge in patients with exacerbations of COPD. *Thorax* 2000; 55: 907–12.

57 Davies L, Wilkinson M, Bonner S, Calverley PMA, Angus RM. Hospital at home versus hospital care in patients with exacerbations of chronic obstructive pulmonary disease: prospective randomised controlled trial. *BMJ* 2000; 321: 1265–8.

58 Nichol KL, Baken L, Nelson A. Relation between influenza vaccination and out patient visits, hospitalisation and mortality in elderly patients with chronic lung disease. *Ann Intern Med* 1999; 130: 397–403.

59 Poole PJ, Black PN. Oral mucolytic drugs for exacerbations of chronic obstructive pulmonary disease: systematic review. *BMJ* 2001; 322: 1271–4.

60 Burge PS, Calverley PMA, Jones PW *et al*. Randomised, double blind, placebo controlled study of fluticasone propionate in patients with moderate to sever chronic obstructive pulmonary disease: the ISOLDE trial. *BMJ* 2000; 320: 1297–303.

61 Paggiaro PL, Dahle R, Bakran I, Frith L, Hollingworth K, Efthimiou J. Multicentre randomised placebo-controlled trial of inhaled fluticasone propionate in patients with chronic obstructive pulmonary disease. *Lancet* 1998; 351: 773–80.

62 Jarad N, Wedzicha JA, Burge PS, Calverley PMA. An observational study of inhaled corticosteroid withdrawal in patients with stable chronic obstructive pulmonary disease. *Respiratory Med* 1999; 93: 161–6.

63 Mahler DA, Donohue JF, Barbee RA *et al*. Efficacy of salmeterol xinafoate in the treatment of COPD. *Chest* 1999; 115: 957–65.

64 Van Noord JA, de Munck DRAJ, Bantje ThA *et al*. Long-term treatment of chronic obstructive pulmonary disease with salmeterol and the additive effect of ipratropium. *Eur Resp J* 2000; 15: 878–85.

65 Vincken W, van Noord JA, Greefhorst APM. Improved health outcomes in patients with COPD during 1 year's treatment with tiotropium. *Eur Respir J* 2002; 19: 209–16.

66 Kanner RE, Anthonisen NR, Connett JE. Lower respiratory illnesses promote FEV_1 decline in current smokers but not ex-smokers with mild chronic obstructive lung disease: results from the Lung Health Study. *Am J Respir Crit Care Med* 2001; 164: 358–64.

67 Donaldson GC, Seemungal TAR, Bhowmik A, Wedzicha JA. The relationship between exacerbation frequency and lung function decline in chronic obstructive pulmonary disease. *Thorax* 2002; 57: 847–52.

16: Which patients with acute COPD exacerbation should receive ventilatory support?

Mrinal Sircar and Mark Elliott

Introduction

An exacerbation of chronic obstructive pulmonary disease (COPD) of sufficient severity to necessitate hospital admission indicates a poor prognosis, carrying a 6–26% mortality [1,2]. In one study, an 11% in-hospital mortality was reported, but this increased over the next 2 months, 6 months, 1 year and 2 years of follow-up to 20%, 33%, 43% and 49%, respectively [3]. Another study found 5-year survival rates of 45% after hospital discharge, but this decreased to 28% with any further episode of hospitalization [4]. Numerous studies have been carried out to identify predictors of mortality during an acute exacerbation of COPD. It has variously been correlated to: age, alveolar–arterial oxygen gradient greater than 5.5 kPa (41 mmHg), ventricular or atrial arrhythmias [4,5], requirement for long-term oxygen therapy, low albumin or sodium, low forced expiratory volume in 1 s (FEV_1) [4,6] and reversibility of hypercapnia [7]. Mortality increases with low body mass index [8] and in the presence of comorbidity, such as other organ failure [9]. The most important predictor of in-hospital mortality [2,10,11] and need for intubation [12] is the level of acidosis. Unsurprisingly, patients admitted to the intensive-care unit (ICU) have a high mortality, for instance Seneff *et al.* [13] reported overall hospital mortality at 24% following admission to the ICU, doubling to 59% at 1 year. Others have reported lower mortality rates after admission to ICU for mechanical ventilation, the ICU and hospital case fatality rates in one study being 1% and 11%, respectively [14]. On the other hand, mortality as high as 88.8% at 2 years after ICU admission has also been reported [15].

Non-invasive ventilation

Following a number of case series of the successful use of non-invasive mechanical ventilation (NIMV) [16–18] in patients with an acute exacerbation of COPD, there has been a great expansion of interest in this area. The obvious attraction of NIMV is the avoidance of intubation and its attendant complications. Patients do not require sedation and can cooperate with physiotherapy and eat normally [19]. Intermittent ventilatory support is practical, and patients can undergo mobilization at an early stage. Furthermore, patients can communicate with medical and nursing staff and with family; this is likely to reduce the feelings of powerlessness and anxiety [13]. However, concerns have been raised that when NIMV is unsuccessful, the delay in intubation may affect the outcome [20,21], that a nasal or face mask is uncomfortable and claustrophobic and that the procedure is more time-consuming for medical and nursing staff [22].

Physiologically, NIMV is little different from invasive mechanical ventilation; positive pressure is delivered to the lungs, but because of difficulties in getting a perfect seal with the mask, it is theoretically less efficient than invasive ventilation. On the other hand, the fact that NIMV is relatively less efficient may be to its advantage. Barotrauma such as pneumothorax is not uncommon with ventilation after intubation, but it has not been reported in any of the major studies of NIMV, perhaps due to the lack of a perfect seal acting as a safety valve preventing high pressures being transmitted to the lungs. NIMV decreases inspiratory muscle effort and respiratory rate and increases tidal volumes and oxygen saturation in stable COPD patients [23] and during an acute exacerbation [24]. Arterial PaO_2 increases while the $PaCO_2$ decreases with NIMV [17,25]. In a study by Celikel $et\ al.$, NIMV significantly improved PaO_2, $PaCO_2$, pH and respiratory rate, while medical treatment achieved only an improvement in respiratory rate [26]. For the same FiO_2, the $AaDO_2$ increases due to a rise in clearance of CO_2 and hence increased respiratory exchange ratio [25]. There is a fall in cardiac output leading to a slight decrease in systemic oxygen delivery, but this is not accompanied by a change in PvO_2. There appears to be no improvement in VA/Q ratio with NIMV [25].

Ventilators usually used for NIMV are either volume-targeted or pressure-targeted. There are theoretical advantages to each mode, but broadly speaking they are comparable in efficacy. Volume-targeted ventilators have been shown to produce more complete off-loading of the respiratory muscles, but at the expense of comfort [27]. In intubated patients however, assist pressure controlled ventilation has been shown to be more effective than assist control volume ventilation at reducing various parameters of respiratory muscle effort, although this difference was only seen at moderate tidal volumes and low flow rates [28]. In stable patients, little difference in gas exchange was seen with different types of ventilator [23,29]. In terms of outcome, Vitacca $et\ al.$ [30] found that there was no difference whether volume-targeted or pressure-targeted machines were used, but pressure-targeted machines were better tolerated by patients. A new mode of proportional assisted ventilation (PAV) improves gas exchange and dyspnoea in stable COPD [31] and has been used successfully in the treatment of acute respiratory failure of various aetiologies [32]. PAV delivers ventilation according to patient demand, which should theoretically be more comfortable, but makes the assumption that the patient with respiratory failure knows best what he or she needs in terms of ventilatory support. PAV using flow assistance and positive end-expiratory pressure (PEEP) achieved greatest improvement in minute ventilation, dypnoea and reduction in pressure–time product per breath of the respiratory muscles and diaphragm in COPD patients with acute respiratory failure [33]. It has been shown to decrease patient effort, work of breathing and neuromuscular drive (P0.1) in COPD patients being weaned off invasive mechanical ventilation [34,35]. Further data are needed comparing PAV with conventional modes of ventilation.

PEEP can be added during NIMV and has beneficial effects, off-loading the respiratory muscles, probably by counterbalancing the inspiratory threshold load imposed by intrinsic PEEP [36] and lavaging carbon dioxide from the mask [37]. In a short-term study in stable patients, the addition of PEEP has been shown to reduce oxygen delivery despite an adequate SaO_2 [38]. Mask continuous positive airway pressure (CPAP) has also been shown to significantly decrease respiratory rate and the subjective sensation of dyspnoea, decreasing $PaCO_2$, increasing PaO_2 [39], significantly improving ventilation [40] and avoiding intubation and mechanical ventilation [41] in exacerbations of COPD. In stable patients, the degree of unloading with CPAP is less than with NIMV [23], but given the lack of randomized controlled data on the use of CPAP in acute exacerbations of COPD, in contrast to NIMV (see below), its use should be confined to centres in which NIMV is not available.

What is the evidence for the clinical usefulness of non-invasive ventilation?

Numerous uncontrolled studies have reported efficacy of NIMV in acute exacerbations of COPD, producing clinical and physiological improvement. Meduri et al. [16] successfully ventilated 10 patients, including six with exacerbations of COPD, using a pressure-control mode delivered through a face mask in 1989 and followed up subsequently with a larger series of 18 patients with hypercapnic respiratory failure, with similar results [42]. Similar results have also been reported by other workers in uncontrolled studies [18,43–47]. However, in a small study, including only three patients with COPD, NIMV was not found to be useful and indeed took up a considerable amount of nursing time [22]. The duration of NIMV required may be brief, suggesting that even short periods of successful ventilation may be sufficient to buy time for other therapies to work. Hilbert et al. [48] found that, using sequential mask bilevel positive airway pressure support, at least 30 min every 3 hours, only 11 patients, compared to 30 of 42 matched historical controls, eventually required intubation. In-hospital mortality was similar, but duration of ventilatory support and length of ICU stay were shortened.

There have been a number of other studies comparing NIMV with historical controls. Brochard et al. [17] reported 13 patients, of whom 12 could be managed with face mask NIMV without requiring intubation. These patients were also weaned off their ventilator faster and spent less time on the intensive-care unit than the controls. In another study, 24 patients treated with NIMV showed more rapid improvement in blood gases and a better pH and respiratory rate at discharge as compared to matched historical controls [49]. Only two patients receiving NIMV required intubation, compared with nine controls. Hospital stays were also shorter in the survivors in the NIMV group, but the in-hospital survival rates were no different. However, long-term survival at 12 months was significantly better in the patients receiving NIMV (71% vs. 50%). Vitacca et al. [50] also found no difference in hospital mortality in patients receiving NIMV compared to historical controls who were intubated and ventilated (20% vs. 26%), but a survival advantage with NIMV became apparent at 3 months (77% vs. 52%) and 12 months (70% vs. 37%).

This longer-term survival advantage with NIMV is intriguing. It has been suggested that it is due to imperfect matching of the control and patient groups [51]. However, there are other possible explanations. If ICU care has been prolonged, and weaning difficult, there may be reluctance on the part of either medical staff or the patients themselves to consider invasive mechanical ventilation (IMV) for a subsequent exacerbation. Secondly, it is possible that IMV has adverse effects that may be significant later; electrophysiological and biopsy evidence of muscle dysfunction has been shown after as little as 1 week of invasive ventilation [52,53]. Such dysfunction of the respiratory muscles will reduce the capacity of the respiratory muscle pump, which may increase the risk of ventilatory failure in subsequent exacerbation. However, these observations are speculative and need to be substantiated in further prospective studies.

The first prospective randomized controlled trial of NIMV in COPD exacerbation was reported in 1993 [54] (Table 16.1). Patients receiving standard medical therapy and NIMV from a volume-cycled ventilator in the assisted control mode had a significantly greater improvement in both the pH and $PaCO_2$ as compared to patients on standard medical therapy alone. On an intention-to-treat basis, there was no difference in survival between NIMV and conventional therapy, but only one out of 26 patients who actually received NIMV died, compared to nine out of 30 patients in the control group ($P = 0.014$). However, the mortality in the control arm was higher than expected from other studies, given that the mean pH at the time of randomization showed only mild acidosis, and in addition few patients who died were offered IMV. In a multicentre study in five European ICUs, Brochard et al. [55]

Table 16.1 Randomized controlled trials of non-invasive mechanical ventilation in acute exacerbations of chronic obstructive pulmonary disease.

Trial	Location for trial	No. of patients (study/control)	Type of ventilator	Baseline pH (NIMV/control)	Outcome (NIMV vs. control)	Comments
Bott 1993	Ward	26/30	Volume-cycled ventilation via nasal mask	7.348/7.331	Mortality 1/26 vs. 9/30 ETI 0/26 vs. 2/30 + 3 NIMV	NIMV + ST vs. ST alone
Kramer 1995	ICU	16/15z (11/12 COPD)	Bilevel via nasal mask	7.28/7.29	Mortality 1/16 vs. 2/15 ETI 5 vs. 11 (COPD 1/11 vs. 8/12 + 3 NIMV)	NIMV + ST vs. ST alone
Brochard 1995	ICU	43/42	Pressure-support ventilation via nasal mask	7.27/7.28	Mortality 4/43 vs. 12/42 ETI 11 vs. 31	NIMV + ST vs. ST alone
Angus 1996	Ward	9/8	Pressure-cycled ventilation via nasal mask	7.31/7.3	Mortality 0/9 vs. 3/8 ETI 0/9 vs. 0/8 + 2 NIMV	NIMV + ST vs. ST + doxapram
Barbe 1996	ED/ward	10/10	Bilevel via nasal mask	7.33/7.33	Mortality 0/10 vs. 0/10 ETI 0/10 vs. 0/10	NIMV + ST vs. ST alone
Wood 1998	ED	16/11	Bilevel via nasal mask	7.35/7.34	Mortality 4/16 vs. 0/11 ETI 7/16 vs. 5/11	NIMV + ST vs. ST alone
Celikel 1998	ICU	16/15	Pressure support + CPAP via face mask	7.27/7.28	Mortality 0 ETI 1/16 vs. 2/15 + 4 NIMV	NIMV + ST vs. ST alone
Plant 2001	Ward	118/118	Bilevel via face or nasal mask	7.32/7.31	Mortality 10% vs. 20% ETI surrogate 15 vs. 27%	

COPD, chronic obstructive pulmonary disease; CPAP, continuous positive airway pressure; ED, emergency department; ETI, endotracheal intubation; ICU, intensive-care unit; NIMV, non-invasive mechanical ventilation; ST, standard medical treatment.

demonstrated a significantly lower rate of endotracheal intubation (11 of 43 vs. 31 of 42), mortality (4 vs. 12) and shorter hospital stays (23 vs. 35 days) in patients on NIMV compared to those only on standard medical therapy. The complication rate, particularly for pneumonia, was much lower in the NIMV group (two vs. seven) and most of the excess of complications and mortality in the control group was attributed to intubation. These data suggest that NIMV may be superior to IMV, but importantly these were highly selected patients, with the majority (70%) of patients with COPD admitted to the ICUs during the study period being excluded from the study. The intubation rate in the control group was higher than that in some other studies, and it has been suggested that over zealous oxygen supplementation precipitated worsening hypercapnia in some patients [51]. Kramer *et al.* [56] reported similar results with non-invasive pressure support ventilation in a mixed group of patients with acute respiratory failure, with a substantial reduction in the need for intubation, which was most marked in the subgroup with exacerbation of COPD (one of 11 patients on NIMV compared to eight of 12 controls). However, the mortality rate was no different (one of 16 vs. two of 15). Another study that used a conventional ICU ventilator to deliver pressure support with CPAP by a face mask also found a decreased need for intubation and decreased length of hospital stay in patients ventilated non-invasively, besides achieving significant physiological improvement [26].

However, not all studies have shown benefit from NIMV. Barbe *et al.* found no benefit from NIMV over conventional treatment [57]. Patients received two sessions of NIMV, using pressure support, of 3 h each for the first 3 days of their admission. None of the patients in either group required intubation or died. In a recent study of unselected patients with respiratory failure of different aetiologies, there was no difference between NIMV and standard medical treatment alone [21]. However, there was a trend to an increased mortality in the NIMV group, which was attributed to a delay in intubation in the NIMV group (4 vs. 26 h). However, the study included only six patients with COPD (two in the NIMV and four in the control group) and the two groups were not well matched, particularly for aetiology of respiratory failure.

Studies performed in the ICU [26,55,56] show that NIMV is feasible and results in more rapid physiological improvement [26,55,56] and that the endotracheal intubation (ETI) rate is substantially reduced [55,56]. In the largest study [55], there was a reduction in mortality with NIMV. By contrast, studies performed outside the ICU (in the emergency room or on a general ward) [21,54,57] have failed to show an advantage for NIMV. A number of factors may explain this difference. Firstly, nurse staffing and doctor-to-patient ratios are likely to be less than those on the ICU, resulting in less time spent adapting the ventilator to the patient. However, physiological improvement was still seen in these studies, suggesting that, at least initially, effective ventilation was provided. In the study by Barbe *et al.* [57], no patient in either group required ETI or died; the mean pH was 7.33 and thus recovery in most patients was likely. Given the small number of patients studied, it is not surprising that no difference was seen between the two groups. Furthermore, NIMV was initiated in the emergency room before other medical therapies had been given time to work. In contrast, the patients treated on the ICU were more ill (more acidotic) and are likely to have failed to improve with initial treatment with bronchodilators, steroids, etc. A recent study has shown that 25% of acidotic patients will correct their pH into the normal range following medical treatment in the emergency room [58].

A multicentre randomized controlled trial of NIMV in 236 patients with acute exacerbations of COPD on general respiratory wards in 13 centres [59] has recently been reported. NIMV was administered with an unsophisticated ventilator and only the level of inspiratory positive airway pressure (IPAP) and expiratory positive airway pressure (EPAP) had to be adjusted by the usual ward staff according to a simple protocol. Patients were randomized to NIMV or conventional therapy if respiratory rate was >23 breaths/min and pH between 7.25 and 7.35 inclusive on arrival on the ward, after a period had elapsed allowing time for treatment initiated in the emergency department to work. 'Treatment failure', a surrogate for the need for intubation, defined by *a priori* criteria, was reduced from 27% to 15% by NIMV ($P<0.05$). In-hospital mortality was also reduced, from 20% to 10% ($P<0.05$). Subgroup analysis [59,60] suggested that the outcome in patients with pH <7.30 after initial treatment was inferior to that in the studies performed in the ICU, suggesting that the use of a very simple ventilator according to protocol on a general ward is only appropriate for those with milder exacerbations.

There is no direct comparison between invasive mechanical ventilation (IMV) and NIMV, and the two techniques should be viewed as complementary, with NIMV being regarded as a means of obviating the need for ETI rather than as a direct alternative. Some patients require intubation from the outset and others after a failed trial of NIMV. Patients with COPD may be difficult to wean from invasive mechanical ventilation [61], and NIMV has been used successfully in weaning [62,63]. A multicentre randomized controlled trial [64] in which 50 patients who failed a 2-h T-piece trial after 48 h invasive mechanical ventilation were randomized to continued endotracheal intubation and weaning using pressure support or extubation onto NIMV, and a similar weaning strategy showed a clear advantage for NIMV. More patients were weaned (88% vs. 68%), and the duration of ventilation (10.2±6.8 vs. 16.6±11.8 days) and ICU stay (15.1±5.4 vs. 24.0±13.7 days) were reduced using NIMV. Ninety-two per cent of patients randomized to NIMV were alive at 60 days, compared with 72% who received continuing invasive mechanical ventilation. There were no episodes of pneumonia in the non-invasive group, but seven in the control group. Girault *et al.* [65], in a further randomized controlled trial involving 33 patients, showed a reduction in the duration of invasive mechanical ventilation (4.6 ± 1.9 vs. 7.7 ± 3.8 days) and a reduced mean daily ventilatory support. However, the study found that there was an increased total duration (11.5 ± 5.2 vs. 3.5 ± 1.4 days) of ventilatory support when the non-invasive approach was used. There was no difference in the percentage of patients successfully weaned, or in complication rates.

A proportion of patients weaned from invasive ventilation subsequently deteriorate and require further ventilatory support. Hilbert *et al.* reported 30 COPD patients who developed hypercapnic respiratory distress within 72 h of extubation [66]. They were treated with mask bilevel pressure support ventilation. Only six of these 30 patients, compared with 20 of 30 historical controls, required reintubation. Although in-hospital mortality was not significantly different, the mean duration of ventilatory assistance and length of intensive-care stay related to the event were significantly shortened by non-invasive ventilation.

Other modes of non-invasive ventilation

The use of other modes of non-invasive ventilation has been reported in patients with COPD exacerbation. In a retrospective uncontrolled study, 105 patients were successfully weaned, and 93 were eventually discharged from hospital after intermittent negative-pressure ventilation by means of an iron lung [67]. Of these 105 patients, 62 were in coma and 43 had a deteriorating level of consciousness at presentation. All patients were initially ventilated continuously for 12–48 h and subsequently received intermittent daytime ventilation until weaned. Any subsequent exacerbation was also treated with negative-pressure ventilation. Survival was 92% and 37% at 1 and 5 years, respectively. A more recent study by the same group was carried out in 150 patients with hypoxic hypercapnic coma (including 79% patients with COPD) [68]. Of the 74 patients with only exacerbation of COPD as cause of coma, treatment failed only in 19 (26%) patients, including 14 (19%) who died.

When should assisted ventilation be started? Is it appropriate in all patients with an exacerbation of COPD?

One of the theoretical advantages of NIMV is that it can be started at an earlier stage in the evolution of ventilatory failure, before invasive ventilation would normally be considered appropriate. It has been suggested that NIMV should be started when the pH is <7.35 and the respiratory rate >30 [69,70]. The data from the Yorkshire non-invasive ventilation (YONIV) trial [59] support these criteria, suggesting it be instituted at an even lower respiratory rate

(>23 breaths/min), but after a period during which the effect of drug treatment, adjustment of oxygen therapy, etc. can be evaluated. Reversing ventilatory failure is likely to be easier at an early stage, when theoretically lower pressures used for shorter periods may improve tolerance [69,70]. NIMV is less likely to be effective in patients with more severe physiological disturbances at the outset, suggesting that once decompensation has become well established, the cycle of deterioration may not be broken with the use of NIMV [55,71]. If NIMV does not improve pH and respiratory rate within the first hour or two, intubation should be considered [55,71,72]. Patients with high Acute Physiology and Chronic Health Evaluation (APACHE) II scores, an inability to minimize the amount of mouth leak (because of lack of teeth, secretions, or breathing pattern) or inability to coordinate with NIMV are poor candidates for NIMV [73]. In another study, patients who failed on NIMV had a significantly higher incidence of pneumonia (38.5% vs. 8.7%), were underweight, had a greater level of neurological deterioration, a higher APACHE II score and reduced compliance with ventilation as assessed by the physician in charge, compared to those who were successfully treated [71]. Although both groups had similar PaO_2/FiO_2 ratios, patients failing on NIMV had a significantly more abnormal $PaCO_2$ and pH before starting NIMV. Only baseline pH was found by logistic regression analysis to be able to predict success or failure of NIMV (mean 7.28 in successful group, versus 7.22 in the failure group) with a sensitivity of 97% and specificity of 71%. Coma or confusion, upper gastrointestinal bleeding, high risk of aspiration, haemodynamic instability or uncontrolled arrhythmia have been suggested as contraindications to NIMV [74]. This is primarily for theoretical reasons, as these patients have been excluded from previous studies, and not because there is any evidence that invasive mechanical ventilation (IMV) is superior in these situations.

The question of which patients should be intubated is difficult. Poor prognostic indicators for patients who are invasively ventilated are: admissions after cardiorespiratory arrest, previous therapy with long-term oral steroids, development of renal or cardiac failure in ICU and high APACHE II scores [75]. However, clinical estimates of survival for the same patient may vary among physicians [76]. Numerous authors have tried to find prediction models that could help in the clinical decision to invasively ventilate patients presenting with acute exacerbation of COPD. Kaelin *et al.* reported that a multivariate analysis including eight parameters (fever greater than 38 °C, FEV_1/forced vital capacity (FVC), age, leucocytosis, $PaCO_2$ when the patient was stable, low-flow oxygen treatment and plasma protein) could differentiate between those likely to survive for more than 6 months with an accuracy of 78% [77]. However, if the decision to intubate and ventilate had been based on this analysis, it would have denied ventilation to 23% of patients who eventually survived for more than 6 months. Stauffer *et al.* [78] also found that a multivariate analysis (including age, diagnosis and duration of mechanical ventilation) could not produce a predicted probability of survival for weaning, ICU discharge, hospital discharge or 1 year post hospital discharge. Another study performed in patients requiring ventilation for more than 3 weeks found that $PaCO_2$ and maximal inspiratory pressure (MIP) could predict weaning success or failure, but not the survival rate [79]. However, this study found that survival to 2 years in those not able to be weaned from the ventilator was very poor compared to those who were eventually weaned (22% vs. 68%). Other authors have found that patients requiring long-term home ventilation (either non-invasively or via tracheostomy) have survival periods no different from those requiring only long-term home oxygen, the mean survival being 3 years [80]. Overall, it appears that predicting the successful long-term survival of patients being considered for invasive ventilation is imprecise, and any prediction model will misclassify a significant proportion of patients who are likely to survive after ventilation.

Mechanical ventilation and end-of-life decisions

The decision to treat patients with severe COPD with mechanical ventilation was previously taken solely by physicians. However, the importance of patients and their families in decisions on instituting such life-sustaining treatments is now well recognized. It has been suggested that decisions regarding life-sustaining interventions should be made by patients educated concerning their disease and treatment options [81]. Shared decision-making is increasingly recognized as an emerging trend in health care [82]. However, this does not mean that the physician should always forfeit his opinion in favour of the patient's preference [83]. The American Thoracic Society has outlined a physician's responsibilities in these situations as follows: firstly, to assess whether the patient has adequate decision-making capacity; secondly, to inform the patient regarding the diagnosis, prognosis, risks, benefits and consequences of the full range of available medical interventions; and thirdly, to provide a professional recommendation [84].

Often, discussions take place once patients have been brought to hospital for an exacerbation, when they are too ill to participate in the decision-making process, and physicians and family members end up taking the decisions on their behalf [85]. Unfortunately, health-care decisions made for a patient frequently do not reflect the patient's own preferences [86]. Physicians for their part consider the patient's quality of life, while taking decisions to provide or withhold life-sustaining treatment options. This involves interpretation of the patient's prior medical experience, the physician's attitudes about medical responsibilities/patient rights and estimates of the patient's survival time [87].

There are definite cultural differences in patient, family and physician attitudes regarding end-of-life medical-care decisions, and in some societies both physicians and family members may regard withholding or withdrawing life-sustaining treatment as abandonment or even killing [88,89]. In a study carried out by Sullivan *et al.* [83], physicians were in favour of prior discussions regarding life-sustaining treatment options, but felt that patients had difficulty in grasping such information and accepting it in a short time. Patient individuality and differing rates of progression of disease add to the difficulty in deciding the optimal time for such a discussion. The use of a living will by individuals with chronic illness is a common practice in some societies and is one way in which patients' views regarding life-sustaining treatments can be determined. Even within such societies, certain sections such as 'black, poorly educated, underinsured, or cognitively impaired' are less likely to prepare a living will [90]. Furthermore, the decisions that patients make are strongly influenced by the way physicians present the options [83,91,92]. In practice, during a crisis several problems are encountered even in patients who have made a living will. They include delay in presenting the advanced directive, conflict between the dictates of the living will and the wishes of the person named in the durable power of attorney, and controversy among health-care providers as to when in the course of disease the spirit of the advanced directive has been met [93]. The legal validity of such an advanced directive also needs to be considered in each country.

Current data suggest that for selected patients, the outcome with NIMV is certainly no worse than with IMV [56] and possibly better [55] and it should therefore be the first-line treatment for most patients. If the patient's wishes about the appropriateness of intervention are unknown, NIMV is less problematic than IMV, because patients can choose to discontinue NIMV subsequently, when they may be better able to make such decisions. Patients retain a higher degree of control over their own destiny than is possible when they have been intubated. It may also buy time for family members to accept that further intervention is not appropriate. Indeed, NIMV has been successfully used in patients refusing endotracheal intubation [94].

A strong case cannot be made on current evidence for denying ventilation, especially NIMV, to any patient presenting with acute respiratory failure due to COPD and requiring ventilatory support. At the same time, it has been aptly stated that 'We have this technology that can, in some cases, save lives and in others prolong dying; we have a greater responsibility to determine when that technology will be used' [95].

What is the cost of NIMV?

In an early report on the use of NIMV in six patients, Chevrolet *et al.* [22]

found that, particularly in patients with obstructive lung disease, the technique was very time-consuming for the nurses and the time was largely wasted, since all of the patients eventually had to be intubated. As with any new technique, there is a learning curve, and the same group have subsequently published more encouraging results [96]. In the ICU, in which there are high nurse-to-patient ratios, any additional work associated with NIMV is unlikely to have a major effect, but the issue of medical and nursing time is very relevant if the technique is to be performed in the ward environment. Nurses and therapists will have responsibility for a much larger number of patients, and any extra work associated with NIMV may mean that other tasks and patients are neglected.

In a randomized controlled trial comparing standard treatment with or without NIMV in a general ward setting, Bott et al. [54] found no difference in nursing care requirements, recorded on a daily basis by asking the senior nurse to record the amount of care needed using a simple visual analogue scale. This may have underestimated the care requirements associated with NIMV, because ventilation was initiated and maintained by staff supernumerary to the normal ward complement. In another study, with more detailed analysis of nursing and therapist activity, Kramer et al. [56] found that the respiratory therapist spent more time with patients in the NIMV group compared to the standard treatment group in the first 8 h, but this difference did not reach statistical significance. The time required in the NIMV group dropped significantly in the second 8-h period. The time demands on the nurses did not differ in the two groups throughout the measurement period, and neither the respiratory therapist nor the nurses considered caring for patients on NIMV as being any more difficult than the control patients. Nava et al. [97] found that in the first 48 h of assisted ventilation, NIMV was no more time-consuming or demanding for staff than invasive mechanical ventilation. However, after the first few days of ventilation, NIMV was significantly less time-consuming for both medical and nursing personnel.

Since most studies report a shorter period of ventilation and ICU and hospital stay, it is has been suggested that NIMV should be cheaper than invasive mechanical ventilation [98,99]. However, patients treated with NIMV do incur substantial financial costs during their hospitalization [100]. Nava et al. [97] found that the total cost per day was comparable for invasive and non-invasive ventilation, although NIMV was performed on a respiratory ICU. In the study by Kramer et al. [56], the total hospital charges were 37.6±7.9 (in thousands of dollars) in patients receiving NIMV vs. 33.9±6.9 in control patients not receiving NIMV, which was not statistically different [56]. In a recent multicentre study from the UK, the incremental cost of NIMV per patient avoiding the 'need for intubation' was £2829. However, the incremental savings per death avoided were £4114, by way of decreased ICU usage, thus providing a strong economic argument for the use of NIMV [101].

How should NIMV be used and by whom? Is it viable in the ordinary district general hospital setting?

Although early experience of NIMV in COPD exacerbation came from the ICU [16,17] it has been shown to be effective in the non-ICU setting [18,54,59,102]. The successful application of NIMV is critically dependent on nursing, therapist and medical staff expertise, and it is vital that all staff involved be adequately trained in the technique. Expertise and skill retention will be facilitated by maximizing exposure of all staff to patients receiving NIMV. The expected throughput of patients is another factor to be considered in deciding on the best location for NIMV. In a recent study in the UK, it has been suggested that for the average general hospital, serving a population of 250 000 and with a standardized mortality rate for COPD of 100, six patients per month with an acute exacerbation of COPD will require NIMV, assuming that ventilation is initiated in patients with a pH < 7.35 after initial treatment [58]. This number excludes patients with other conditions requiring NIMV and those who require it later in their hospital stay, e.g. for weaning, etc. With relatively small numbers of patients per month, NIMV is best performed in a single-sex location, to facilitate staff training and to maximize throughput and skill retention. In areas with a higher prevalence of COPD or hospitals serving larger populations, an NIMV service could reasonably be provided in more than one location.

A proportion of patients will fail with NIMV, requiring intubation and invasive ventilation; it is important that personnel and the facility for intubation be rapidly available if needed, if the trend to increased mortality with NIMV, as reported by Wood *et al.*, is to be avoided [21]. It could be argued that for patients with a high likelihood of failing (e.g. severe acidosis, severe hypercapnia, initiating event unlikely to be rapidly reversible, etc.) [71], NIMV should be initiated on the ICU and once stabilized the patient could be transferred to the ward normally providing NIMV.

In any discussion about the location of an NIMV service, it is important to note that the model of hospital care differs from country to country and that 'ICU', 'high-dependency unit' (HDU) and 'general ward' will have different levels of staffing, facilities for monitoring, etc. [103–105]. Care must therefore be taken in the extrapolation of results obtained in one environment to other hospitals and countries.

In summary, staff training and experience are more important than location, and adequate numbers of staff, skilled in NIMV, must be available throughout the 24-h period. Because of the demands of looking after these acutely ill patients, and to aid training and skill retention, NIMV is usually best carried out in one single-sex location, with one nurse responsible for no more than three to four patients in total.

Is there still a role for ventilatory stimulants?

In acute respiratory failure due to COPD, respiratory drive is usually high [106]. Despite this, respiratory stimulants have been used in exacerbations of COPD and may obviate the need for intubation [2,107,108]. Of a number of respiratory stimulants (doxapram, ethamivan, amiphenazole, prethcamide and nikethamide), only doxapram produced a significant increase in minute volume [109], and it also increased sputum production. It is also the only respiratory stimulant licensed for use in the UK. In a double-blind cross-over trial in eight patients with an acute exacerbation of COPD on controlled oxygen therapy, three patients had a rise in $PaCO_2$ on placebo, which was reversed with doxapram [110]. A double-blind study compared 40 patients on a doxapram infusion with 38 patients on placebo over a 2-h period [111]. There was a significantly higher pH and lower $PaCO_2$ in the doxapram group at all time points. However, intubation and death rates were not affected. One patient on doxapram developed a psychosis. In a randomized controlled study, patients with exacerbation of COPD and type II respiratory failure, who were not improving on conventional treatment, received either non-invasive ventilation or doxapram [112]. Both groups of patients had an improvement in PaO_2, but the level was higher and the peak level was sustained at 4 h only in the NIMV group. Similarly, $PaCO_2$ decreased in both groups of patients, but was sustained at 4 h only in those on NIMV. In the early part of the study, three patients in the doxapram group died. Subsequently, the protocol was modified and two further patients deteriorating on doxapram received NIMV and survived to discharge. Another respiratory stimulant, almitrine, is effective in improving both PaO_2 and $PaCO_2$ levels when infused in COPD patients with chronic respiratory failure, by increasing ventilation and improving the ventilation–perfusion relationship [113]. A comparison of almitrine 0.5 mg/kg infusion with doxapram 1 mg/kg found that the former was significantly better in increasing PaO_2 and decreasing $PaCO_2$ in patients with chronic type II respiratory failure [114]. However, a randomized controlled trial against placebo in acute exacerbations of COPD revealed no benefit from almitrine [115].

Respiratory stimulants in acute exacerbations of COPD have been shown to have a short-term physiological effect, but there are no data to show that this translates into an improved outcome. Such evidence as there is suggests that NIMV is superior to doxapram. Respiratory stimulants may have a role when NIMV is not available or not tolerated.

Conclusion

Patients with an acute exacerbation of COPD place a major burden on health services. There is now good evidence from a number of randomized controlled trials that there is a major role for NIMV and that it should be introduced early, if acidosis persists after initial therapy in the emergency room. NIMV should be considered as a means of avoiding intubation rather than as a substitute for invasive ventilation, and the two techniques should be viewed as complementary. With regard to location, successful NIMV has been reported in the ICU, respiratory ICU and on the ward; the best location will vary from hospital to hospital and is largely dependent on staff training and expertise. Most patients with COPD will die of their disease, and better data are needed to inform the decision-making process regarding the appropriate use of non-invasive and invasive ventilation in acute exacerbations of COPD, if unnecessary suffering and prolongation of the act of dying are to be avoided.

References

1 Martin TR, Lewis SW, Albert RK. The prognosis of patients with chronic obstructive pulmonary disease after hospitalization for acute respiratory failure. *Chest* 1982; **82**: 310–14.
2 Jeffrey AA, Warren PM, Flenley DC. Acute hypercapnic respiratory failure in patients with chronic obstructive lung disease: risk factors and use of guidelines for management. *Thorax* 1992; **47**: 34–40.
3 Connors AF Jr, Dawson NV, Thomas C *et al.* Outcomes following acute exacerbation of severe chronic obstructive lung disease. The SUPPORT investigators. *Am J Respir Crit Care Med* 1996; **155**: 959–67.
4 Vestbo J, Prescott E, Lange P, Schnohr P, Jenson G. Vital prognosis after hospitalization for COPD: a study of a random population sample. *Respir Med* 1998; **92**: 772–6.
5 Fuso L, Incalzi R, Pistelli R *et al.* Predicting mortality of patients hospitalized for acutely exacerbated chronic obstructive pulmonary disease. *Am J Med* 1995; **98**: 272–7.
6 Anon JM, Garcia de Lorenzo A, Zarazaga A, Gomez-Tello V, Garrido G. Mechanical ventilation of patients on long-term oxygen therapy with acute exacerbation of chronic obstructive

pulmonary disease: prognosis and cost-utility analysis. *Intensive Care Med* 1999; **25**: 452–7.
7 Costello R, Deegan P, Fitzpatrick M, McNicholas WT. Reversible hypercapnia in chronic obstructive pulmonary disease: a distinct pattern of respiratory failure with a favorable prognosis. *Am J Med* 1997; **102**: 239–44.
8 Schols AM, Slangen J, Volovics L, Wouters EF. Weight loss is a reversible factor in the prognosis of chronic obstructive pulmonary disease. *Am J Respir Crit Care Med* 1998; **157**: 1791–7.
9 Antonelli Incalzi R, Fuso L *et al.* Co-morbidity contributes to predict mortality of patients with chronic obstructive pulmonary disease. *Eur Respir J* 1997; **10**: 2794–800.
10 Warren PM, Flenley DC, Millar JS, Avery A. Respiratory failure revisited: acute exacerbation of chronic bronchitis between 1961 and 68 and 1970–76. *Lancet* 1980; i: 467–70.
11 Kamat SR, Heera S, Potdar PV *et al.* Bombay experience in intensive respiratory care over 6 years. *J Postgrad Med* 1989; **35**: 123–34.
12 Braghiroli A, Zaccaria S, Ioli F, Erbetta M, Donner CF. Pulmonary failure as a

cause of death in COPD. *Monaldi Arch Chest Dis* 1997; **52**: 170–5.

13 Seneff MG, Wagner DP, Wagner RP, Zimmerman JE, Knaus WA. Hospital and 1-year survival of patients admitted to intensive care units with acute exacerbation of chronic obstructive pulmonary disease. *JAMA* 1995; **274**: 1852–7.

14 Moran JL, Green JV, Homan SD, Leeson RJ, Leppard PI. Acute exacerbation of chronic obstructive pulmonary disease and mechanical ventilation: a reevaluation. *Crit Care Med* 1998; **26**: 71–8.

15 Driver AG, McAlevy MT, Smith JL. Nutritional assessment of patients with chronic obstructive pulmonary disease and acute respiratory failure. *Chest* 1982; **82**: 568–71.

16 Meduri GU, Conoscenti CC, Menashe P, Nair S. Noninvasive face mask ventilation in patients with acute respiratory failure. *Chest* 1989; **95**: 865–70.

17 Brochard L, Isabey D, Piquet J *et al.* Reversal of acute exacerbations of chronic obstructive lung disease by inspiratory assistance with a face mask. *N Engl J Med* 1990; **323**: 1523–30.

18 Elliott MW, Steven MH, Phillips GD, Branthwaite MA. Non-invasive mechanical ventilation for acute respiratory failure. *BMJ* 1990; **300**: 358–60.

19 Pingleton SK. Complications of acute respiratory failure. *Am Rev Respir Dis* 1988; **137**: 1463–93.

20 Ambrosino N. Noninvasive mechanical ventilation in acute respiratory failure. *Eur Respir J* 1996; **9**: 795–807.

21 Wood KA, Lewis L, Von Harz B, Kollef MH. The use of noninvasive positive pressure ventilation in the emergency department. *Chest* 1998; **113**: 1339–46.

22 Chevrolet JC, Jolliet P, Abajo B, Toussi A, Louis M. Nasal positive pressure ventilation in patients with acute respiratory failure. *Chest* 1991; **100**: 775–82.

23 Elliott MW, Aquilina R, Green M, Moxham J, Simonds AK. A comparison of different modes of noninvasive ventilatory support: effects on ventilation and inspiratory muscle effort. *Anaesthesia* 1994; **49**: 279–83.

24 Girault C, Richard J, Chevron V *et al.* Comparative physiological effects of noninvasive assist-control and pressure support ventilation in acute hypercapnic respiratory failure. *Chest* 1997; **111**: 1639–48.

25 Diaz O, Iglesia R, Ferrer M *et al.* Effects of noninvasive ventilation on pulmonary gas exchange and hemodynamics during acute hypercapnic exacerbations of chronic obstructive pulmonary disease. *Am J Respir Crit Care Med* 1997; **156**: 1840–5.

26 Celikel T, Sungur M, Ceyhan B, Karakurt S. Comparison of noninvasive positive pressure ventilation with standard medical therapy in hypercapnic acute respiratory failure. *Chest* 1998; **114**: 1636–42.

27 Girault C, Richard JC, Chevron V *et al.* Comparative physiologic effects of noninvasive assist-control and pressure support ventilation in acute hypercapnic respiratory failure. *Chest* 1997; **111**: 1639–48.

28 Cinnella G, Conti G, Lofaso F *et al.* Effects of assisted ventilation on the work of breathing: volume-controlled versus pressure-controlled ventilation. *Am J Respir Crit Care Med* 1996; **153**: 1025–33.

29 Meecham Jones DJ, Wedzicha JA. Comparison of pressure and volume preset nasal ventilator systems in stable chronic respiratory failure. *Eur Respir J* 1993; **6**: 1060–4.

30 Vitacca M, Rubini F, Foglio K, Scalvini S, Nava S, Ambrosino N. Non-invasive modalities of positive pressure ventilation improve the outcome of acute exacerbations in COLD patients. *Intensive Care Med* 1993; **19**: 450–5.

31 Ambrosino N, Vitacca M, Polese G *et al.* Short-term effects of nasal proportional assist ventilation in patients with chronic hypercapnic respiratory insufficiency. *Eur Respir J* 1997; **10**: 2829–34.

32 Patrick W, Webster K, Ludwig L *et al.* Non-invasive positive-pressure ventilation in acute respiratory distress without prior respiratory failure. *Am J Respir Crit Care Med* 1996; **153**: 1005–11.

33 Ranieri VM, Grasso S, Mascia L *et al.* Effects of proportional assist ventilation on inspiratory muscle effort in patients

with chronic obstructive pulmonary disease and acute respiratory failure. *Anaesthesiology* 1997; **86**: 79–91.

34 Wrigge H, Golisch W, Zinserling J *et al.* Proportional assist versus pressure support ventilation: effects on breathing pattern and respiratory work of patients with chronic obstructive pulmonary disease. *Intensive Care Med* 1999; **25**: 790–8.

35 Appendini L, Purro A, Gudjonsdottir M *et al.* Physiological response of ventilator-dependent patients with chronic obstructive pulmonary disease to proportional assist ventilation and continuous positive airway pressure. *Am J Respir Crit Care Med* 1999; **159**: 1510–17.

36 Appendini L, Patessio A, Zanaboni S *et al.* Physiologic effects of positive end-expiratory pressure and mask pressure support during exacerbations of chronic obstructive pulmonary disease. *Am J Respir Crit Care Med* 1994; **149**: 1069–76.

37 Ferguson GT, Gilmartin M. CO_2 rebreathing during BiPAP ventilatory assistance. *Am J Respir Crit Care Med* 1995; **151**: 1126–35.

38 Ambrosino N, Nava S, Torbicki A *et al.* Haemodynamic effects of pressure support and PEEP ventilation by nasal route in patients with stable chronic obstructive pulmonary disease. *Thorax* 1993; **48**: 523–8.

39 de Lucas P, Tarancon C, Puente L, Rodriguez C, Tatay E, Monturiol JM. Nasal continuous positive airway pressure in patients with COPD in acute respiratory failure: a study of the immediate effects. *Chest* 1993; **104**: 1694–7.

40 Dottorini M, Baglioni S, Eslami A, Todisco T, Fiorenzano G. N-CPAP in patients with COPD in acute respiratory failure. *Chest* 1995; **107**: 585–6.

41 Miro AM, Shivaram U, Hertig I. Continuous positive airway pressure in COPD patients in acute hypercapnic respiratory failure. *Chest* 1993; **103**: 266–8.

42 Meduri GU, Abou-Shala N, Fox RC *et al.* Noninvasive face mask mechanical ventilation in patients with acute hypercapnic respiratory failure. *Chest* 1991; **100**: 445–54.

43 Marino W. Intermittent volume cycled mechanical ventilation via nasal mask in patients with respiratory failure due to COPD. *Chest* 1991; **99**: 681–4.

44 Benhamou D, Girault C, Faure C, Portier F, Muir JF. Nasal mask ventilation in acute respiratory failure. *Chest* 1992; **102**: 912–17.

45 Fernandez R, Blanch L, Valles J, Baigorri F, Artigas A. Pressure support ventilation via face mask in acute respiratory failure in hypercapnic COPD patients. *Intensive Care Med* 1993; **19**: 456–61.

46 Conway JH, Hitchcock RA, Godfrey RC, Carroll MP. Nasal intermittent positive pressure ventilation in acute exacerbation of chronic obstructive pulmonary disease: a preliminary study. *Respir Med* 1993; **87**: 387–94.

47 Confalonieri M, Aiolfi S, Gandola L *et al.* Severe exacerbation of chronic obstructive pulmonary disease treated with BiPAP by nasal mask. *Respiration* 1994; **61**: 310–16.

48 Hilbert G, Gruson D, Gbikpi-Benissan G, Cardinaud JP. Sequential use of noninvasive pressure support ventilation for acute exacerbations of COPD. *Intensive Care Med* 1997; **23**: 955–61.

49 Confalonieri M, Parigi P, Scartabellati A *et al.* Noninvasive mechanical ventilation improves the immediate and long-term outcome of COPD patients with acute respiratory failure. *Eur Respir J* 1996; **9**: 422–30.

50 Vitacca M, Clini E, Rubini F *et al.* Non-invasive mechanical ventilation in severe chronic obstructive lung disease and acute respiratory failure: short-and long-term prognosis. *Intensive Care Med* 1996; **22**: 94–100.

51 Shneerson JM. The changing role of mechanical ventilation in COPD. *Eur Respir J* 1996; **9**: 393–8.

52 Coakley JH, Nagendran K, Honavar M, Hinds CJ. Preliminary observations on the neuromuscular abnormalities in patients with organ failure and sepsis. *Intensive Care Med* 1993; **19**: 323–8.

53 Coakley JH, Nagendran K, Ormerod IE, Ferguson CN, Hinds CJ. Prolonged neurogenic weakness in patients requiring mechanical ventilation for acute airflow limitation. *Chest* 1992; **101**: 1413–16.

54 Bott J, Carroll MP, Conway JH et al. Randomised controlled trial of nasal ventilation in acute ventilatory failure due to chronic obstructive airways disease. Lancet 1993; 341: 1555–7.

55 Brochard L, Mancebo J, Wysocki M et al. Noninvasive ventilation for acute exacerbations of chronic obstructive pulmonary disease. N Engl J Med 1995; 333: 817–22.

56 Kramer N, Meyer TJ, Meharg J, Cece RD, Hill NS. Randomized, prospective trial of noninvasive positive pressure ventilation in acute respiratory failure. Am J Respir Crit Care Med 1995; 151: 1799–806.

57 Barbe F, Togores B, Rubi M et al. Noninvasive ventilatory support does not facilitate recovery from acute respiratory failure in chronic obstructive pulmonary disease. Eur Respir J 1996; 9: 1240–5.

58 Plant PK, Owen J, Elliott MW. One year period prevalence study of respiratory acidosis in acute exacerbation of COPD: implications for the provision of non-invasive ventilation and oxygen administration. Thorax 2000; 55: 550–4.

59 Plant PK, Owen JL, Elliott MW. A multicentre randomised controlled trial of the early use of non-invasive ventilation for acute exacerbations of chronic obstructive pulmonary disease on general respiratory wards. Lancet 2000; 355: 1931–5.

60 Plant PK, Owen JL, Elliott MW. Non-invasive ventilation in acute exacerbations of chronic obstructive pulmonary disease: long term survival and predictors of in-hospital outcome. Thorax 2001; 56: 708–12.

61 Grassino A, Comtois N, Galdiz HJ, Sinderby C. The unweanable patient. Monaldi Arch Chest Dis 1994; 49: 522–6.

62 Udwadia ZF, Santis GK, Steven MH, Simonds AK. Nasal ventilation to facilitate weaning in patients with chronic respiratory insufficiency. Thorax 1992; 47: 715–18.

63 Restrick LJ, Scott AD, Ward EM et al. Nasal intermittent positive-pressure ventilation in weaning intubated patients with chronic respiratory disease from assisted positive-pressure ventilation. Respir Med 1993; 87: 199–204.

64 Nava S, Ambrosino N, Clini E et al. Noninvasive mechanical ventilation in the weaning of patients with respiratory failure due to chronic obstructive pulmonary disease: a randomized, controlled trial. Ann Intern Med 1998; 128: 721–8.

65 Girault C, Daudenthun I, Chevron V et al. Noninvasive ventilation as a systematic extubation and weaning technique in acute-on-chronic respiratory failure: a prospective, randomized controlled study. Am J Respir Crit Care Med 1999; 160: 86–92.

66 Hilbert G, Gruson D, Porel L et al. Noninvasive pressure support ventilation in COPD patients with post extubation hypercapnic respiratory insufficiency. Eur Respir J 1998; 11: 1349–53.

67 Corrado A, Bruscoli G, Messori A et al. Iron lung treatment of subjects with COPD in acute respiratory failure: evaluation of short- and long-term prognosis. Chest 1992; 101: 692–6.

68 Corrado A, De Paola E, Gorini M et al. Intermittent negative pressure ventilation in the treatment of hypoxic hypercapnic coma in chronic respiratory insufficiency. Thorax 1996; 51: 1077–82.

69 Elliott MW. Noninvasive ventilation in chronic obstructive pulmonary disease. N Engl J Med 1995; 333: 870–1.

70 Baldwin DR, Allen MB. Non-invasive ventilation for acute exacerbations of chronic obstructive pulmonary disease. BMJ 1997; 314: 163–4.

71 Ambrosino N, Foglio K, Rubini F et al. Non-invasive mechanical ventilation in acute respiratory failure due to chronic obstructive airways disease: correlates for success. Thorax 1995; 50: 755–7.

72 Meduri GU, Turner RE, Abou-Shala N, Wunderink R, Tolley E. Noninvasive positive pressure ventilation via face mask: first-line intervention in patients with acute hypercapnic and hypoxemic respiratory failure. Chest 1996; 109: 179–93.

73 Soo Hoo GW, Santiago S, Williams AJ. Nasal mechanical ventilation for hypercapnic respiratory failure in

chronic obstructive pulmonary disease. determinants of success and failure. *Crit Care Med* 1994; **22**: 1253–61.

74 Ambrosino N. Noninvasive mechanical ventilation in acute on chronic respiratory failure: determinants of success and failure. *Monaldi Arch Chest Dis* 1997; **52**: 73–5.

75 Hill AT, Hopkinson RB, Stableforth DE. Ventilation in a Birmingham intensive care unit, 1993–95: outcome for patients with chronic obstructive pulmonary disease. *Respir Med* 1998; **92**: 156–61.

76 Pearlman RA. Variability in physician estimates of survival for acute respiratory failure in chronic obstructive pulmonary disease. *Chest* 1987; **91**: 515–21.

77 Kaelin RM, Assimacopoulos A, Chevrolet JC. Failure to predict six-month survival of patients with COPD requiring mechanical ventilation by analysis of simple indices: a prospective study. *Chest* 1987; **92**: 971–8.

78 Stauffer JL, Fayter NA, Graves B *et al.* Survival following mechanical ventilation for acute respiratory failure in adult men. *Chest* 1993; **104**: 1222–9.

79 Nava S, Rubini F, Zanotti E *et al.* Survival and prediction of successful ventilator weaning in COPD patients requiring mechanical ventilation for more than 21 days. *Eur Respir J* 1994; **7**: 1645–52.

80 Chailleux E, Fauroux B, Binet F, Dautzenberg B, Polu J. Predictors of survival in patients receiving domiciliary oxygen therapy or mechanical ventilation: a 10-year analysis of ANTADIR observatory. *Chest* 1996; **109**: 741–9.

81 Deber RB. Physicians in health care management, 7: the patient–physician partnership—changing roles and the desire for information. *Can Med Assoc J* 1994; **151**: 171–6.

82 Denger LF, Sloan JA. Decision making during illness: what role do patients really want to play? *J Clin Epidemiol* 1992; **45**: 941.

83 Sullivan KE, Hebert PC, Logan J, O'Connor AM, McNeely PD. What do physicians tell patients with end-stage COPD about intubation and mechanical ventilation? *Chest* 1996; **109**: 258–64.

84 American Thoracic Society. Withholding and withdrawing life sustaining therapy. *Ann Intern Med* 1991; **115**: 478–85.

85 Nommos D, Dubler N. *Ethics on Call: Taking Charge of Life and Death Choices in Today's Health Care System.* New York: Random House, 1993.

86 Uhlmann RF, Peralman RA, Cain KC. Physicians and spouses predictions of elderly patients resuscitation preferences. *J Gerontol* 1988; **43**: 115–21.

87 Pearlman RA, Jonsen A. The use of quality-of-life considerations in medical decision making. *J Am Geriatr Soc* 1985; **33**: 344–52.

88 Asai A, Fukuhara S, Inoshita O *et al.* Medical decisions concerning the end of life: a discussion with Japanese physicians. *J Med Ethics* 1997; **23**: 323–7.

89 Prendergast TJ, Claessens MT, Luce JM. A national survey of the end-of-life care for critically ill patients. *Am J Respir Crit Care Med* 1998; **158**: 1163–7.

90 Hanson LC, Rodgman E. The use of living wills at the end of life: a national study. *Arch Intern Med* 1996; **13**: 1018–22.

91 Malloy TR, Wigton RS, Meeske J, Tape TG. The influence of treatment descriptions on advance medical directive decisions. *J Am Geriatr Soc* 1992; **40**: 1255–60.

92 McNeely PD, Hebert PC, Dales REO *et al.* Deciding about mechanical ventilation in end-stage chronic obstructive pulmonary disease: how respirologists perceive their role. *Can Med Assoc J* 1997; **156**: 177–83.

93 Ewer MS, Taubert JK. Advance directives in the intensive care unit of a tertiary cancer centre. *Cancer* 1995; **76**: 1268–74.

94 Meduri GU, Fox RC, Abou-Shala N, Leeper KV, Wunderink R. Noninvasive mechanical ventilation via face mask in patients with acute respiratory failure who refused endotracheal intubation. *Crit Care Med* 1994; **22**: 1584–90.

95 Adler DC. The ethics of technology. *Chest* 1986; **5**: 765–6.

96 Chevrolet JC, Jolliet P. Workload on non-invasive ventilation in acute respiratory failure. In: Vincent JL, ed.

Yearbook of Intensive and Emergency Medicine. Berlin: Springer, 1997: 505–13.

97   Nava S, Evangelisti I, Rampulla C *et al.* Human and financial costs of noninvasive mechanical ventilation in patients affected by COPD and acute respiratory failure. *Chest* 1997; **111**: 1631–8.

98   Vitacca M, Clini E, Porta R, Sereni D, Ambrosino N. Experience of an intermediate respiratory intensive therapy in the treatment of prolonged weaning from mechanical ventilation. *Minerva Anestesiol* 1996; **62**: 57–64.

99   Anderer W, Kunzle C, Dhein Y, Worth H. [Noninvasive ventilation in the acute care hospital: a cost factor?]. *Med Klin* 1997; **92** (Suppl. 1): 119–22.

100 Criner GJ, Kreimer DT, Tomaselli M, Pierson W, Evans D. Financial implications of noninvasive positive pressure ventilation (NPPV). *Chest* 1995; **108**: 475–81.

101 Plant PK, Owen J, Elliott MW. A cost effectiveness analysis of non-invasive ventilation (NIV) in acute exacerbations of COPD [abstract]. *Thorax* 1999; 54 (Suppl. 3): A11.

102 Servera E, Perez M, Marin J, Vergera P, Castano R. Noninvasive nasal mask ventilation beyond the ICU for an exacerbation of chronic respiratory insufficiency. *Chest* 1995; **108**: 1572–6.

103 Elliott MW, Baudouin SV. Respiratory intensive care in Europe: lessons for the UK. *Thorax* 1998; **53**: 725–6.

104 Nava S, Confalonieri M, Rampulla C. Intermediate respiratory intensive care units in Europe: a European perspective. *Thorax* 1998; **53**: 798–802.

105 Parikh CR, Karnad DR. Quality, cost, and outcome of intensive care in a public hospital in Bombay, India. *Crit Care Med* 1999; **27**: 1754–9.

106 Appendini L, Purro A, Patessio A *et al.* Partitioning of inspiratory muscle workload and pressure assistance in ventilator-dependent COPD patients. *Am J Respir Crit Care Med* 1996; **154**: 1301–9.

107 Kerr HD. Doxapram in hypercapnic chronic obstructive pulmonary disease with respiratory failure. *J Emerg Med* 1997; **15**: 513–15.

108 Hirshberg AJ, Dupper RL. Use of doxapram hydrochloride injection as an alternative to intubation to treat chronic obstructive pulmonary disease patients with hypercapnia. *Ann Emergency Med* 1994; **24**: 701–3.

109 Edwards G, Leszczynski SO. A double blind trial of five respiratory stimulants in patients in acute ventilatory failure. *Lancet* 1967; i: 226–9.

110 Riordan JF, Sillett RW, McNichol MW. A controlled trial of doxapram in acute respiratory failure. *Br J Dis Chest* 1975; **69**: 57–62.

111 Moser KM, Luchsinger PC, Adamson JS *et al.* Respiratory stimulation with intravenous doxapram in respiratory failure: a double-blind co-operative study. *N Engl J Med* 1973; **288**: 427–31.

112 Angus RM, Ahmed AA, Fenwick LJ, Peacock AJ. Comparison of acute effects on gas exchange of nasal ventilation and doxapram in exacerbation of chronic obstructive pulmonary disease. *Thorax* 1996; **51**: 1048–50.

113 Powles AC, Tuxen DV, Mahood CB, Pugsley SO, Campbell EJ. The effect of intravenously administered almitrine, a peripheral chemoreceptor agonist, on patients with chronic air-flow obstruction. *Am Rev Respir Dis* 1983; **127**: 284–9.

114 Marcq M, Gepts L, Erven W, Minette A. [Effect of almitrine on arterial gases in patients with chronic respiratory insufficiency: comparison with doxapram—preliminary results.] *Rev Inst Hyg Mines (Hasselt)* 1979; **34**: 141–9.

115 Bardsley PA, Tweney J, Morgan N, Howard P. Oral almitrine in treatment of acute respiratory failure and cor pulmonale in patients with an exacerbation of chronic obstructive airways disease. *Thorax* 1991; **46**: 493–8.

17: Outcome measures in COPD — what is success?

Wisia Wedzicha and Mike Pearson

Why is there a need for a variety of outcome measures in COPD?

Chronic obstructive pulmonary disease (COPD) is characterized by a progressive decline in lung function that leads to dyspnoea on exertion and eventually to death. However, there is considerable variability in the rate of decline of forced expiratory volume in 1 second (FEV_1) in different patients. A number of guidelines have been produced for the management of COPD, including those from the European Thoracic Society [1], American Thoracic Society [2], British Thoracic Society [3] and the Word Health Organization's Global Initiative for Chronic Obstructive Lung Disease (GOLD) guidelines [4]. All of these guidelines agree on the point that the most accurate way to diagnose the condition is with measurement of FEV_1 by spirometry and that the FEV_1 also gives an indication of the severity of the disease. However, FEV_1 is only part of the explanation for the symptoms. In addition to the effect on lung function, there are important effects on physical disability and psychological function that impact on the quality of life experienced by the patient. Examples include the systemic effect in more severe COPD, leading to muscle wasting, that may progress and have direct effects on exercise capacity.

The levels of disability for a particular level of FEV_1 can therefore vary markedly; one patient with an FEV_1 of 40% predicted may be less breathless than a patient with an FEV_1 of 60% predicted. Studies of health status in patients with COPD have shown that there is variability in the relation between health status and FEV_1 [5,6] (Fig. 17.1). Two patients with the same degree of impairment of FEV_1 may therefore have a different level of health status or quality of life. Clinical studies have also shown that some therapeutic agents, such as long-acting bronchodilators, may have a relatively small effect on FEV_1 but a greater effect on health status [7]. Evaluation of new therapeutic agents thus requires a wider range of outcome measures, including measures of health status, exercise capacity and daily activities.

Symptoms, health status, exercise capacity and the exacerbation rate have all been proposed as additional outcome measures to the FEV_1, but because

227

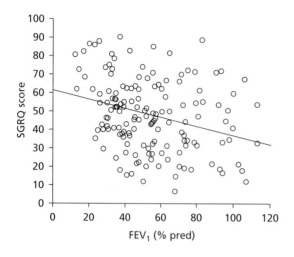

Fig. 17.1 The St George's Respiratory Questionnaire (SGRQ) is related to the level of forced expiratory volume in 1 s (FEV$_1$), but the relationship is such that almost any level of SGRQ can be associated with almost any level of FEV$_1$. From [6].

they may change differently with various interventions—e.g. exercise capacity changes by a much greater extent after a course of pulmonary rehabilitation [8] than after home ventilatory support [9]—the outcome must be specifically chosen in relation to the particular intervention being tested. But if a clinician is to interpret these different measures, it is essential to understand how the measurements relate to stable populations, how they behave in different types of COPD and how they vary over time. There is a further problem in that definitions for each of these vary between studies: 'acute exacerbation' has been defined in many ways, ranging from relatively mild exacerbations that may require a visit to the general practitioner to a severe attack that requires hospitalization.

Perhaps the most difficult aspect is that of time. Doctors treating asthma problems are used to observing dramatic changes in function within hours or days and are able to use these to make decisions about treatment that are understandable to the patient and more important are often confirmed to be correct in the longer term. By comparison, COPD is a chronic, slowly evolving disorder in which there are few short-term changes and even fewer that can be easily or reliably measured. This makes assessment and treatment planning difficult and has often been used as an excuse for negativism. However, the work that has been performed on outcomes in COPD in recent years would suggest that it is possible to record outcomes in COPD and that many changes are perceived favourably by patients and their relatives. This chapter addresses some of the outcomes in more detail.

What outcome measures are useful in COPD?

Symptoms

Symptoms are what the patient experiences and thus arguably are the most important effect of COPD. The commonest are dyspnoea on exertion, and cough (with or without sputum). Wheeze is often noted by the physician, but less commonly complained of by the patient. Symptoms are by definition subjective and therefore prone to interpretation. Many factors affect reporting, such as the ability to estimate distance; thus 'I can walk 100 m without stopping' is dependent on how far the individual thinks 100 m, is and few people are able to estimate distance reliably. Relating a symptom to a specific activity such as climbing stairs can help standardize the work requirement, but still leaves a subjective interpretation that relates to the person's ability to perceive 'load' and to their depression status. Depressed patients will report more symptoms than non-depressed ones, and sensitive 'wimps' may report more than more tolerant 'stoics', who are inclined to keep going and 'make the best of it'.

Thus, no one has yet derived a successful symptom score with which to evaluate all COPD patients. Some have attempted to produce scores. A Dutch group [10] used a modified Delphi process to ask a series of experts to derive a 10-question score of the most important symptoms. This remains under evaluation, but it is doubtful whether busy clinicians will find time to ask 10 questions at each clinic visit, and moreover the utility and reliability of the score have not yet been established. Most practical clinicians rely on recording a few basic symptoms from the patient, based on activities that the patient actually does. The same specific activities can then be asked about on subsequent visits — i.e. using the patient as his or her own control and assessing the change in a particular lifestyle.

Breathlessness

Validated research measures that have been used include the Borg score and visual analogue scores that require patients to estimate how breathless they are in relation to a prompt. These scores are of limited value in estimating individual experience at any point in time, because of the substantial interindividual variability mentioned above, and they do not have much utility in the clinical context. However, they do have value when applied to measuring short-term changes in breathlessness in the individual, or in assessing the overall effect in groups of patients. Such measures have been used to document improvement in breathlessness in response to a number of interventions in

COPD such as physical training, bronchodilators and ambulatory oxygen therapy [8,11,12].

While the limitations of interpreting breathlessness data for the individual are legion, the picture when studying groups is much more encouraging. The Medical Research Council (MRC) dyspnoea score [13] set out a scale for grading disability in populations in the 1960s that has stood the test of time. This scale runs from 1 (breathless only with strenuous exercise) to 5 (too breathless to leave the house). Studies have shown that with increasing MRC grade, there are reductions in exercise capacity, daily activities and health status, and thus this scale can be used to select patients for pulmonary rehabilitation [14]. There was much enthusiasm at the Royal College of Physicians Edinburgh Consensus COPD conference [15], suggesting that all doctors should record a simple measure like this as a marker case-mix variable to help evaluate responses to interventions such as rehabilitation. It has not been used in many studies, and there is concern that it may not be capable of responding to change. Few if any patients will respond to an intervention sufficient to move a whole point on the scale, and thus it is unlikely to be useful to evaluate the effects of interventions.

Cough and sputum

The next most important symptoms in COPD are cough and sputum production; these symptoms may occur in the early stages of COPD. Fletcher and Peto [16] suggested that cough and sputum did not relate to mortality or progression of COPD and that they therefore reflected a separate process in the lung. More recently, Vestbo *et al.* [17] have suggested that those with cough and sputum do have a worse outcome, but the predictive value in individuals is weak.

As with dyspnoea, there are many factors that affect the reporting and recording of cough and sputum. The recent GOLD guidelines have suggested an early stage (stage 0) of COPD, in which cough and sputum are present (bronchitis), but without any change in airflow obstruction [4]. Some may debate whether or not this stage is really a stage of COPD, since the 'O' in the acronym is not satisfied. If patients do not notice that a productive cough is abnormal, because they expect it as a 'smoker's cough' — a normal response to smoking — then they may not report it. And how should the symptoms be recorded with regard to the severity of COPD? Consider the smoker who has a regular cough during mild and moderate phases of COPD and who then develops severe disease and sufficient symptoms that he is persuaded to quit smoking. The productive cough will often abate or disappear with the smoking cessation, but the severity of the COPD remains high. It is therefore possible to record more symptoms in mild disease than in severe—making it hard to interpret either individual or group data.

Other symptoms

The same problems apply to wheeze, which is a common but variable symptom in COPD. Weight loss, which is an important symptom in severe COPD and predictive of early mortality, is only of value in the most severe cases [18].

Thus, the symptoms have so far proved to be of limited value in outcome assessments, because we have not yet developed ways in which to evaluate symptoms that are consistent enough across individuals to be incorporated easily into clinical assessments or into clinical trials. This is a factor in the move toward quality-of-life measures, or more accurately health-status tools, described below.

Physiological measurement

The accelerated decline in FEV_1 over many years is characteristic of COPD, and the measurement of FEV_1 is key to both diagnosis and the staging of severity [16]. It is effort-independent and thus a reproducible measure of airflow limitation, and many studies have shown that FEV_1 (particularly the post-bronchodilator FEV_1) is closely linked to the prognosis in COPD [19]. Theory would suggest that interventions should aim either to improve FEV_1 or at least to reduce the loss of function over time.

Improving FEV_1

In groups of patients, it is possible to show improvements in FEV_1 with a number of interventions, such as bronchodilators [20] and some anti-inflammatory therapies [21]. The changes are often relatively small and difficult to distinguish from the natural variability of the FEV_1 measurement. When applied to individuals, there has been considerable debate about the use of FEV_1 short-term reversibility to bronchodilators. The day-to-day variation in reversibility test results and the difficulty of separating a real variation from chance mean that unless changes are large (i.e. of a level that indicates that the diagnosis is more likely to be asthma), there is little value in clinical practice. Short-term responses are not predictive of later responses to therapy [22].

It is also possible to have improvement in functioning without a change in the FEV_1, for example in the response to physical interventions such as exercise training or oxygen therapy [8,12].

Measuring a reduced rate of decline of FEV_1

Any intervention that purports to alter the eventual natural history of the disease must be associated with a change in the rate of loss of FEV_1. Smoking cessation unequivocally produces a reduction in FEV_1 decline [20,23]. But the problems of measurement are even more difficult than for short-term responses. The average rate of decline of FEV_1 in healthy subjects is between 20 and 30 mL/year, and the average rate of decline in smokers is approximately double this. The average covers a wide range, with a few individuals (almost all of them smokers) losing FEV_1 at a rate of more than 100 mL/year. Distinguishing a difference between an average of 50 mL/year and 25 mL/year while using a measurement that has a natural variability between repeated measures of 170 mL [24] is clearly difficult. The slow change of FEV_1 means that it is not possible to make realistic estimates of rate of decline in an individual unless there are repeated measures over 3–5 years. In groups, it is possible to show change over shorter periods [20], and it will remain an important outcome goal of large-scale therapeutic and epidemiological studies.

However, day-to-day clinical practice demands outcomes that can be measured on a much shorter time scale, and FEV_1 is of almost no value in measuring the effectiveness of daily clinical practice. It is probably worth recording in order to be able to record the mean rate of decline over time to inform the prognosis, but there are no published data to support such an assertion.

Measurements of peak expiratory flow rate (PEFR) have been used much less in COPD, as isolated measurements cannot distinguish COPD from other types of lung disease, whether obstructive or restrictive. PEFR is much less reproducible than FEV, but it too can be of value in large-scale group data. Recently, the Copenhagen City Lung Study suggested that PEFR may be valuable as a predictor of overall mortality in COPD [25]. One study of the long-acting anticholinergic bronchodilator tiotropium has also shown significant effects of tiotropium on peak flow, compared to placebo [26].

Exercise capacity

Measurement of exercise capacity provides an indication of the patient's functional limitation. Although generally there is a relation between FEV_1 and exercise capacity, this is variable in the individual patient, and exercise capacity cannot be predicted from the level of the FEV_1 [27]. The complex exercise tests—requiring specialized equipment, with measurement of ventilation and maximum oxygen consumption and with considerable physiological expertise being needed for interpretation—are usually kept as research tools. They have been replaced by much simpler walking tests, such as the 6-min walking test, which are probably as informative. Asking patients to walk at their own pace for 6 min is much more typical of daily living and does not require any complex equipment. Such tests, despite their simplicity, have been shown to be reproducible, as long as correct procedures are followed and practice walks are performed [28]. A variant is the shuttle walk test [29], which is an externally paced maximum walking test, requiring the patient to walk between two cones placed 10 m apart. Walking tests have been shown to be very useful for assessing the outcome after pulmonary rehabilitation, and physical training is one of the few interventions that has been shown to increase exercise capacity to date [30].

However, as with symptoms and FEV_1, these are changes that can be detected in groups of patients, and the value of the measures in assessing the progress of an individual patient is less well documented.

Quality of life/health-status questionnaires

Health status is a concept that has grown in importance over the last 15 years. It attempts to measure the overall effect of a disease on the individual and to make allowance for factors such as depression by estimating function in a series of domains, of which physical functioning is but one. There are generic health-status questionnaires, such as the SF36 or the Sickness Impact Profile (SIP), that can be applied in any condition, but which were found to be generally insensitive to change in patients with COPD. Two important disease specific questionnaires were introduced: the Chronic Respiratory Questionnaire (CRQ) [31] and the St George's Respiratory Questionnaire (SGRQ) [32]. Both of these questionnaires have been shown to be sensitive to interventions in COPD. The CRQ is based on the symptom of dyspnoea, while the SGRQ consists of three components—symptoms, activities and impacts—that are summed to provide a total score for health status.

These are now among the most important outcome measures in COPD and have been shown to be improved by a variety of measures, including pulmonary rehabilitation and pharmacological therapies such as bronchodilators and inhaled steroids. Health status has been shown to deteriorate with progressive COPD and is closely linked to exacerbation rates [33,34]. Their importance has been recognized by regulatory authorities, such as the Commission on the Safety of Medicines in the UK, for demonstrating efficacy—i.e. improved quality of life is a valid outcome. This might sound obvious, but until these instruments were devised, there was no way of demonstrating such effects.

Although the SGRQ provides a score for activities, there are other questionnaires that have been developed to assess daily activities. The Nottingham Extended Activities of Daily Living (NEADL) has been used in COPD [35], although it is of more use in describing disability in a population and is not sensitive to change after an intervention such as rehabilitation. One reason for the lack of sensitivity is that daily activities are only affected significantly in more severe COPD, e.g. MRC dyspnoea scores 4 and 5 [14]. The London Chest Activity of Daily Living Questionnaire (LCADL) has been developed for use in this population with more severe disability, although experience with its use in interventions is limited to date [36].

A novel feature of these health-status scores is that they have made it possible to determine the magnitude of change that is likely to be noticeable by the individual patient. A change of four points on the SGRQ scale is likely to be observable by the individual patient [7], and changes that exceed this threshold in a group study can thus be inferred to be noticeable by more than half the group. This considerably helps those who have to interpret the various studies and is a major improvement on the long history of clinical studies demonstrating highly statistically significant, but very clinically insignificant, changes in function. With justification, clinicians have questioned the relevance of small changes that an individual would be unable to perceive and have asked whether the cost of the intervention could be justified. However, there is a significant caution that must be borne in mind before accepting these new measures as definitive—the fact that they are significantly influenced by non-COPD factors such as mood and depression [37].

The weakness of health-status questionnaires is their relative length and thus their impracticability for routine clinical use. However, as they provide information on the likely health needs of the patient group and on their likely future health costs, it seems probable that use will increase. The process of developing newer and simpler versions is likely to accelerate this process.

Exacerbations (see also Chapter 15)

Recently, exacerbations of COPD have been shown to be a major outcome measure in COPD. The frequency of exacerbations is directly related to health status, and has important health-economic implications [38]. It is also cited by patients as one of the features that concerns them most. There is also some recent evidence that exacerbations may have an effect on disease progression in COPD, and thus it is essential to define and detect exacerbations accurately [39,40]. Exacerbations are unusual in mild to moderate COPD and are too infrequent to be of value as an outcome indicator. In the Inhaled Steroids in Obstructive Lung Disease in Europe (ISOLDE) study [41], the population were divided up into tertiles and it was only in the tertile with the lowest FEV_1 ($<1.25\,L$) that there was a significant alteration in the exacerbation rate in response to drugs. This was in part because only in this group were exacerbations sufficiently frequent that there were enough numbers to achieve comparisons.

An exacerbation refers to a worsening of symptoms, especially of the major symptoms of dyspnoea, increased sputum volume and sputum purulence. Exacerbations are associated with physiological change and increased inflammatory markers in the sputum, although these measures are too variable to be of use in diagnosis [42]. The exacerbation frequency refers to the number of exacerbations per year, and in group studies, a number of pharmacological interventions have been shown to reduce exacerbation frequency [33]. However, to estimate exacerbation frequency, a whole year of data must be collected. Other exacerbation measures that can be used over shorter periods have therefore been devised, such as time to the first exacerbation [43]. But this is of limited value, as it is dependent on season and withdrawal of medication before the study.

Exacerbations are not easy to measure. Not only does the definition above include a subjective interpretation of 'worsening', but also a significant number of exacerbations are not reported to health-care professionals. Collecting complete data from patients in the community who have elected not to attend hospital is a challenge.

Other possible outcomes in COPD

A number of other outcomes have been proposed, although experience with them and with the effects of interventions is still limited.

• Changes in sputum inflammatory markers, e.g. the levels of leukotriene B_4 (LTB_4) can occur in response to treatment and resolution of an exacerbation [44], although the use of such markers in clinical practice to follow exacerbations has not been evaluated. Further work is required on the longer-term changes in sputum inflammatory markers and relationships to disease progression.

• There is relatively little information on the use of bronchial biopsies in COPD. A relationship has been shown between the number of CD8 lymphocytes in the biopsies and FEV_1, but to date only patients with relatively mild COPD have been studied [45]. There is also little information on the relationship between sputum examination and changes in bronchial biopsies. Thus, the use of bronchial biopsies is currently limited to research studies in COPD.

• Other outcomes such as computed tomography (CT) scanning may have a role in the future, both to diagnose COPD and follow changes after interventions, although experience is limited to date.

So what is success?

Much of the discussion above has focused on the limitations of the various outcome measures, and this remains a major challenge for those who wish to treat COPD more aggressively and with more success. Much depends on what can realistically be expected.

Long-term epidemiology

The FEV_1 remains the best marker of the rate of long-term decline of FEV_1, and any therapy for which a disease-modifying role can be claimed will need to show that it can slow the rate of decline. So far, only smoking cessation is known to alter the long-term outcome measured in this way. Therapies that can reduce exacerbation frequency also may affect disease progression.

Shorter-term clinical outcomes

Once COPD has become established, the damage cannot at present be repaired; improvements in lung function with therapy are small and are rarely of value in individuals.

In patients with more severe COPD, the reduction in the exacerbation frequency is probably the most sensitive measure of response and moreover is one that has clear economic benefits and that is instantly appreciated by patients.

The disease-specific health-status measures apply to both severe and moderate stages of disease and have been shown to be responsive to a range of supportive treatments, including long-acting bronchodilators and rehabilitation programs. Again, these can be quantified, and the proportion of patients experiencing noticeable changes can be calculated. Unfortunately, measurement often takes too long for busy clinicians to use any of these in routine practice.

Routine practice is still dependent on the subjective recording of symptoms and the very subjective 'Do you feel better?' approach—and a challenge for researchers is to improve on this weak armamentarium.

Success for the patient or success by the doctor?

In the modern world, physicians are expected not only to provide treatment, but also to demonstrate that their treatments work. In a condition in which little can be expected to change over a period of years in the individual, the patient outcomes discussed above are of little value when trying to determine whether a doctor is providing good or bad care. This is a problem common to many, if not all, chronic diseases and has led to attempts to examine the process of care rather than just the outcome. If the process measures are chosen to have some potential to predict outcome, then there is purpose to the exercise, and this has been shown to have merit in cardiology [46].

A recent audit of care provided in 46 UK hospitals collected data on 1400 acute admissions with an acute exacerbation and examined a series of standards derived from current COPD management guidelines, a number of severity indicators (to control for case mix) and the 3-month mortality. Care standards varied very widely between hospitals and so too did the 3-month mortality. For most factors measured, the care ranged from acceptable to appalling—few units scored consistently well. It is difficult to justify the management provided for many aspects of care. As an example, spirometry is recommended as essential for making the diagnosis by all national and international guidelines, and the audit accepted any measurement made either in the 5 years prior to or the 3 months after the index admission. Even with this latitude, only half the patients (51%) had their diagnosis confirmed [47]. There were three strong statistically significant predictors of death within 3 months—the performance score (as used in cancer studies), severe acidosis on admission and the presence of bilateral ankle oedema. Even after controlling for these three predictors, there was a more than twofold difference in deaths between large and small hospitals, which raises worrying questions about the service being offered [48].

The marked differences in the process of care between hospitals shown in the above study are mirrored in other national audits of other conditions as disparate as stroke [49], incontinence [50], and blood transfusions [51]. Professionals are often unwilling to admit that the care they provide is anything less than excellent—until faced with figures that tell a different story. Defining target outcomes for COPD is clearly an important step forward, but those targets are unlikely to be attained if the processes of care within our hospital units are so variable and so far below the optimal levels set out in management guidelines.

COPD has been a Cinderella condition for many years—that is, one in which the professions acknowledge the patients' existence, but take little interest in their problems and provide even less in the way of health-care resources. Part of this has been due to the feeling that in part COPD is the patient's fault—a self-inflicted disability due to their cigarette-smoking habit. But society does not impose similar criticism on those who develop heart disease following over-indulgence in fatty foods. And even if it were possible for cigarettes to be banned now, those with airflow limitation will still be with us for many years and will still require treatment.

The last decade has witnessed a marked change. Firstly, it has been recognized that even if the damage done cannot be reversed, the quality of life for COPD patients can be significantly improved and in some cases their life expectancy can be improved too. Secondly, the research world has woken up to the possibilities, and the burgeoning number of sessions allocated to COPD at international meetings is evidence of the amount of new effort being devoted to the disease. And thirdly, the pharmaceutical industry has developed a range of products that are now of proven benefit—with more on the way.

We hope that those who read this book will be left with an enthusiasm that COPD is not a 'no-hope' disorder. Much can and should be done that will benefit not only the patients directly, but also their families and thus society. But if we are to succeed, we need not only to recognize what can be done, but also to put into place systems that ensure it really is done.

References

1 Siafakas NM, Vemeire P, Pride NB *et al.* Optimal assessment and management of chronic obstructive pulmonary disease (COPD). The European Respiratory Society Task Force. *Eur Respir J* 1995; **8**: 1398–420.

2 American Thoracic Society. Standards for the diagnosis and care of patients with chronic obstructive pulmonary disease. *Am J Respir Crit Care Med* 1995; **152**: 77–120.

3 [Anon.] BTS guidelines for the management of chronic obstructive pulmonary disease. The COPD Guidelines Group of the Standards of Care Committee of the BTS. *Thorax* 1997; **52** (Suppl. 5): S1–28.

4 Global Initiative for Chronic Obstructive Lung Disease. *NHLBI/WHO Workshop Report: Global Strategy for the Diagnosis, Management, and Prevention of COPD.* Bethesda, MD: National Heart, Lung and Blood Institute, 2001 (NIH Publication No. 2701).

5 Jones PW, Quirk FH, Baveystosk CM, Littlejohns P. A self-complete measure of health status for chronic airflow limitation: the St George's Respiratory Questionnaire. *Am Rev Respir Dis* 1992; **145**: 1321–7.

6 Wijkstra PJ, Jones PW. Quality of life in patients with COPD. In: Postma DS, Siafakas NM eds. *Management of COPD* (ERS monograph) 1998; 3(Monograph 7): 238.

7 Jones PW, Bosh TK. Quality of life changes in COPD patients treated with salmeterol. *Am J Respir Crit Care Med* 1997; **155**: 1283–9.

8 Wedzicha JA, Bestall J, Garnham R *et al.* Randomised controlled trial of pulmonary rehabilitation in patients with severe chronic obstructive pulmonary disease stratified for disability. *Eur Respir J* 1998; **12**: 363–9.

9 Meecham Jones DJ, Paul EA, Jones PW, Wedzicha JA. Nasal pressure support ventilation plus oxygen compared with oxygen therapy alone in hypercapnic COPD: a randomised controlled study. *Am J Respir Crit Care Med* 1995; **152**: 538–44.

10 van der Molen T, Juniper EF, Schokker S, Steege M, Postma DS. How can we measure COPD symptom control? The development of a COPD symptom control questionnaire *Am J Respir Crit Care Med* 1999; **159**: A832.

11 Spence DPS, Hay JG, Carter J *et al.* Oxygen desaturation and breathlessness during corridor walking in chronic obstructive pulmonary disease. *Thorax* 1993; **48**: 1145–50.

12 O'Donnell D, D'Arsigny C, Webb KA. Effects of hyperoxia on ventilatory limitation during exercise in advanced chronic obstructive pulmonary disease. *Am J Respir Crit Care Med* 2001; **163**: 892–8.

13 Medical Research Council. Definition and classification of chronic bronchitis for medical and epidemiological purposes. *Lancet* 1965; i: 775–9.

14 Bestall JC, Paul EA, Garrod R *et al.*

Usefulness of the Medical Research Council (MRC) dyspnoea scale as a measure of disability in patients with chronic obstructive pulmonary disease. *Thorax* 1999; **54**: 581–6.

15 Consensus statement on Management of Chronic Obstructive Pulmonary Disease. March 2001. www.rcpe.ac.uk/esd/consensus/COPD-.01.html.

16 Fletcher C, Peto R. The natural history of chronic airflow obstruction. *BMJ* 1977; i: 1645–8.

17 Vestbo J, Prescott E, Lange P, CCHS Group. Association of chronic mucus hypersecretion with FEV_1 decline and chronic obstructive pulmonary disease morbidity. *Am J Respir Crit Care Med* 1996; **153**: 1530–5.

18 Schols AM, Slangen J, Volovics L, Wouters EF. Weight loss is a reversible factor in the prognosis of chronic obstructive pulmonary disease. *Am J Respir Crit Care Med* 1998; **157**: 1791–7.

19 Anthonisen NR. Prognosis in chronic obstructive pulmonary disease results from multi-center clinical trials. *Am Rev Respir Dis* 1989; **40**: S95–S99.

20 Anthonisen NR, Connett JE, Kiley JP, *et al.* Effects of smoking intervention and the use of an inhaled anticholinergic bronchodilator on the rate of decline of FEV_1. The Lung Health Study. *JAMA* 1994; **272**: 1497–505.

21 Compton CH, Gubb J, Nieman R *et al.* Cilomilast, a selective phosphodiesterase-4 inhibitor for treatment of patients with COPD: a randomised, dose-ranging study. *Lancet* 2001; **358**: 265–70.

22 O'Driscoll BR, Kay EA, Taylor RJ, Bernstein A. Home nebulisers: can optimal therapy be predicted by laboratory studies? *Respir Med* 1990; **84**: 471–7.

23 Anthonisen N, Connett J, Kiley J *et al.* Effects of smoking intervention and the use of an inhaled anticholinergic bronchodilator on the rate of decline of FEV_1. *JAMA* 1994; **272**: 1497–505.

24 Tweedale PM, Alexander F, McHardy GJR. Short-term variability in FEV_1 and bronchodilator responsiveness in patients with chronic obstructive ventilatory defects *Thorax* 1987; **42**: 487–90.

25 Hansen EF, Vestbo J, Phanareth K, Kok-Jensen A. Peak flow as predictor of overall mortality in asthma and chronic obstructive pulmonary disease. *Am J Respir Crit Care Med* 2001; **163**: 690–3.

26 Casaburi R, Briggs DD, Donohue JF *et al.* The spirometric efficacy of once-daily dosing with tiotropium in stable COPD. *Chest* 2000; **118**: 1294–302.

27 Swinburn CR, Wakefield JM, Jones PW. Performance, ventilation and oxygen consumption in three different types of exercise tests in patients with chronic obstructive lung disease. *Thorax* 1985; **40**: 581–6.

28 Butland RJA, Pang J, Gross ER, Woodcock AA, Geddes DM. Two-, six- and twelve-minute walking tests in respiratory disease. *BMJ* 1982; **284**: 1607–8.

29 Singh SJ, Morgan DL, Scott S, Walters D, Hardman AE. Development of a shuttle walking test of disability in patients with chronic airways obstruction. *Thorax* 1992; **47**: 1019–24.

30 Lacasse Y, Wong E, Guyatt G, Cook D, Goldstein R. Meta-analysis of respiratory rehabilitation in chronic obstructive pulmonary disease. *Lancet* 1996; **348**: 1115–19.

31 Guyatt GH, Berman LB, Townsend M, Pugsley SO, Chambers LW. A measure of quality of life for clinical trials in chronic lung disease. *Thorax* 1987; **42**: 773–8.

32 Jones PW, Quirk FH, Baveystock CM, Littlejohns P. A self-complete measure of health status for chronic airflow limitation. *Am Rev Respir Dis* 1992; **145**: 1321–7.

33 Burge PS, Calverley PM, Jones PW *et al.* Randomized placebo-controlled study of fluticasone propionate in patients with moderate to severe chronic obstructive pulmonary disease: the ISOLDE trial. *BMJ* 2000; **320**: 1297–303.

34 Seemungal TAR, Donaldson GC, Paul EA *et al.* Effect of exacerbation on quality of life in patients with chronic obstructive pulmonary disease. *Am J Respir Crit Care Med* 1998; **157**: 1418–22.

35 Okubadejo AA, O'Shea L, Jones PW, Wedzicha JA. Home assessment of activities of daily living in patients with severe chronic obstructive pulmonary disease on long term oxygen therapy. *Eur Respir J* 1997; **10**: 1572–55.

36 Garrod R, Paul EA, Wedzicha JA. An evaluation of the reliability and sensitivity

of the London Chest Activity of Daily Living Scale (LCADL). *Respir Med* [in press].

37 Okubadejo AA, Jones PW, Wedzicha JA. Quality of life in patients with COPD and severe hypoxaemia. *Thorax* 1996; **51**: 44–7.

38 Seemungal TAR, Donaldson GC, Paul EA *et al*. Effect of exacerbation on quality of life in patients with chronic obstructive pulmonary disease. *Am J Respir Crit Care Med* 1998; **157**: 1418–22.

39 **Kanner RE, Anthonisen NR, Connett JE.** Lower respiratory illnesses promote FEV_1 decline in current smokers but not ex-smokers with mild chronic obstructive pulmonary disease: results from the Lung Health Study. *Am J Respir Crit Care Med* 2001; **164**: 358–64.

40 Donaldson GC, Seemungal TAR, Bhowmik A, Wedzicha JA. The relationship between exacerbation frequency and lung function decline in chronic obstructive pulmonary disease. *Thorax* 2002 [in press].

41 Burge PS, Calverley PM, Jones PW *et al*. Randomised, double blind, placebo-controlled study of fluticasone propionate in patients with moderate to severe chronic obstructive pulmonary disease: the ISOLDE trial. *BMJ* 2000; **320**: 1297–330.

42 Bhowmik A, Seemungal TAR, Sapsford R, Donaldson GC, Wedzicha JA. Relation of sputum inflammatory markers to symptoms and physiological changes at COPD exacerbations. *Thorax* 2000; **55**: 114–20.

43 Seemungal TAR, Donaldson GC, Bhowmik A, Jeffries DJ, Wedzicha JA. Time course and recovery of exacerbations in patients with chronic obstructive pulmonary disease. *Am J Respir Crit Care Med* 2000; **161**: 1608–13.

44 Crooks SW, Bayley DL, Hill SL, Stockley RA. Bronchial inflammation in acute bacterial exacerbations of chronic bronchitis: the role of leukotriene B_4. *Eur Respir J* 2000; **15**: 274–80.

45 O'Shaughnessy TC, Ansari TW, Barnes NC, Jeffery PK. Inflammation in bronchial biopsies of subjects with chronic bronchitis: inverse relationship of CD8+ T lymphocytes with FEV_1. *Am J Respir Crit Care Med* 1997; **155**: 852–7.

46 Mant J, Hicks N. Detecting differences in quality of care: how sensitive are process and outcome measures in the treatment of acute myocardial infarction? *BMJ* 1995; **311**: 793–6.

47 Roberts CM, Ryland I, Lowe D *et al*. Audit of acute admissions of COPD. standards of care and management in the hospital setting. *Eur Respir J* 2001; **17**: 343–9.

48 Roberts CM, Ryland I, Lowe D *et al*. Predictors of outcome following admission to hospital with acute COPD in the UK National Audit. *Thorax* 1997; **57**: 137–41.

49 Rudd A, Irwin P, Rutledge Z *et al*. The national sentinel audit of stroke a tool for raising standards of care. *J R Coll Phys Lond* 1999; **33**: 460–5.

50 Georgiou A, Potter J, Brocklehurst JC, Lowe D, Pearson MG. Measuring the quality of urinary continence care in long term care facilities: an analysis of outcome indicators. *Age Ageing* 2001; **30**: 63–6.

51 Murphy MF, Wilkinson J, Lowe D, Pearson M. National audit of the Blood Transfusion Process in the UK. *Transfus Med* 2001; **11**: 363–70.

Index

Notes: As the subject of this book is chronic obstructive pulmonary disease (COPD), all entries in this index refer specifically to COPD unless otherwise stated. The entries are given in letter-by-letter order and page numbers in *italics* and **bold** represent figures and tables respectively.